APPLIED POPULATION HEALTH APPROACHES FOR ASIAN AMERICAN COMMUNITIES

APPLIED POPULATION HEALTH APPROACHES FOR ASIAN AMERICAN COMMUNITIES

EDITED BY

SIMONA C. KWON
CHAU TRINH-SHEVRIN
NADIA S. ISLAM
STELLA S. YI

FOREWORD BY MARJORIE KAGAWA-SINGER

AFTERWORD BY SHOBHA SRINIVASAN AND RINA DAS

JB JOSSEY-BASS™
A Wiley Brand

Registered Office
John Wiley & Sons, Inc., 111 River Street, Hoboken, NJ 07030, USA

Editorial Office
111 River Street, Hoboken, NJ 07030, USA

For details of our global editorial offices, customer services, and more information about Wiley products visit us at www.wiley.com.

Wiley also publishes its books in a variety of electronic formats and by print-on-demand. Some content that appears in standard print versions of this book may not be available in other formats.

Limit of Liability/Disclaimer of Warranty

Library of Congress Cataloging-in-Publication Data applied for

Paperback ISBN: 9781119678564

Cover Design: Wiley
Cover Image: © RODINA OLENA/Shutterstock

Set in 10.5/12.5 pt and Times LT Std by Straive, Chennai

SKY10037004_101922

CONTENTS

PART ONE: CONTEXT

PART TWO: MEASURES

PART THREE: APPROACHES

FIGURES AND TABLES

FIGURES

FOREWORD

You Don't Count If You Are Not Counted

In the mid-1960s, the only option I had on any demographic data forms to describe my racial and ethnic heritage was "Other." Even when I began my research career in Asian American health during the 1980s, a scan of published work in the health field showed a dearth of articles on Asian Americans. Usability of published data was further limited by the aggregation of all Asian American groups into the single category, "Oriental," which held on as the aggregate term used to describe our multicultural populations. When founding the Asian American Political Alliance in 1968, followed rapidly by the establishment of the Asian American Studies Center at the University of California at Los Angeles (UCLA) in 1968, Yuji Ichioka coined the term "Asian American," noting, "we are not carpets." Yet years passed before this more meaningful term came into common use.

Due to the perseverance of Asian American researchers and community advocates, recognition of the enormous and growing diversity of our population groups, both by culture as well as immigration history, has become widespread. There is now a clearer picture of who we are, how our health beliefs and needs differ, and the best ways to obtain data describing us to inform the development of effective programs to provide health education and proactive health practices to our communities in culturally consonant and compelling ways.

In 2022, with the publication of this book, *Applied Population Health Approaches for Asian Americans*, we can clearly demonstrate the heterogeneity of this population group. Asian Americans are and have been in the United States since Filipinos arrived with the Spanish in the late 1500s. The major wave of Asians arrived on the West Coast of the United States in the mid-1800s and, now, the US Asian American population likely includes representation from every Asian population in the world. Importantly, for scientific inquiry, we now have a growing body of disaggregated data to document threats to health and well-being in our highly diverse communities so that we can more effectively work with these communities to improve outcomes.

Notably, this volume also highlights the concerted efforts of a cohesive team of Asian American scholars and community leaders who donated their time and expertise to write these chapters. It also highlights the work of their colleagues around the country conducting the community-based research that informed the innovative and essential theoretical grounding and methodological expertise required in the field of public health to effectively address the needs of this highly heterogeneous population group.

Obtaining funding for research in our communities has been an arduous ordeal. Significantly, the director of the National Institutes of Health (NIH), Dr. Francis Collins, apologized for the structural racism that has blocked funding for health research among communities of color in the United States.[1] Along with leaders representing the various institutes and centers of NIH, Dr. Collins recently published a framework for ending structural racism in biomedical research.[2] In that article, leaders acknowledged and committed to ending structural racism "in the criteria used to fund scientific inquiry at the NIH, developing robust health disparities/equity research, and improving the internal culture so that diversity, equity, and inclusion are reflected in funded research and the biomedical workforce." This acknowledgment and the promise of change in biomedical research represent a remarkable milestone but we must also demand that NIH address the role of structural racism in limiting the funding for and progress in behavioral research among communities of color. NIH must be accountable to both domains of health research.

The authors contributing to this volume have worked in partnership with their communities for many years and describe what they know to be the truths in these communities. Notably, many of the researchers are also members of these communities and, therefore, know the essential nuances of communication within them. Most importantly, they have gained the trust of community leaders and members, allowing them to effectively inform communities of various health issues and challenges and craft solutions in partnership with them. To achieve this progress, these researchers have worked tirelessly with community leaders and members to negotiate and establish mutually acceptable intervention designs and evaluation measures that are useful to both the community and the researchers. Although this process is recognized as essential in community health efforts, NIH's criteria for funding to date have not been accommodating or supportive of the additional time required for these steps. Naïve communities or refugee populations have well-warranted wariness of "government programs" asking personal questions. Given the history of "research" in the African American and Native American communities, in particular, researchers of color well know the valid wariness of these communities. Many of our Asian American populations have fled war-torn countries and are equally wary of "government" efforts, rendering the trust-building process a time- and effort-intensive one for researchers aiming to partner with and improve outcomes for these communities.

The chapters in this book clearly illustrate the sophistication of this team of authors in overcoming these barriers and building trust with a diverse array of communities across the country, as well as demonstrating the scientific expertise of these researchers. For example, in Chapters 4 and 5, the authors identified the dual challenges of generating population-based samples and interfacing with federal requirements for data collection. In the lessons learned sections, the authors identify the strengths and challenges of carrying out truly partnered work with communities, including ensuring that study designs are consciously inclusive of cultural differences in communication, social forces, and specific health needs of different Asian American populations. Notably, the authors also address the pros and cons of "fit" for different types of study designs to meet the cultural, social, and health needs of diverse Asian American populations, using multiple theoretical lenses to develop scientifically rigorous and culturally compatible and respectful methodologies to maximize intervention success.

This textbook presents lessons learned from research conducted in partnership with population groups that have been – as Dr. Moon S. Chen Jr., the renowned national expert in cancer and health disparities, was wont to say – not "hard to reach," but rather, "hardly reached." When applied, these lessons learned can improve the science of working in partnership with communities to enhance and support the health and well-being of vastly diverse Asian American populations. As NIH Director Collins indicated in the report referenced above, our science needs to be more inclusive of diversity. This textbook can guide community health sciences to more effectively reach the communities that have been, heretofore, "hardly reached."

Marjorie Kagawa-Singer, PhD, MN, RN
Professor Emerita, School of Public Health and
Department of Asian American Studies,
University of California Los Angeles

NOTES

1. NIH stands against structural racism in biomedical research, National Institutes of Health, March 1, 2021, https://www.nih.gov/about-nih/who-we-are/nih-director/statements/nih-stands-against-structural-racism-biomedical-research.

2. F. S. Collins, A. B. Adams, C. Aklin, et al., Affirming NIH's commitment to addressing structural racism in the biomedical research enterprise, *Cell* 184 (12) (June 10, 2021): 3075–3079, https://www.cell.com/cell/fulltext/S0092-8674(21)00631-0.

THE EDITORS

SIMONA C. KWON, DrPH, MPH is associate professor in the Departments of Population Health and Medicine, director of the Section for Health Equity, and vice chair for Diversity, Equity, and Inclusion in the Department of Population Health at NYU Grossman School of Medicine. Kwon is the director and multi-principal investigator of the National Institute on Minority Health and Health Disparities (NIMHD)-funded Center of Excellence, the NYU Center for the Study of Asian American Health (CSAAH). Kwon also co-leads the Community Outreach and Engagement Core of the NYU Langone Perlmutter Cancer Center, a National Cancer Institute–designated Comprehensive Cancer Center, and serves as the community engagement and dissemination lead for the Centers for Disease Control and Prevention (CDC)-funded NYU BOLD Public Health Center of Excellence on Early Detection of Dementia.

She is a socio-behavioral epidemiologist with extensive experience in the use of, among other methods, community-based participatory research, mixed methods (qualitative and quantitative) approaches, evidence-based strategies, dissemination and implementation science, and multidisciplinary teams to address community-level health disparities. Kwon works in collaboration with multisector coalitions made up of local and national community-based organizations, governmental agencies, service delivery organizations, and researchers from discrete disciplines.

Kwon's research examines the social and cultural factors that influence health and health outcomes in racial and ethnic communities, with a particular focus on Asian Americans. She employs a social determinants of health framework to implement and evaluate evidence-based strategies in community settings, focusing on cultural relevance and impact and finding more effective channels through which to translate research into practice. Her work is grounded in applying social marketing principles and community- and culture-centered approaches to culturally tailor meaningful messages and adapt evidence-based strategies to engage and reach racial/ethnic minority and immigrant communities.

Kwon was awarded her master of public health in epidemiology from Yale University and her doctorate in the Division of Sociomedical Sciences from the Mailman School of Public Health, Columbia University. She served as a W.K. Kellogg Community Scholars postdoctoral Fellow at the Johns Hopkins Bloomberg School of Public Health in the Department of Health Behavior & Society.

■ ■ ■

CHAU TRINH-SHEVRIN, DrPH is professor in the Departments of Population Health and Medicine, director of the Division of Health and Behavior, vice chair for Research in the Department of Population Health, and Institutional Review Board chair at NYU Grossman School of Medicine. For over 20 years, her research has focused on the rigorous development and evaluation of multi-level strategies to reduce health disparities and advance health equity.

Trinh-Shevrin is multi-principal investigator (MPI) of a National Institute on Minority Health and Health Disparities (NIMHD) Center of Excellence, the NYU Center for the Study of Asian American Health (CSAAH), and a National Institute on Aging (NIA) Engagement in Longevity and Medicine Research Collaborative. Trinh-Shevrin also led a Centers for Disease Control and Prevention (CDC) Research Center for over a decade and currently leads a CDC Cancer Prevention and Control Research Network Center. Building on her expertise in community-based participatory research and longstanding relationships with national and local community partners, she is MPI of a National Institutes of Health (NIH) Community Engagement Alliance to End COVID-19 Disparities and associate director of Community Outreach and Engagement for the Perlmutter Cancer Center, a National Cancer Institute-designated Comprehensive Cancer Center.

Trinh-Shevrin is dedicated to mentoring junior faculty and students in minority and health disparities research. She is involved in many NIH-funded research training and education programs and leads an NIA Academic Leadership Award to support mentored research opportunities in healthy aging and health disparities research.

Trinh-Shevrin earned her doctorate in public health from the Mailman School of Public Health, Columbia University, and masters in health policy and management at the State University of New York at Albany. She has co-authored more than 130 peer-reviewed publications and is co-editor of two textbooks, *Asian American Communities and Health* (Jossey-Bass, 2009) and *Empowerment and Recovery: Confronting Addiction during Pregnancy with Peer Counseling* (Praeger Press, 1998).

NADIA S. ISLAM, PhD, is a medical sociologist, associate professor in the Department of Population Health, and associate director of the Institute for Excellence in Health Equity at NYU Grossman School of Medicine. Her research focuses on developing culturally relevant community-clinical linkage models to reduce cardiovascular disease and diabetes disparities in disadvantaged communities.

Islam leads, as principal investigator, several National Institutes of Health (NIH) and Centers for Disease Control and Prevention (CDC)-funded initiatives evaluating the impact of community health worker intervention on chronic disease management and prevention in diverse populations.

Islam also directs the cardiovascular disease and diabetes research track for the National Institute on Minority Health and Health Disparities (NIMHD)-funded Center of Excellence, the NYU Center for the Study of Asian American Health (CSAAH), which is dedicated to reducing health disparities facing Asian American communities. Islam is also research director at the NYU-CUNY Prevention Research Center and principal investigator of a CDC-funded Racial and Ethnic Approaches to Community Health (REACH) program project.

Islam's work has been featured in the *American Journal of Public Health, Diabetes Care,* and numerous other peer-reviewed journals. She is co-editor of *Asian American Communities and Health* (Jossey-Bass, 2009).

Islam received her doctorate in the Division of Sociomedical Sciences from the Mailman School of Public Health, Columbia University. She currently serves on the American Diabetes Association task force on Asian American, Native Hawaiian, and Pacific Islanders. Islam previously served on the board of the Public Health Association of New York City and as chair of the Asian and Pacific Islander Caucus for Public Health of the American Public Health Association.

STELLA S. YI, PhD, MPH, is a cardiovascular epidemiologist and associate professor in the Department of Population Health's Section for Health Equity at NYU Grossman School of Medicine. Her work focuses on improving lifestyle behaviors for reducing chronic disease risk and improving data disaggregation and reporting practices through multi-sector collaborations and community-partnered research for both the New York City population at large and for Asian American and immigrant communities, specifically. Prior to joining the faculty at NYU in 2014, she worked for six years at the NYC Department of Health and Mental Hygiene (DOHMH) leading research and evaluation efforts of city nutrition policies and community-clinic initiatives. Given these experiences, she possesses a unique viewpoint on health, policy and research that encompasses a citywide perspective paired with an understanding of unique health needs of disparity subgroups.

Within the Section, Yi leads the Applied Research and Evaluation Unit, the purpose of which is to utilize mixed methods, community-partnered systems science, and implementation science methods to improve the health of diverse populations. In this vein, Yi leads several National Institutes of Health (NIH) and Centers for Disease Control and Prevention (CDC)-funded initiatives that utilize participatory systems science, epidemiology, and quantitative methods to inform research policy and practice in real-world settings to address health equity. She is committed to improving the scientific evidence base to accurately reflect the diversity of the United States through the application of rigorous methods and improving data collection and reporting systems at the institutional, city, state, and federal levels.

Yi received her master of public health in Chronic Disease Epidemiology/Social Behavioral Sciences at the Yale School of Public Health and her doctorate in epidemiology from the Johns Hopkins Bloomberg School of Public Health.

THE CONTRIBUTORS

GULNAHAR (NAHAR) ALAM, has been an organizer in the United States and Bangladesh for 28 years. She works towards a vision in which all workers are treated with respect and their rights are enforced. She has been organizing South Asian immigrant workers in New York City since 1993 through several grassroots Asian-Pacific Islander community organizations. Alam was instrumental in founding Andolan in 1998, a community group focusing on organizing low-wage South Asian women workers. She provides presentations and trainings to workers, law students and other organizations serving the community. Alam represented Andolan at the World Conference against Racism in South Africa (2001) and Switzerland (2005). She received the Susan B. Anthony Award from NOW (1996). In June 2010, New York State passed a Domestic Workers Bill of Rights with the advocacy of Andolan. Since 2008, Alam has worked as a ommunity health worker at the NYU Center for the Study of Asian American Health (CSAAH) at NYU Grossman School of Medicine on interventions to improve diabetes management and breast cancer screening. She participates in mentorship and training opportunities with her peers to share best practices and provide social support.

SHAHMIR H. ALI, BA, is a doctoral student in the Department of Social and Behavioral Sciences at the NYU School of Global Public Health. His current research focuses on interpersonal and community level factors involved in the eating behaviors of young and second-generation Asian Americans, and how these factors can be integrated into innovative intervention designs to address non-communicable disease disparities. His past publications and work have spanned projects in the United States, Australia, Pakistan, and China on topics ranging from innovative approaches in health promotion (such as mHealth) and understanding cultural, environmental, and social influences on health. Ali completed his bachelor's degree in public health and political science at Johns Hopkins University where he was a recipient of the Woodrow Wilson research fellowship. During this time, he was employed with the Johns Hopkins Bloomberg School of Public Health (US), Griffith University Centre for Environment and Population Health (Australia), and George Institute for Global Health (China) on various research projects.

LARISSA R. BURKA, BSN, RN, is a registered nurse currently working in New York City. She graduated from New York University with degrees in Nursing and Global Public Health. Her research has focused on health disparities among immigrant populations and language barriers in the healthcare field. During the COVID-19 pandemic, she served on the frontlines and is currently involved in several research projects associated with the psychological impact of the pandemic on healthcare workers. She is presently serving as the EU Coordinator on a global COVID team project. She plans to pursue a Master's in Public Health and a PhD in the near future.

ANDREA CARACOSTIS, MD, MPH, has been the Chief Executive Officer at the Asian American Health Coalition dba HOPE Clinic since 2007. HOPE Clinic is a Federally Qualified Health Center that provides care at four locations to the large multicultural and multilingual community in southwest and northeast Houston. A unique characteristic of HOPE Clinic is its capacity to provide services in more than 25 languages, including Mandarin, Cantonese, Vietnamese, Korean, Burmese, Arabic and Spanish. Caracostis' career has centered on quality healthcare access and passion for eliminating disparities and improving the health status of minorities and other underserved communities. She has made tremendous contributions to HOPE Clinic's success, and her important work has made a transformative difference to the community. Caracostis has served as a board member of the Susan G. Komen Medical Board, the Asian American Pacific Islander Community Health Centers, and the MD Anderson Institutional Review Board. She is currently a board member of Harris Health System and the Texas Association of Community Health Centers.

NADINE L. CHAN, PhD, MPH, is the Assistant Chief of Assessment, Policy Development, and Evaluation at Public Health - Seattle and King County and a Clinical Assistant Professor of Epidemiology at the University of Washington School of Public Health. She has over 20 years of experience using participatory approaches to evaluate multi-level and multi-sector strategies to improve health equity. Chan is currently a co-Principal Investigator of the Racial Ethnic Approaches to Community Health and a co-Principal Investigator of a mixed-methods evaluation of Seattle's sweetened beverage tax. She previously was a co-investigator of several community health interventions funded by the Centers for Disease Control and Prevention as well as a natural experiment of the King County menu labeling policy. She leads a team of senior level epidemiologists and social research scientists and launched a study team to develop the evaluation for the Best Starts for Kids Initiative, which includes the Communities of Opportunity initiative, a public/private partnership with The Seattle Foundation. Chan previously served as Chair, Program Chair, and Secretary for the Asian Pacific Islander Caucus for Public Health.

PERLA CHEBLI, PhD, MPH, is a postdoctoral researcher at NYU Grossman School of Medicine, Section for Health Equity. Her research leverages community engagement strategies to explore cancer disparities in underserved immigrant communities and facilitate the adaptation and implementation of evidence-based interventions. Her current work includes examining cultural and contextual determinants of HPV vaccine acceptance and hesitancy in Arab and Mexican communities in New York City to inform the development of a culturally adapted multilevel campaign. Chebli is a Social Determinants of Health Emerging Scholar with the Robert Wood Johnson Foundation-funded training program at Scholars Strategy Network and a Dissemination and Implementation Scholar with the Cancer Prevention and Control Network. She earned her master's in public health at New York University and PhD in public health sciences at the University of Illinois at Chicago.

IONA CHENG, PhD, MPH, is a Professor in the Department of Epidemiology and Biostatistics at the University of California, San Francisco. She is a cancer and genetic epidemiologist, and Principal Investigator of multiple NIH- and foundation-funded projects aimed at examining genetics, lifestyle factors, and neighborhood characteristics in relation to cancer risk. Cheng has an extensive research program investigating racial/ethnic differences in cancer risk and has expertise in leading population-based cancer surveillance studies that document the variation in cancer incidence and mortality patterns across race/ethnicity.

JOHN J. CHIN, PhD, is a Professor in the Department of Urban Policy and Planning at Hunter College, City University of New York. His research focuses on access to social and health services for under-served urban communities, including immigrant communities and communities of color. His NIH-funded research has examined the role of immigrant-led community institutions in delivering HIV prevention and stigma-reduction messages. He recently completed an NIH-funded study of HIV risk, working conditions, and experiences with law enforcement for Asian immigrant women working in sexually oriented massage parlors. Prior to his academic career, Chin helped to found the Asian & Pacific Islander Coalition on HIV/AIDS (now a Federally Qualified Health Center known as Apicha Community Health Center), where he served as Deputy Executive Director. Chin was a member of the National Institutes of Health Office of AIDS Research Advisory Council and is currently the chair of the National Advisory Committee for the Robert Wood Johnson Foundation's Health Policy Research Scholars Program. Chin has a PhD in Urban Planning from Columbia University, an MS in Urban Policy Analysis from the New School for Social Research, and a BA from Cornell University.

MATTHEW K. CHIN, MPH, is a Research Coordinator at the NYU Center for Study of Asian American Health (CSAAH) at NYU Grossman School of Medicine. His work entails conducting community-centered research projects that examine disparities among Asian American subgroups and other underserved racial and ethnic minority groups in order to inform policy and programs. His recent projects have entailed investigating the impacts of the COVID-19 pandemic on Asian American subgroups, conducting a community needs assessment for older adult immigrants in New York City, and exploring methods for retrospectively improving race/ethnicity classification in secondary datasets. Previously he worked at the Charles B. Wang Community Health Center, where he conducted research and evaluation projects to improve culturally tailored care and services for the Chinese American community. Chin completed his MPH with a concentration in epidemiology and biostatistics at the Johns Hopkins Bloomberg School of Public Health as a Bloomberg American Health Initiative Fellow and earned his BA in Health, Behavior & Society and History of Medicine at the University of Rochester.

JULIET K. CHOI, JD, is the president and Chief Executive Officer of the Asian & Pacific Islander American Health Forum (APIAHF), a national health justice organization which influences policy, mobilizes communities, and strengthens programs and organizations to improve the health of Asian Americans, Native Hawaiians and Pacific Islanders. She served in the Obama administration as the former chief of staff and senior advisor of two federal agencies: U.S. Citizenship and Immigration Services (USCIS) at the U.S. Department of Homeland Security; and the Office for Civil Rights (OCR) at the U.S. Department of Health and Human Services. Prior to her political appointments, Choi led disaster relief operations and strategic partnerships at the American Red Cross as a member of the disaster leadership team. She has previously worked at the Partnership for Public Service, Asian American Justice Center, Mental Health America, and a Fortune 500 corporation. Choi received her law school's Alumni Association Award for Leadership and Character and Rising Star Alumnus Award. Currently, she serves on the boards of the NAPABA Law Foundation and national YWCA USA.

RINA DAS, PhD, is the Director of Division of Integrative Biological and Behavioral Sciences at National Institute on Minority Health and Health Disparities (NIMHD), NIH. She focuses on promoting research to understand and address the various factors that play a role in health disparities in different underserved populations, including Asian American, Native Hawaiian and Pacific islanders. Das lends her expertise to a wide array of NIMHD programs that seek to improve minority health and health disparities, including translational sciences, behavioral sciences, cancer health disparities, research on the integration of biological and social sciences, social epigenomics, sleep health disparities, and immigrant health. At NIMHD she initiated the Immigrant health program to improve our understanding of the complex factors for health advantages and health disparities among immigrant populations and to develop intervention to address the health disparities. Prior to joining NIMHD,

Das served as a Program Director at the Center to Reduce Cancer Health Disparities at the National Cancer Institute managing programs on cancer health disparities research that focused on community-based interventions and grants to improve diversity in the research workforce.

MINDY C. DeROUEN, PhD, MPH, is a research scientist in the Department of Epidemiology and Biostatistics at the University of California San Francisco. DeRouen completed her doctoral training in Cancer Biology from Stanford University in 2010 and earned a Masters of Public Health in Epidemiology from UC Berkeley in 2014. She also studied Politics, Philosophy, and Economics at the University of Oxford (Hertford College). Her ongoing research efforts are focused on cancer prevention and control and address cancer disparities due to multi-level determinants, especially social determinants of health. DeRouen has experience with pooling and harmonizing complex multi-level data, including contextual-level data and data from electronic health records, from disparate sources and designing studies of multi-level data to study cancer disparities. She is a member of UCSF's DREAM Lab and an associate member of the Helen Diller Family Comprehensive Cancer Center.

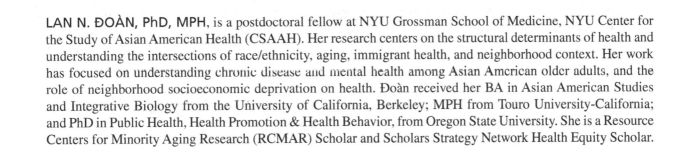

LAN N. ĐOÀN, PhD, MPH, is a postdoctoral fellow at NYU Grossman School of Medicine, NYU Center for the Study of Asian American Health (CSAAH). Her research centers on the structural determinants of health and understanding the intersections of race/ethnicity, aging, immigrant health, and neighborhood context. Her work has focused on understanding chronic disease and mental health among Asian American older adults, and the role of neighborhood socioeconomic deprivation on health. Đoàn received her BA in Asian American Studies and Integrative Biology from the University of California, Berkeley; MPH from Touro University-California; and PhD in Public Health, Health Promotion & Health Behavior, from Oregon State University. She is a Resource Centers for Minority Aging Research (RCMAR) Scholar and Scholars Strategy Network Health Equity Scholar.

MARY ANNE FOO, MPH, is the executive director and founder of the Orange County Asian and Pacific Islander Community Alliance (OCAPICA), a nonprofit organization in California with over 100 staff who serve more than 50,000 community members in 26 different languages on an annual basis. She has been working for over 30 years with underserved populations in the areas of health, mental health, youth leadership and development, workforce development, housing, and civic engagement. Foo's previous positions have been with organizations including, Association of Asian Pacific Community Health Organizations (AAPCHO), Asian Pacific Health Care Venture (APHCV), Orange County Health Care Agency, CalOptima, and Families in Good Health/ St Mary Medical Center. Foo has served as Principal Investigator and co-PI on numerous community based participatory research programs including a CDC National Centers of Excellence. She also serves as a trustee on several boards including a local hospital and foundation. Foo received her Bachelor of Science from the University of California, Davis and her Master in Public Health from the University of California, Los Angeles.

CHANDAK GHOSH, MD, MPH, a board-certified ophthalmologist and Captain in the U.S. Public Health Service, is with the Health Resources and Services Administration (HRSA), an agency within the U.S. Department of Health and Human Services. A nationally-recognized expert in health equity, he stands committed to the health needs of underserved populations and keeps focus on the impact of economic downsizing on quality of care. The findings of his research and publications have been presented before the U.S. Congress and the White House and have energized collaborations among foundations, community-based groups, government, and academia. He worked on the design and implementation of the Affordable Care Act and the development of the National Performance Review Protocol, utilized to improve quality at all Federal health grantees, including hospitals, universities, and community health centers. The U.S. Public Health Service has awarded Ghosh a rare Meritorious Service Medal, among its highest honors, for "influencing progress towards health equity on a national scale." He holds degrees from Yale University, Medical College of Virginia, and Harvard School of Public Health.

SCARLETT LIN GOMEZ, PhD, MPH, is Professor in the Department of Epidemiology and Biostatistics and Co-Leader of the Cancer Control Program of the Helen Diller Family Comprehensive Cancer Center, at the University of California, San Francisco. She is Director of the Greater Bay Area Cancer Registry, a participant in the NCI SEER (Surveillance, Epidemiology, End Results) program and the California Cancer Registry. Her research focuses on cancer health disparities and aims to understand the multilevel drivers, particularly the social determinants, of those disparities. Gomez has enhanced the capability of population-level cancer surveillance data to examine the roles of immigration, ethnic enclave, and institutional and neighborhood-level factors, with attention to providing empirical cancer statistics for disaggregated populations defined by race/ethnicity, nativity, and other social determinants. A central focus of this work has been on the Asian American populations.

HAE-RA HAN, PhD, RN, FAAN, is a professor of nursing and public health and the Elsie M. Lawler Endowed Chair at the Johns Hopkins University. She is also Associate Dean for Community Programs and Initiatives at the School of Nursing. In this role, she oversees community nurse-led health centers and wellness programs in Baltimore, Maryland. Her interdisciplinary research focuses on promoting health equity in chronic care among people of color, particularly those with limited health literacy and limited English proficiency. Her program of research has advanced thinking from the traditional paradigm of knowledge transfer from provider-to-patients to developing health literacy skills of patients to traverse the landscape of health screening and patient self-care to reduce health inequities. Han served multiple terms on the American Journal of Public Health editorial board while assuming leadership roles including vice chair and chair of the board. She has received multiple honors and awards from national and international organizations such as American Public Health Association, National Coalition of Ethnic Minority Nurse Associations, and Sigma Theta Tau-International.

MARJORIE KAGAWA-SINGER, PhD, MN, RN, is Professor Emerita in the School of Public Health and Department of Asian American Studies at the University of California Los Angeles (UCLA). She has a master's degree in nursing and a master's and doctorate in anthropology, all from UCLA. Her research has focused on the etiology and elimination of disparities in physical and mental health care outcomes primarily with the Asian American and Pacific Islander communities. Kagawa-Singer was principal investigator of the Los Angeles site for the national Asian American Network on Cancer Awareness, Research and Training and is the UCLA Minority Training Program for Cancer Control Research, funded by the UCLA Comprehensive Cancer Center. She was also a member of the UCLA School of Public Health Center for Health Policy Research.

LIZA KING, MPH, is a research scientist at the New York City Department of Health and Mental Hygiene. King is passionate about data disaggregation and committed to the health of marginalized populations. At the Bureau of Epidemiology Services, King is producing a report to highlight the health of Asian and Pacific Islander New Yorkers. In 2018, she also authored a data brief on Health Disparities among Asian New Yorkers.

KATHY KO CHIN, MS, is a strategic advisor to those in philanthropy and nonprofits. From 2010 - 2020, she served as president & CEO of the Asian & Pacific Islander American Health Forum. The daughter of immigrants from China, Ko Chin's 40-year career has been committed to building community institutions that contribute to a just and multiracial society, which led the American Public Health Association to honor her with the prestigious Helen Rodriguez-Trias Social Justice Award in 2020. Ko Chin, a renowned voice in AA, NH, and PI communities, has served on and chaired the boards of numerous nonprofit organizations at the national, California state, and local levels. From 2014 to 2017, she served as a member of the President's Advisory Commission on Asian Americans and Pacific Islanders. She joined The Kresge Foundation Board of Trustees in 2017. She earned a master's degree in health policy and management from the Harvard T.H. Chan School of Public Health and a bachelor's degree in economics from Stanford University.

CHRISTINA Y. LEE, MPH, is an Overdose Prevention Coordinator with the New York City Department of Homeless Services, where she implements substance use treatment and access programs. Previously, she worked at the NYU Center for the Study of Asian American Health (CSAAH) at NYU Grossman School of Medicine, where she researched gender-based violence among Asian American, Native Hawaiian, and Pacific Islander populations, and at the NYC Department of Health and Mental Hygiene, where she developed a community-engagement framework for a report on the health of Asians and Pacific Islanders in NYC. Lee received her bachelor's degree in Psychobiology from UCLA and earned her master's in Sociomedical Sciences and Health Promotion from Columbia University Mailman School of Public Health, where she authored a thesis on consent and sexual assault experiences among Asian American undergraduate women. She has extensive public health program planning experience for youth and young adults, and her other academic interests include menstrual equity and the effect of state violence on health. Lee currently organizes in NYC to end the criminalization of domestic and sexual violence survivors.

MATTHEW LEE, DrPH, MPH, is an Associate Research Scientist at NYU Grossman School of Medicine in the Department of Population Health's Section for Health Equity and the NYU Center for the Study of Asian American Health (CSAAH). Matthew earned a bachelor's degree in Anthropology and English Literature from Washington University in St. Louis, a master's of public health degree with a certificate in Health Promotion Research and Practice from the Columbia University Mailman School of Public Health, and a doctor of public health degree from the Columbia University Mailman School of Public Health. Matthew was also a pre-doctoral fellow in the Robert Wood Johnson Foundation Health Policy Research Scholars program and is currently an associate member of the New York Academy of Medicine. As a health equity researcher and community-engaged implementation scientist, Lee's research applies participatory approaches and mixed methods to examine the equitable reach, impact, and sustainability of evidence-based interventions within underserved communities.

YAN LI, PhD, is an Associate Professor in the Departments of Population Health Science and Policy, and Obstetrics, Gynecology, and Reproductive Science at the Icahn School of Medicine at Mount Sinai. He is also the Director of the Health Policy Modeling Laboratory and a member of the Blavatnik Family Women's Health Research Institute at Mount Sinai. He is a Fellow of the New York Academy of Medicine. Li and his team at Mount Sinai have developed a broad range of innovative simulation tools that can be used to simulate disease progression, evaluate the cost-effectiveness of prevention and treatment interventions, and improve public health practices and healthcare management. These projects have led to more than 70 publications in high-quality academic journals in both systems engineering and public health fields. His research has been supported by multiple funding agencies such as the National Institutes of Health, Robert Wood Johnson Foundation, European Commission, and American Heart Association.

SAHNAH LIM, PhD, MPH, MIA, is an assistant professor who is leading the Gender Equity scientific track at NYU Grossman School of Medicine's Department of Population Health's Section for Health Equity. As a health disparities researcher, Lim conducts applied, community-engaged studies that seek to address gender-related health issues among hard-to-reach populations such as sex workers and immigrant survivors of gender-based violence. Her research uses intersectionality and syndemics frameworks to understand how multiple marginalization impacts mental and sexual health outcomes. Lim is a mixed-methods researcher, with expertise in psychosocial statistics and survey methods.

SUNGWOO LIM, DrPH, MA, MS, is a director of research and evaluation unit at Bureau of Epidemiology Services, New York City Department of Health and Mental Hygiene. He is trained as a statistician/epidemiologist, and leading a team of 12 statisticians, epidemiologists, and a geographer. Lim and his team have been leading projects to improve the utility and quality of large administrative data as a tool to assess effectiveness of public health programs and answer public health questions. In particular, collaborating with academic partners and city agencies, he has developed expertise in data matching, causal inference techniques, and program evaluation for large scale public health programs such as supportive housing for people with homelessness and jail-based methadone treatment program. These methodological works, along with program evaluation reports, have been presented and published, contributing to advancing public health practices and statistical methods. Lim received his MA in international trade and investment policy from George Washington University, his MS in survey methodology from University of Michigan, and DrPH in epidemiology from City University of New York Doctor of Public Health program.

SHINU MAMMEN, MPH, is a Senior Project Coordinator in the Department of Population Health at NYU Grossman School of Medicine. She works on implementing lifestyle and behavior change interventions for the South Asian community that focus on diabetes prevention and management. In her role, she developed expertise in customizing provider registry lists to enhance better follow-up for patients with diabetes. She also enhanced the utilization of electronic health record (EHR) clinical decision support tools to increase provider adherence to screening guidelines for diabetes. Mammen works closely with community-based organizations serving New York City South Asian communities to disseminate culturally salient health information. She is passionate about advancing health equity for underserved immigrant communities and providing communities the resources needed to manage their health. She formerly worked on the Mediators of Atherosclerosis in South Asians Living in America (MASALA) Study, the first longitudinal cohort study to assess risk factors for heart disease in South Asians living in the United States. Mammen holds a BS from Loyola University Chicago and a MPH from Benedictine University.

SARA S. METCALF, PhD, is a geography professor who uses systems science approaches in urban health and sustainability research projects to identify and implement feedback mechanisms with dynamic simulation models. She applies system dynamics to guide simulation experiments informing potential pathways toward community health, equity, and sustainability. Her educational background includes a doctorate in geography, master's degrees in management and chemical engineering, and bachelor's degrees in biochemistry and chemical engineering. Metcalf has worked with agent-based models since her doctoral research on disparities in urban networks, incorporating insights from system dynamics that she learned as a master's student at MIT as a means of mathematically and visually representing feedback and delays embedded in social structures underlying problematic behavior over time. Metcalf has leveraged systems modeling, including group model building processes as well as simulation experiments, in research to identify ways of promoting societal benefits such as health equity, food justice, and ecosystem resilience. As a research investigator, she has been funded by the NIH/NIDCR in projects addressing oral health disparities in minority populations, including Asian Americans.

DEBORAH K. MIN, MPH, is a Project Coordinator at the NYU Center for the Study of Asian American Health (CSAAH) within the Department of Population Health's Section for Health Equity at NYU Grossman School of Medicine. She is also a doctoral student in the Health Equity and Social Justice track at the Johns Hopkins Bloomberg School of Public Health. Broadly, her research interests include culturally-relevant community-engaged projects that confront health disparities and advance health equity within and across Asian American communities. She received her BA in Psychology at Wheaton College (IL) and MPH from Columbia University's Mailman School of Public Health, Department of Sociomedical Sciences with a concentration in Child, Youth, and Family Health.

SARAH M. MINER, RN, PhD, is an Assistant Professor of Community Health Nursing at St. John Fisher College in Rochester, NY. She received her doctoral degree from the University of Rochester and has over 20 years of experience working as a community health nurse with non-English speaking populations. She has worked both nationally and abroad on NIH funded research projects, and received numerous awards for her community-engaged work with non-English speaking populations. Miner is currently a faculty fellow of the St. John Fisher Social Innovation Academy which aims to build the leadership capacity, community engagement efforts and social innovation capabilities of community leaders, community staff, and neighborhood residents, alongside the faculty, staff, and students of St. John Fisher College. Her program of research aims to understand and address health disparities among non-English speaking older adult populations in home and community-based settings, particularly in the areas of chronic illness and medication literacy.

SADIA MOHAIMIN, BA, is a Project Coordinator at the NYU Center for the Study of Asian American Health (CSAAH) within the Department of Population Health, NYU Grossman School of Medicine. In her role, she coordinates community-engaged research projects focused on improving health and chronic disease management among South Asian patients in primary care settings. Mohaimin also provides support for gender equity studies that seek to address health issues among South Asian survivors of gender-based violence. She is committed to engaging underserved and disadvantaged communities in ways that are culturally and contextually relevant; she has organized in-language community workshops and forums on a number of topics including nutrition, mental health, and vaccine hesitancy, and has led culturally-tailored dance exercise sessions for South Asian seniors. Mohaimin graduated from New York University in 2018 where she studied Psychology. Mohaimin is an aspiring physician who hopes to practice preventive care in primary care settings and apply evidence-based strategies for prevention and self-management to reduce health disparities. Outside of work, she likes to dance and spend time with her family.

SHAARANYA PILLAI, BA, is the Deputy Director of India Home. Before joining India Home's development team in 2018, Shaaranya worked in academia at her alma mater of New York University, facilitating and administering courses at the Child and Adolescent Mental Health Studies department, through which she grew a passion for integrating cultural competency in service settings. Since joining the organization, Pillai has taken the organization through several successful community outreach projects, capital grant processes, and development efforts. She has also helped the organization make key partnerships including with NYC Census and the NYC Test & Trace Program. Pillai also contributed towards India Home's research paper on mental health needs in South Asian older adults, which was published in 2021 in the International Journal of Geriatric Psychiatry. In 2017, Pillai presented at the Tamil Studies Symposium at York College (Ontario, CA) on mental health in diasporic Sri Lankan Tamil youth. Pillai was also a recipient of the prestigious LankaCorps Fellowship in 2016, through which she worked for nonprofits in Sri Lanka for psychosocial needs and reconciliation efforts.

NINEZ A. PONCE, PhD, MPP (BS UC Berkeley; MPP Harvard; PhD UCLA), is Professor in the UCLA Fielding School of Public Health and Director of its Center for Health Policy Research. She leads the California Health Interview Survey, the nation's largest state health survey. A health economist, her research focuses on implementing population-based health surveys in diverse populations and examining the intersection of social factors and health policy. Ponce was honored in 2019 by Asian Health Services, a nationally-accolaed community-health center, awarded the 2020 UCLA Don T. Nakanishi Award for Outstanding Engaged Scholarship, and received the 2020 inaugural Data Equity award by Asian Pacific Partners for Empowerment, Advocacy and Leadership. In 2019 Ponce received the top prize in her field from Academy Health that recognized the impact of her work in population health measurement to inform public policies. She is an elected member of the National Academy of Social Insurance, board member for AcademyHealth, and is a Commissioner for the 2021 Robert Wood Johnson Foundation's National Commission to Transform Public Health Data Systems.

MARGUERITE J. RO, DrPH, is the Chief of the Assessment, Policy Development, and Evaluation (APDE) unit and Director of the Chronic Disease and Injury Prevention (CDIP) section of Public Health – Seattle & King County. Ro has focused her efforts on working with diverse communities to achieve health equity for our nation's most at-risk populations. As Deputy Director of the Asian & Pacific Islander American Health Forum (a national health advocacy organization), she played a leadership role in Health Through Action, a groundbreaking partnership program to close health gaps for Asian Americans, Native Hawaiians, and Pacific Islanders. During her time at Columbia University as an assistant professor, Ro also served as senior policy analyst for the W.K. Kellogg Foundation's Community Voices initiative, a national demonstration project to improve access to care for vulnerable populations. She is the 2018 recipient of the Washington State Public Health Association's Public Health Leadership Award. Ro obtained her masters and doctorate from the Johns Hopkins University School of Public Health.

RIENNA G. RUSSO, MHS, is a project coordinator in the Section for Health Equity at NYU Grossman School of Medicine, Department of Population Health and PhD student in the Department of Epidemiology at the Harvard T.H. Chan School of Public Health. Her research interests include investigating the operationalization of race/ethnicity in datasets and clinical algorithms, as well as evaluating how structural racism drives social determinants of health and cardiovascular disease disparities. Russo received her Masters of Health Science in Epidemiology from Johns Hopkins Bloomberg School of Public Health.

RACHEL SACKS, MPH, is an independent public health consultant specializing in scientific and technical writing. Prior to establishing her consulting business in 2006, she served in managerial positions with non-profit organizations, a university-based research center, and a public health department in Bangkok, Thailand; Mumbai, India; and New York City, USA. She received her bachelor's degree at Tufts University in International Relations and French and her master's degree in public health at Yale University School of Medicine in the Division of International Health.

TINA R. SADARANGANI, PhD, RN, ANP-BC, GNP-BC, is a PhD-prepared board-certified adult and gerontological nurse practitioner with expertise in managing older adults with complex health and social needs. Her work is rooted in a commitment to improving the health of vulnerable populations, specifically older immigrants, by leveraging the strengths of community-based organizations. She is currently an Assistant Professor at NYU, and a principal investigator on two studies funded by the National Institutes of Health. To date, her research career has blended her in-depth knowledge of anthropology and nursing science. She is interested in how social, cultural, and policy factors contribute to health. Her work, which incorporates principles of design thinking, focuses on developing multicomponent interventions involving individuals, families, and communities to meet the needs of older adults. Sadarangani was recently recognized as a Rising Star and Woman of Distinction in Long-term Care, by McKnight's, a national leader in long-term news. She is also a leading member of the National Adult Day Services Research committee, shaping research priorities for home and community-based services across the United States.

RITI SHIMKHADA, PhD, MPH, is a senior research scientist at the UCLA Center for Health Policy Research. She is an epidemiologist with interest and experience in health policy. She is a member of the faculty task force for the California Health Benefits Program and has extensive research experience in examining state policies. She is an author of "Federal Policies and Health" in Immigrant California: Understanding the Past, Present, and Future of U.S. Policy (2021). She has recently led and published analyses of social media data. She has also been involved in research on disaggregated data for Asian populations as well as for American Indian/Alaska Native groups. As the daughter of Nepali immigrants, Shimkhada is involved with Nepali diaspora groups and has a special concern for small South Asian populations.

SELVIA SIKDER, MA, is a nonprofit and government sector professional and passionate advocate for the senior community. She is currently working for the New York City government. Her passion for underrepresented immigrant communities led her to begin her career in the U.S. with the Bangladeshi American Community Development and Youth Services (BACDYS). Afterward, she joined India Home Inc., a Queens-based nonprofit organization serving South Asian seniors, where she served over three years, beginning as Case Manager and ultimately as Program Director. Sikder pursued her Master's degree in the Study of the Americas Program at the City College of New York, CUNY, focusing her research on South Asian Immigrants in the United States. She has a Bachelor's and Master's degree in International Relations from the Jahangirnagar University of Bangladesh. As she continues to work in the public sector, she hopes to use her passion to improve the lives of older adults living in New York City

SHOBHA SRINIVASAN, PhD, is a sociologist and the Senior Advisor for Health Disparities in the Office of the Director, Division of Cancer Control and Population Sciences (DCCPS), National Cancer Institute (NCI). She currently coordinates activities across DCCPS, NCI, the National Institutes of Health, and with other federal and non-governmental agencies to develop programs and initiatives to address health disparities and promote health equity. Through these NCI-funded programs she promotes the building of partnerships between communities and universities to address various health challenges in underserved and immigrant communities. Previously, Srinivasan has taught and conducted research at various universities, and has worked as a research director at a community-based health advocacy organization. Her research focuses primarily on social determinants of health, place, poverty, and resulting inequities, including challenges in the utilization and access to health services. In all these projects, the goal is largely to inform health policy at the local, state, and national levels regarding health and health care for underserved and underrepresented populations.

SABIHA SULTANA, BSW, is a community health worker at the NYU Center for the Study of Asian American Health (CSAAH), within the Department of Population Health at NYU Grossman School of Medicine. Sabiha is fluent in Bengali/English and is dedicated to serving her community. Within her role at NYU, she works closely with the New York City (NYC) South Asian community. She has experience helping patients from NYC primary care practices to prevent and manage cardiovascular diseases, such as diabetes and hypertension, by providing in-language and culturally-appropriate health education and lifestyle coaching. She has also built strong relationships with women's groups in the Bangladeshi community in Brooklyn and Queens for the NYU Community Service Plan. Sultana is also a certified health navigator and assists in enrolling patients into health insurance plans. Sabiha graduated from the City University of New York (CUNY) at York College with a Bachelor's degree in Social Work and a Bachelor's degree in Social Welfare from National University of Dhaka, Bangladesh, and thus, has extensive experience and skill providing social services. Previously she's worked as a case work liaison and outreach services specialist, providing services within New York City. In her free time, Sultana enjoys doing arts and crafts, gardening and cooking up healthy Bangladeshi dishes.

MD TAHER, MPH, is a Project Coordinator at the NYU Center for Study of Asian American Health (CSAAH) at NYU Grossman School of Medicine where he provides research support for the studies designed to reduce the burden of diabetes, hypertension, and other chronic illnesses among the members of the South Asian and Arab American communities living in New York City through education and empowerment. Taher is a passionate community health advocate. He is well connected to the South Asian and Arab American community groups in New York City. Taher has over 10 years of experience working at CSAAH where he plays a key role in building and fostering partnerships with diverse community and faith-based organizations. Taher earned his Bachelor of Science in Community Health Education from Hunter College of the City University of New York, and his MPH with a concentration in Community and International Health from New York University.

■ ■ ■

LOIS M. TAKAHASHI, MS, PhD, is Houston Flournoy Professor of State Government at the University of Southern California Sol Price School of Public Policy, and Director of USC Price in Sacramento. Prior to joining USC Price, she was Interim Dean (2015-2016) and Associate Dean for Research (2014-2015) at the UCLA Luskin School of Public Affairs, Chair of the UCLA Department of Urban Planning (2011-2013), and Director of the University of California Asian American and Pacific Islander Policy Multicampus Research Program (UC AAPI Policy MRP; 2009-2013). She was President of the Association of Collegiate Schools of Planning (2015-2017). Her current funded research includes the effects of community violence on African American adolescent development (Dexter Voisin/PI, University of Toronto), and violence experiences of transgender women of color

(Karin Tobin/PI, Johns Hopkins University). Takahashi is also working with Cambria Solutions on Project 19th, a social media tool to increase the number of women who consider running for US elected office. With John Chin, Hunter College, she continues research examining the spatial configuration of the massage parlor industry in Los Angeles and New York City.

YI-LING TAN, MPH, is a Program Manager at the NYU Center for the Study of Asian American Health (CSAAH) at NYU Grossman School of Medicine in New York City. She implements and manages community-based participatory research studies and projects focused on reducing health disparities in the Asian American community, ranging from chronic disease prevention to uptake of vaccines and screening programs. Tan works with a team of Chinese-speaking community health workers to deliver evidence-based and culturally adapted health education interventions, sessions and resources. She also serves on the board of managers for the Chinatown YMCA. She received her MPH in Forced Migration and Health at the Columbia University Mailman School of Public Health.

WINSTON TSENG, PhD, is research scientist of community health sciences at University of California, Berkeley (UCB) and associate director of research at UCB Health Research for Action. Tseng's participatory action research has focused on underserved and immigrant communities, particularly Asian American & Pacific Islanders (AA&PIs) (e.g., Chinese, Hmong, Korean, Samoan, Vietnamese), to understand community assets and needs, and design and implement community-defined interventions to strengthen community health infrastructure. His research focus areas included health equity, health literacy, building community capacity, chronic conditions, healthy aging, and behavioral health. Tseng serves on the AAPI Standing Committee under the UCB Office of Equity & Inclusion. He served as Chair (2012–2014) of the Community Health Planning & Policy Development Section of the American Public Health Association (APHA). The APHA Asian Pacific Islander Caucus recognized Tseng in 2012 for the Best Published Paper: "Reshaping Data and Research through the Affordable Care Act: Opportunities for Asian American, Native Hawaiian and Pacific Islander Health." He received his PhD in Medical Sociology from UC San Francisco and his BA in Biology from Johns Hopkins University.

MD JALAL UDDIN, BS, MS, is a Research Data Associate in the Department of Population Health within NYU Grossman School of Medicine. He graduated with a Masters degree in Data Science from the CUNY School of Professional Studies in 2019. He holds a Bachelors degree in Statistics from Hunter College. In his role, he provides health education and coaching in Bengali/English as part of a community health worker intervention to improve diabetes prevention and management in the South Asian community. He works closely with primary care practices participating in the intervention, and assists with data collection and technical assistance for optimizing use of electronic health records (EHR). As a fellow immigrant himself, Uddin uses his understanding of the South Asian community and community resources to assist community members to achieve their goals for a better life. He enjoys motivating community members to change their food and physical activity behaviors to improve their health, as well as assisting community members with unemployment, health insurance and immigration processes. In his free time, he enjoys listening to music, reading and playing badminton.

JENNIFER A. WONG, MPH, is a Senior Program Coordinator at the Section for Health Equity within the Department of Population Health at NYU Grossman School of Medicine where she coordinates and oversees strategic partnerships and community engagement efforts at the NYU Center for the Study of Asian American

Health (CSAAH). Her work centers the use of community-based participatory research approaches to deliver collaborative and culturally responsive training, education, and dissemination. She received her undergraduate degree at Bryn Mawr College and earned a Master of Public Health degree in Health Promotion Research and Practice at the Department of Sociomedical Sciences at the Mailman School of Public Health, Columbia University.

YOUSRA YUSUF, PhD, MPH, is a Postdoctoral Fellow at NYU Grossman School of Medicine, Section for Health Equity. Her current research focuses on the intersection of structural determinants of health around COVID-19 vaccine uptake, nutrition decisions, and cancer management. Her background is on reproductive health through the life course among individuals in underserved, immigrant communities. She uses mixed methods in community-engaged research to explore gender equity in racial/ethnic and religious minority groups in the United States. Yusuf serves as the President of the South Asian Public Health Association, a national nonprofit that aims to promote the health and well-being of South Asian communities in the United States. She sits on several nonprofit boards serving Asian American communities in New York and internationally. Yusuf completed her Masters in Public Health at the SUNY Downstate School of Public Health with a specialization in Epidemiology and a research focus in maternal health and her PhD in women's and maternal health with a certificate in health communications from the Johns Hopkins Bloomberg School of Public Health.

SIDRA ZAFAR, BS, is a Community Health Representative at the NYU Center for the Study of Asian American Health (CSAAH) at NYU Grossman School of Medicine. Zafar received her Bachelor of Science in Health Administration and Services at the City University of New York (CUNY) where she was the recipient of the Emerging Scholar Award. She currently works on the Diabetes Research Education and Action for Minorities (DREAM) Initiative providing a culturally tailored health education intervention for prediabetes and diabetes patients. She is fluent in Urdu, Hindi and Punjabi. Zafar has previously worked on projects focusing on improving hypertension management and breast cancer screening in the South Asian and Arab American communities, respectively. Zafar is a strong patient advocate, and follows up with her patients' physicians regarding medication questions, prescription refills, and specialist referrals in order to improve management of their health. She connects community members to housing, employment and SNAP benefits as well as provides vaccination scheduling. She is also a certified patient navigator providing assistance to community members with health insurance enrollment.

JENNIFER ZANOWIAK, MA, is a Program Manager for the Section for Health Equity, Department of Population Health at NYU Grossman School of Medicine. She coordinates research and implementation science projects involving the translation and adaptation of evidence-based community and clinical linkage strategies to reduce cardiovascular disease and diabetes disparities in diverse racial, ethnic and minority communities in New York City. She works in partnership with community health workers, primary care provider practices, and community- and faith- based groups. She received a BA in Metropolitan Studies and Psychology from New York University, and an MA in International Affairs from The New School. While completing her graduate studies, she worked as a consultant on projects in New York City and Mumbai in the areas of public health, HIV/AIDs, and gender equality.

ACKNOWLEDGMENTS

This book was supported in part by the National Institutes of Health (NIH) National Institute on Minority Health and Health Disparities (NIMHD) Award Number U54MD000538. The content is solely the responsibility of the authors and does not necessarily represent the official views of the NIMHD.

We would also like to thank the NYU Center for the Study of Asian American Health (CSAAH) community and scientific advisory groups for their continued guidance and support of our health disparities research efforts.

CSAAH's National Advisory Committee on Research (NAC)

- Therese R. Rodriguez, CEO, Apicha Community Health Center
- Layal Rabat, MA, Programs Director, Asian Pacific Community in Action
- Chaiwon Kim, President & CEO, Center for Pan Asian Community Services
- Mujtaba Ali, Programs Director, Council Of Peoples Organization
- Warren W. Chin, MD, Executive Director, Chinese American Medical Society
- Andrea Caracostis, MD, MPH, CEO, HOPE Clinic
- Vasundhara Kalasapudi, Executive Director, India Home
- Emerson Ea, PhD, DNP, APRN, CNE, Chairman, Kalusugan Coalition
- Sheri-Ann Daniels, EdD, Executive Director, Papa Ola Lōkahi
- Linda Lee, MS, Executive Director, Korean Community Services of Metropolitan NY
- O. Fahina Tavake-Pasi, MS, Executive Director, National Tongan American Society
- Mary Anne Foo, MPH, Executive Director, Orange County Asian Pacific Islander Community Alliance
- Sudha Acharya, MS, Executive Director, South Asian Council for Social Services
- Hardayal Singh, Executive Director, UNITED SIKHS

CSAAH's Scientific Committee (SC)

- Daphne Kwok, Vice President of Multicultural Markets & Engagement, Asian American & Pacific Islander Audience, AARP
- Tina J. Kauh, PhD, MS, Senior Program Officer, Research-Evaluation-Learning Unit, Robert Wood Johnson Foundation
- Scarlett Lin-Gomez, PhD, MPH, Professor, Department of Epidemiology and Biostatistics, University of California San Francisco
- Nia Aitaoto, PhD, MPH, MS, Research Associate Professor, Nutrition & Integrative Physiology, University of Utah, Utah Center for Pacific Islander Health
- Dorothy Castille, PhD, Project Officer for the U54 Grant, Division of Scientific Programs, Community Health and Population Sciences, National Institute on Minority Health and Health Disparities National Institutes of Health
- Benyam Hailu, MD, MPH, Project Scientist, Division of Scientific Programs, Community Health and Population Sciences, National Institute on Minority Health and Health Disparities National Institutes of Health.

ABOUT THE COMPANION WEBSITE

This book is accompanied by a companion website:

www.wiley.com/go/kwon/asianamerican

This website includes:

- Test Banks
- Lecture PowerPoint Slides

PART

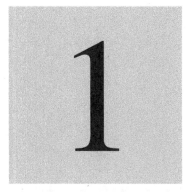

CONTEXT

CHAPTER

1

THE ASIAN AMERICAN POPULATION IN THE UNITED STATES

WINSTON TSENG, LAN N. ĐOÀN

LEARNING OBJECTIVES:

By the end of this chapter, the reader will be able to:

- Describe the social and legal history of Asian Americans.
- Describe the social demographic characteristics of Asian Americans.
- Identify and articulate the root causes of health and health care inequities among Asian Americans.

INTRODUCTION

This chapter provides an overview of the political and social factors that affect the health of Asian Americans. To better understand the root causes of health disparities among Asian Americans today, it is important to consider the historical and structural context within which these disparities have emerged as well as the social and demographic characteristics of the Asian American population today. In addition, the phenomenal population growth of the Asian American population since 1965 and the projected potential growth over the next decades have made Asian Americans and their health concerns a matter of increasing national significance.

Applied Population Health Approaches for Asian American Communities, First Edition. Edited by Simona C. Kwon, Chau Trinh-Shevrin, Nadia S. Islam, and Stella S. Yi.
© 2023 John Wiley & Sons, Inc. Published 2023 by John Wiley & Sons, Inc.
Companion Website: www.wiley.com/go/kwon/asianamerican

BACKGROUND AND HISTORY OF ASIAN AMERICANS

The history of Asian Americans is situated within the greater historical context of the United States, a nation of immigrants (Chan, 1991; Lai & Arguelles, 2003; Takaki, 1998). Like other U.S. immigrants, Asian immigrants came in search of the "American dream," with hope for a brighter future. Uprooted and transplanted, each wave of Asian immigrants has undergone dramatic social, economic, and cultural transitions from their native countries. Through resilience, perseverance, and solidarity, Asian immigrants struggled to survive and prosper in U.S. society. However, the outcomes of this struggle have often been less successful than initially expected. Across many generations in the United States, Asian American experiences have revealed an alternative immigration history, within which voices fell silent, hopes were dashed, and dreams went unfulfilled. The racialized constructions of Asians as a "model minority" and posing a "yellow peril" unveil deeper ethnic and racial tensions that continue to plague new Asian immigrants as well as subsequent generations of Asian Americans. Feelings of victimization, discrimination, and exclusion are frequent themes central to the history of Asian Americans.

Political and Legal History of Asian Immigration

Eight major historical periods inform the racialized political history of Asian Americans: (1) colonial period (1609–1775); (2) American Revolutionary period (1776–1840); (3) old immigration period (1841–1882); (4) regulation period (1882–1920); (5) restriction and exclusion period (1921–1952); (6) partial liberalization period (1952–1965); (7) liberalized policy period (1965–1999); and (8) growing restriction and exclusion period (2000–present) (Kim, 1994).

These historical periods comprise a critical lens through which to examine the political and legal dynamics of the history of Asian immigration to the United States. From this examination, three principal patterns have emerged:

1. *Institutional racism was exerted by the judicial system.* Early American judicial practices and court decisions based on institutional racism have long excluded immigrants from the fundamental privileges of citizenship, civil rights, and property.

2. *Congressional immigration and naturalization laws discriminated against Asian immigrants.* Congressional immigration laws were passed that reflect the founding concept of non-Hispanic White (White) racial and cultural supremacy and exclusivity, thereby restricting U.S. immigration from Asia.

3. *Racial ideology and societal values penetrated all levels, from the personal to the institutional.* Racial ideologies and ethnocentric values persist and continue to significantly limit the acceptance of diversity, including Asian Americans, in all levels of the American social structure (Kim, 1994).

Colonial Period The first immigration from the British Isles to North America occurred during the colonial period (1609–1775). It defined and set the tone for subsequent colonial immigration processes and policies, ranging from race/ethnicity, social class, religion, and other social dynamics (Kim, 1994).

Revolutionary Period The founding fathers of the Revolutionary period (1776–1840) held strong anti-foreign values that influenced the definition and process of individuals eligible for American citizenship. The qualities of people suitable for American citizenship (free White persons) came to be legally defined in this period under the Nationality Act of 1790.

Old Immigration Period Federal ethnocentric immigration policies against Asian immigrants evolved through a process of judicial and public actions during the old immigration period (1841–1882) (Hing, 1994; Kim, 1994). The 1870 revision of the Nationality Act of 1790 extended naturalization rights to persons of African descent, but the law continued to exclude Asian aliens from naturalization. Although Chinese merchants, students, and teachers were allowed entry into the United States for short stays, there was great anti-immigrant and yellow peril sentiments that "dirty" Chinese laborers would contaminate the U.S. cultural roots and its workforce. As a result, the Immigration Act of 1882 and the Chinese Exclusion Act of 1882 barred the entry of Chinese laborers to the country and denied permanent residence to Chinese already in the United States. The Chinese Exclusion Act of 1882 was the first law passed of its kind: it specifically excluded persons from political citizenship based on race/ethnicity. The act was not repealed until 1943 when the United States became allied with China during the Pacific conflicts. However, these restrictions on Chinese immigrants prior to 1943 opened the door for Japanese, Filipino, Korean, and Asian Indian laborers in the late nineteenth and early twentieth centuries to fill the void in the low-cost foreign labor market that Chinese laborers left behind.

Regulation Period During the regulation period (1882–1920), immigration regulation and control became an important component of national policy. The legislative and judicial branches took further actions to restrict and halt the flow of Asian immigration to the United States, particularly of those who were perceived as a threat to native capital and labor interests (Kim, 1994). It was during this period that the quantity of immigrants came to be federally controlled for the first time. The anti-immigration judicial and legislative processes of the regulation period led to the Nationality Origins Act of 1921 and 1924, or Quota Immigration Laws. These laws were significant in that they gave preferential political status and social privileges to certain European immigrant groups; based the annual quota for immigration of non-European immigrant groups on the 2 percent of the existing Asian and other immigrant populations already in the United States by 1890; and specifically excluded Chinese, Japanese, and Koreans from the new immigration quota system.

As a result of the Quota Immigration Laws, trans-Pacific Asian immigration to the United States was dramatically restricted through the end of World War II. There were two notable exceptions. Filipinos were recognized as U.S. nationals between 1902 and 1946 due to the colonization of the Philippines by the United States. In addition, a small and select group of Asian Indian laborers, merchants, and scholars emigrated (fewer than 7,000 total), primarily Sikhs from the Punjab region. These immigrants came to the United States between 1881 and 1917, when good international relations existed between the United States and the British colonial government in India (Hing, 1994). However, the Immigration Act of 1917 (also known as the Asiatic Barred Zone Act) quickly halted Indian immigration flows.

Restriction and Exclusion Period During the restriction and exclusion period (1921–1952), the Tydings-McDuffie Act of 1934 ended the Philippines colonial relationship and proposed to provide Philippine independence. It also served to close the door to future Filipino immigrants in the United States (Kim, 1994). During this same period, major Supreme Court cases continued to deny citizenship to Asian resident aliens based on race. The most notable example of restriction and exclusion of Asian Americans occurred at this time – the internment of Japanese Americans during World War II. Japanese Americans were politically imprisoned and their civil rights were stripped from them in the name of national security.

After World War II, there was a dramatic change in American policy that led to a shift from ethnic and racial exclusion of Asian groups toward a more open immigration policy, particularly for racial and ethnic groups belonging to countries who had political alliances with the United States. Three factors contributed to the shift in immigration policy: the rising status of the United States as a superpower in the post–World War II landscape; increasing American political and economic involvement in Asia, such as in China and India; and growing recognition of the importance of alliances and resources in Asia. The Luce-Celler Act of 1946 reopened immigration to the Philippines and India, and immigrants from those countries were allowed to naturalize as American citizens (1946 Indian and Filipino Immigration and Naturalization (Aka Luce-Celler Act), 1946). However, this act also established an annual legal immigration quota of only 100 Asian Indian immigrants.

Partial Liberalization Period The partial liberalization period (1952–1965) was characterized by major global and national restructuring. American involvement against communist regimes in Asia, such as in China and Korea, led to the passage of more inclusive laws that gave resident aliens from Asia the right to become naturalized (Kim, 1994). These processes initiated new flows of limited Asian immigration to the United States, especially for those Asian individuals married to American military personnel or members of groups allied with the U.S. military during conflicts.

The new international political landscape after World War II led to the Immigration Act of 1952, which opened the doors to displaced persons or refugees from allied groups. As the United States assumed increased political responsibility to assist refugees, it also lifted naturalization restrictions based on ethnicity and race. However, the national origin quotas for immigrants continued to be maintained and limited the annual legal immigration quota to 105 immigrants for China, to 185 immigrants for Japan, and to 100 immigrants each for the other Asian countries. As an alternative, non-quota immigration from family reunification provided another channel for Asian immigrants, who were immediate relatives of U.S. citizens, to emigrate to the United States.

Liberalized Policy Period As part of the civil rights period, the Immigration Act of 1965 led to a liberalized policy period (1965–1999). The policy intentions of the Act aimed to be more inclusive and open to the diversity of European immigrants admitted to the United States. The Act abolished European national origin preferences and other ethnic/racial exclusion laws. More significantly, it redefined the rights to national citizenship based on a new multicultural framework (Hing, 1994; Kim, 1994). No longer was the country of origin the defining or limiting factor in influencing immigration patterns. These new immigration regulations admitted immigrants based on occupational skills, family reunification, and flight from persecution for political and religious reasons.

At the time, it was anticipated that immigrant flows from non-European regions would account for a relatively small percentage of the total future immigration. During this period, non-European residents had accounted for only a small proportion of the total U.S. population. However, that prediction proved incorrect.

The Immigration Act of 1965 gave equal annual quota limits of 20,000 per country irrespective of the migration pattern. As an unintended consequence, the policy essentially opened the doors for larger numbers of Asian and other non-Western European immigrants to enter the United States. As more and more immigrants came from Asia and other non-European countries, Congress once again passed laws, such as the Immigration Reform Law of 1986 and the Immigration Act of 1990, to selectively curb and control the immigration flow from Asia and other non-European countries.

The Immigration Act of 1990 prioritized professionals who had advanced degrees and were highly skilled, like workers in the technology sector (Lee, 2016). The Personal Responsibility and Work Opportunity Reconciliation Act of 1996 (also known as the Welfare Reform Act) was an assault on immigrants' eligibility for public benefits and excluded noncitizen immigrants and legal permanent residents from using public resources like Supplemental Security Income (SSI) and the Supplemental Nutrition Assistance Program (SNAP, commonly referred to as food stamps) (Fujiwara, 1998). The Welfare Reform Act barred immigrants from accessing public benefits, placing them in increasingly precarious situations and having a particularly extreme impact on those who were poor, older adults, and/or disabled. The subsequent passage of the Illegal Immigration Reform and Immigrant Responsibility Act of 1996 strengthened the justification for detention and deportation of undocumented immigrants who committed crimes, including minor and nonviolent convictions in the United States, and imposed greater restrictions on gaining citizenship (Fujiwara, 1998).

Growing Restriction and Exclusion Period During the growing restriction and exclusion period (2000–present), U.S. immigration policies were tied increasingly to national security policy in following the terrorist attacks of September 11, 2001 (9/11 attacks), within the context of the war on terrorism. The USA Patriot Act, Enhanced Border Security and Visa Entry Reform Act, and the Homeland Security Act were passed immediately following the 9/11 attacks and were augmented with additional measures to increase surveillance and border security protocols. These new laws have reduced immigration overall, but they have particularly slowed the flow of Arab, Muslim, and South Asian immigrants (Nguyen, 2005). In 2003, the Immigration and Naturalization Service (INS) agency was moved from the Department of Justice to the Department of Homeland Security and split into three new offices: U.S. Citizenship Immigration Services (USCIS), U.S. Immigration and Customs Enforcement (ICE), and U.S. Customs and Border Protection (CBP) (Nguyen, 2005).

In the last decade, immigration has come to the forefront of American politics once again, with concerns related to terrorism, border security, and economic insecurity driving policy changes. Undocumented immigrants have come under increased scrutiny, with calls for deportation or imprisonment of vast numbers of individuals. Although typically considered in relation to immigrants from Mexico and Central and South America, actions against undocumented immigrants also impact the Asian American community. For example, of those eligible for the Deferred Action for Childhood Arrivals (DACA), an executive action passed in 2012, 120,000 (about 10 percent) were Asian, with significant numbers from Korea, China, and India. DACA was a policy that protected individuals who entered the United States as undocumented children and allowed them to apply for a driver's license, social security number, and work permit. However, DACA individuals were not eligible for health coverage under the Affordable Care Act (ACA) or federally subsidized health programs like Medicaid (Brindis et al., 2014). Since its passage, there have been several attempts to repeal or undermine the DACA program including rejecting new applications to the DACA program and decreasing the time period of protection from two years to one year (Immigrant Legal Resource Center, 2021).

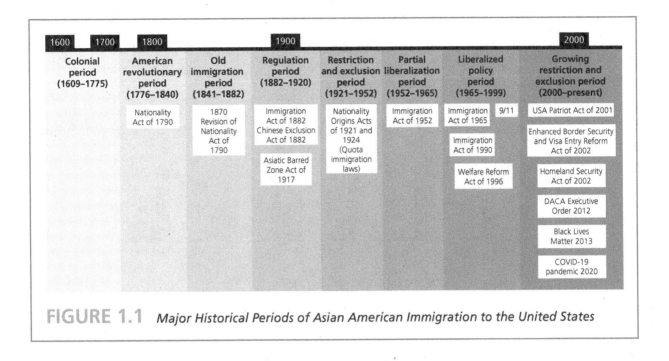

FIGURE 1.1   *Major Historical Periods of Asian American Immigration to the United States*

The Black Lives Matter (BLM) movement was triggered by incidents of racism and violence, including the deaths of Trayvon Martin in Oakland, California, in 2012, Michael Brown in Ferguson, Missouri, in 2014, Eric Garner in Staten Island, New York, in 2014, and George Floyd in Minneapolis, Minnesota, in 2020. BLM has ushered in an overdue reckoning of systemic racism at the societal level, including an acknowledgment that racism is widespread in laws that have disproportionately impacted non-Hispanic Black (Black) and structurally marginalized populations, including Asian Americans (García & Sharif, 2015). Synchronously, the racialized discourse around the novel coronavirus (COVID-19) pandemic as the "Chinese virus" and "Kung Flu" has refueled anti-Asian xenophobia and anti-immigrant rhetoric against Chinese communities, as well as the broader Asian American community (Le et al., 2020).

Figure 1.1 provides a graphical illustration of the major historical periods pertaining to Asian Americans.

Social and Demographic Context of Asian Immigration and Asian Americans

Before 1965, the major immigration sources came from European countries (Arnold et al., 1987). From 1841 to 1960, Pacific migrations from Asia accounted for less than two percent of the total immigration to the United States (See Figure 1.2) (Barringer et al., 1993). The first major wave of Asian immigrants to the United States occurred in the nineteenth century when Chinese, Indian, and Filipino individuals migrated to the Pacific Coast as demand for cheap labor sources for agricultural, mining, railroad, fishing, service, and other labor markets grew. Also, Chinese, Japanese, Korean, and Filipino plantation workers migrated to Hawaii during the mid-nineteenth and early twentieth centuries (Chan, 1991; Takaki, 1998). These first Asian immigrants, who were predominantly men, stayed in the United States for a limited time before returning to their native countries. Over time, a small percentage of these early Asians immigrants stayed, many united with other family members from their native countries and formed new, extended families in the United States. Their U.S.-born offspring consequently took on American roots and were shaped by American values and ideology.

Since 1965, the percentage of European immigrants to the United States has drastically declined. In 1960, 80 percent of immigrants came from Europe (Arnold et al., 1987). By 1984, European immigrants accounted for only 18 percent of the total immigrants to the United States, and the top 10 immigrant groups came from non-European countries.

In contrast, the proportion of Asian immigrants since the 1960s has risen dramatically (U.S. Immigration and Naturalization Service, 1960, 1979). Asian immigrants accounted for approximately 9 percent of all U.S.

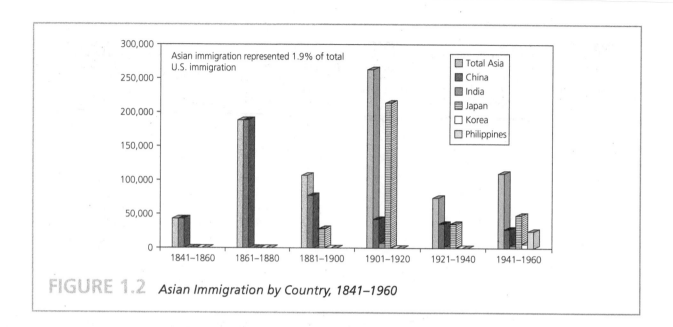

FIGURE 1.2 *Asian Immigration by Country, 1841–1960*

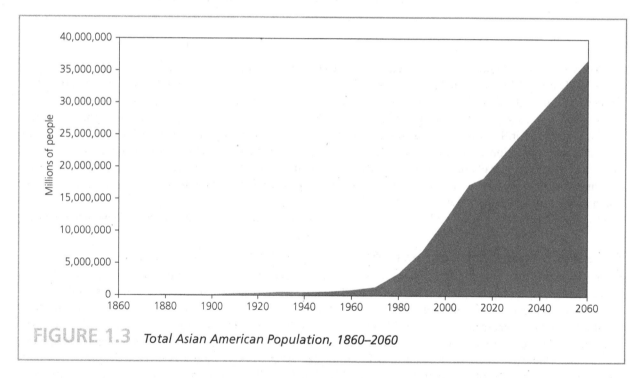

FIGURE 1.3 *Total Asian American Population, 1860–2060*

immigrants in 1960, 20 percent in 1970, and 44 percent by 1980. The last two decades have seen continued immigration to the United States, with Asian immigrants accounting for 22 percent of new immigrants in 2000, 37 percent in 2018, and estimated to reach 38 percent in 2065 (Budiman, 2020). Asian immigrants are projected to make up the largest share of U.S. immigrants in 2055, surpassing the number of Hispanic immigrants (Budiman, 2020).

American policy makers did not expect Asians to migrate to the United States in such large numbers (Reimers, 1992). In 1960, there were 877,000 Asian Americans, representing about 0.5 percent of the total U.S. population (Barringer et al., 1993) (see Figure 1.3). From 1960 to 2015, Asian immigrants increased from 338,328 to 12.1 million people (Pimienti & Polkey, 2019). From 2016 to 2060, the Asian immigrant population is projected to increase 63.5 percent, from 11.9 million to 19.5 million people (Vespa et al., 2020). Asian Americans are the fastest-growing racial group in terms of population growth and the Asian American population is estimated to more than double between 2016 and 2060, rising from 18.3 million to a projected 36.8 million and comprising more than 9 percent of the total U.S. population (Vespa et al., 2020).

In 1960, Japanese (53 percent), Chinese (27 percent), and Filipino (20 percent) Americans represented the largest Asian American ethnic groups and accounted for almost 100 percent of the total Asian American population (Barringer et al., 1993). Since that time, there has been a substantial shift in the demographic composition of the Asian American population, resulting in greater diversity. In 2019, Chinese (22 percent), Asian Indian (20 percent), Filipino (18 percent), Vietnamese (9 percent), Korean (8 percent), and Japanese (6 percent) Americans represented the largest Asian American groups and account for almost 85 percent of the total Asian American population (see Table 1.1) (U.S. Census Bureau, 2020). Other major Asian American populations today include Pakistani, Hmong, Cambodian, Thai, Laotian, Bangladeshi, Taiwanese, Burmese, and Nepalese.

Following historical trends of settlement, Asian Americans continue to settle in or near their Asian ethnic communities or reside near their work sites. Asian Americans today have mainly settled in California, Hawaii, other West Coast states, and a few other states across the nation such as New York, Texas, New Jersey, and Illinois. In 1970, 70 percent of the Asian Americans lived in the Western part of the United States (U.S. Census Bureau, 1973). However, by 1990, as Asian Americans became more geographically dispersed, only 56 percent lived in the West (U.S. Census Bureau, 1993).

By 2019, nearly 71 percent of all Asians lived in 10 states, including California (31 percent), New York (9 percent), Texas (8 percent), New Jersey (5 percent), Illinois (4 percent), Washington (4 percent), Florida

TABLE 1.1 **Asian American Population in 2010 and 2019, by Ethnic Group**

	Asian alone (one detailed Asian group reported)			
	2010 Estimates[1]	% Total Asian	2019 Estimates[2]	% Total Asian
Total U.S.	308,745,538	4.8%	324,697,795	5.5%
Total Asian	14,867,426		17,918,525	
Asian Indian	2,843,391	19.1%	3,995,755	22.3%
Bangladeshi	128,792	0.9%	177,778	1.0%
Bhutanese	15,290	0.1%	25,240	0.1%
Burmese	91,085	0.6%	168,851	0.9%
Cambodian	231,616	1.6%	257,994	1.4%
Chinese, except Taiwanese	3,347,229	22.5%	4,113,299	23.0%
Filipino	2,555,923	17.2%	2,875,514	16.0%
Hmong	247,595	1.7%	293,056	1.6%
Indonesian	63,383	0.4%	74,683	0.4%

(Continued)

TABLE 1.1 (Continued)

	Asian alone (one detailed Asian group reported)			
	2010 Estimates[1]	**% Total Asian**	**2019 Estimates[2]**	**% Total Asian**
Japanese	763,325	5.1%	770,798	4.3%
Korean	1,423,784	9.6%	1,455,185	8.1%
Laotian	191,200	1.3%	201,675	1.1%
Malaysian	16,138	0.1%	20,366	0.1%
Mongolian	14,366	0.1%	19,860	0.1%
Nepalese	51,907	0.3%	160,391	0.9%
Okinawan	2,753	0.0%	3,210	0.0%
Pakistani	363,699	2.4%	472,610	2.6%
Sri Lankan	38,596	0.3%	51,224	0.3%
Taiwanese	196,691	1.3%	172,329	1.0%
Thai	166,620	1.1%	205,145	1.1%
Vietnamese	1,548,449	10.4%	1,809,361	10.1%
Other Asian, not specified	218,922	1.5%	155,755	0.9%
Two or more Asian	346,672	2.3%	438,446	2.4%

[1] U.S. Census Bureau. (2012). *The Asian Population: 2010*. Washington, DC: U.S. Census Bureau.
[2] U.S. Census Bureau, 2015–2019 American Community Survey 5-Year Estimates.
Note: This table includes people who reported the specific Asian ethnicity only and is a more conservative estimate of the Asian American population in the U.S. (compared to the 'Asian alone or in combination with another race' grouping). People who reported multiple Asian responses such as Asian Indian and Japanese; or Vietnamese, Chinese and Hmong are listed under 'Two or more Asian'. This table does not detail the growing multiracial population, which included people who reported being more than one racial group, such as Asian and White.

(3 percent), Virginia (3 percent), Hawaii (3 percent), and Massachusetts (3 percent) (See Table 1.2). (Pew Research Center, 2021). The states with the largest concentration of Asian Americans were Hawaii (36 percent), California (15 percent), New Jersey (10 percent), Washington (9 percent), New York (9 percent), and Nevada (8 percent) (Pew Research Center, 2021). The Asian American population expanded in new directions as well. States that experienced substantial Asian American population growth rates between 2000 and 2019 include North Dakota (241 percent), South Dakota (203 percent), Indiana (183 percent), Nevada (175 percent), and North Carolina (175 percent) (See Table 1.2). (Pew Research Center, 2021). Most Asian Americans tend to settle

TABLE 1.2 **Asian American Population Change by State, 2000 and 2019**

In thousands (unless otherwise specified)

State	2000			2019				
	Population	% of Asian population	% of state population	Population	% of Asian population	% of state population	Pop. change, '00–'19	% pop. change, '00–'19
Alabama	32	0.3%	0.7%	72	0.4%	1.5%	40	125.3%
Alaska	25	0.2%	4.1%	47	0.2%	6.4%	21	83.0%
Arizona	93	0.9%	1.8%	249	1.3%	3.4%	157	168.9%
Arkansas	21	0.2%	0.8%	49	0.3%	1.6%	28	136.3%
California	3.751	35.8%	11.0%	5.869	31.0%	14.9%	2.118	56.5%
Colorado	97	0.9%	2.2%	193	1.0%	3.3%	96	99.5%
Connecticut	85	0.8%	2.5%	172	0.9%	4.8%	87	102.1%
Delaware	17	0.2%	2.1%	39	0.2%	4.0%	22	134.8%
D.C.	16	0.1%	2.7%	31	0.2%	4.3%	15	96.5%
Florida	274	2.6%	1.7%	610	3.2%	2.8%	336	122.5%
Georgia	178	1.7%	2.2%	454	2.4%	4.3%	276	154.5%
Hawaii	500	4.8%	41.2%	516	2.7%	36.4%	16	3.1%
Idaho	12	0.1%	0.9%	26	0.1%	1.4%	14	113.9%
Illinois	433	4.1%	3.5%	732	3.9%	5.8%	299	69.0%
Indiana	61	0.6%	1.0%	171	0.9%	2.5%	111	182.6%
Iowa	38	0.4%	1.3%	83	0.4%	2.6%	45	120.1%
Kansas	48	0.5%	1.8%	91	0.5%	3.1%	43	89.2%
Kentucky	30	0.3%	0.7%	70	0.4%	1.6%	39	130.1%

(Continued)

TABLE 1.2 *(Continued)*

State	2000			2019				
	Population	% of Asian population	% of state population	Population	% of Asian population	% of state population	Pop. change, '00–'19	% pop. change, '00–'19
Louisiana	56	0.5%	1.2%	82	0.4%	1.8%	26	46.3%
Maine	9	0.1%	0.7%	17	0.1%	1.3%	8	83.6%
Maryland	217	2.1%	4.1%	399	2.1%	6.6%	182	84.0%
Massachusetts	246	2.4%	3.9%	490	2.6%	7.1%	244	99.0%
Michigan	181	1.7%	1.8%	332	1.8%	3.3%	151	83.6%
Minnesota	146	1.4%	3.0%	289	1.5%	5.1%	142	97.3%
Mississippi	19	0.2%	0.7%	32	0.2%	1.1%	13	71.0%
Missouri	63	0.6%	1.1%	131	0.7%	2.1%	68	107.3%
Montana	5	<0.05%	0.5%	9	<0.05%	0.9%	5	100.0%
Nebraska	22	0.2%	1.3%	51	0.3%	2.7%	29	130.2%
Nevada	92	0.9%	4.6%	254	1.3%	8.3%	162	175.5%
New Hampshire	16	0.2%	1.3%	40	0.2%	2.9%	23	142.8%
New Jersey	493	4.7%	5.9%	870	4.6%	9.8%	377	76.4%
New Mexico	19	0.2%	1.0%	33	0.2%	1.6%	14	72.7%
New York	1,097	10.5%	5.8%	1,713	9.1%	8.8%	617	56.2%
North Carolina	117	1.1%	1.5%	323	1.7%	3.1%	206	175.4%
North Dakota	4	<0.05%	0.6%	13	0.1%	1.6%	9	241.4%
Ohio	136	1.3%	1.2%	287	1.5%	2.5%	152	111.7%

Oklahoma	47	0.5%	1.4%	91	0.5%	2.3%	44	92.3%
Oregon	103	1.0%	3.0%	199	1.1%	4.7%	95	92.3%
Pennsylvania	225	2.2%	1.8%	472	2.5%	3.7%	246	109.3%
Rhode Island	25	0.2%	2.4%	38	0.2%	3.6%	13	51.6%
South Carolina	37	0.4%	0.9%	91	0.5%	1.8%	55	148.2%
South Dakota	4	<0.05%	0.6%	13	0.1%	1.5%	9	202.7%
Tennessee	58	0.6%	1.0%	130	0.7%	1.9%	72	124.1%
Texas	575	5.5%	2.7%	1,458	7.7%	5.0%	883	153.6%
Utah	38	0.4%	1.7%	82	0.4%	2.5%	44	114.4%
Vermont	5	0.1%	0.9%	12	0.1%	1.9%	6	118.9%
Virginia	269	2.6%	3.8%	579	3.1%	6.8%	310	115.4%
Washington	329	3.1%	5.6%	712	3.8%	9.3%	382	116.1%
West Virginia	10	0.1%	0.5%	14	0.1%	0.8%	5	49.3%
Wisconsin	91	0.9%	1.7%	172	0.9%	3.0%	81	89.2%
Wyoming	3	<0.05%	0.6%	6	<0.05%	1.1%	3	122.5%

Note: Population estimates are as of July 1, 2019. Asians include those who report only being one race and are not Hispanic. Population figures rounded to nearest 1,000.
Source: Pew Research Center analysis of U.S. intercensal population estimates for 2000, and U.S. Census Bureau Vintage 2019 estimates for 2019.

in or near ethnic enclaves in urban and suburban regions. Few settle in rural regions unless they were initially resettled there when they first immigrated. Furthermore, the residential settlement patterns are polarized with affluent Asian Americans settling in suburban areas and less socioeconomic mobile Asian Americans residing in urban ethnic ghettos (Min, 2006c).

The top 10 U.S. metropolitan areas with the highest number Asian Americans has also changed slightly between 2010 and 2019 (see Table 1.3).

TABLE 1.3 **Ten U.S. Places with the Largest Number of Asian Americans, 2010 and 2019**

	2010			2019	
Rank	Place	Estimates[1]	Rank	Place	Estimates[2]
1	New York, NY	1,038,388	1	New York, NY	2,166,784
2	Los Angeles, CA	426,959	2	Los Angeles, CA	2,122,263
3	San Jose, CA	303,138	3	San Francisco, CA	1,226,901
4	San Francisco, CA	267,915	4	San Jose, CA	704,685
5	San Diego, CA	207,944	5	Washington DC	630,663
6	Honolulu, HI	184,950	6	Chicago, IL	624,101
7	Chicago, IL	147,164	7	Seattle, WA	532,270
8	Houston, TX	126,378	8	Honolulu, HI	528,096
9	Fremont, CA	108,332	9	Houston, TX	504,598
10	Philadelphia, PA	96,405	10	Dallas, TX	420,093
11	Sacramento, CA	85,503	11	San Diego, CA	394,742
12	Seattle, WA	84,215	12	Boston, MA	383,691

[1] U.S. Census Bureau. (2012). *The Asian Population: 2010.* Washington, DC: U.S. Census Bureau.
[2] U.S. Census Bureau, 2015-2019 American Community Survey 5-Year Estimates. Place geography defined using the "All Metropolitan Statistical Areas/Micropolitan Statistical Areas within United States."
Note: This table includes people who reported the specific Asian ethnicity only and is a more conservative estimate of the Asian American population in the U.S. (compared to the "Asian alone or in combination with another race" grouping).

Chinese The Chinese have also come to the United States in significant numbers in the liberalized era since 1965. According to USCIS statistics, from 1961 to 2011, approximately 1,650,411 immigrants came from China, 215,814 immigrants came from Taiwan, and 364,934 immigrants came from Hong Kong (Migration Policy Institute, 2013). Many Chinese immigrants during this period were socially advantaged (Oh, 1977; Wang, 1993). The majority had high occupational standing and special relationships with American economic and professional organizations.

The largest Chinese migration stream during the early part of this new liberalized period originated from urban parts of Taiwan, Hong Kong, and other parts of the Chinese diaspora (Chan, 1991). Only a minority of Chinese refugees also came from the People's Republic of China (PRC), which was closed to the outside world during the leadership of Chairman Mao Zedong (1949–1976). However, with the opening of China's markets from the late 1970s and early 1980s under Chairman Deng Xiaoping's economic and political reform policies and the breaking of political ties between the United States and Taiwan in 1979, the annual Chinese immigration quota of 20,000 per year was revised in 1981 (Hing, 1994; Wong, 2006). The revision allowed 20,000 immigrants per year (not counting non-quota immigration) for Chinese immigration from both the PRC and from Taiwan, doubling the Chinese immigration quota. Chinese immigrants from Taiwan and China were counted separately for the first time in the INS immigration statistics from 1982 (Min, 1995b).

Since the 1980s, Chinese immigrants from the PRC have become the major Chinese migration current to the United States, although immigration from Taiwan and Hong Kong continues to be significant (Arnold et al., 1987). Chinese immigrants started with relatively lower occupational and educational standing, as compared to their counterparts from Taiwan and Hong Kong, working first as cheap laborers for entrepreneurs in Chinatowns and Chinese American suburban enclaves (Ong et al., 1994). Strategic American political and economic alliances with China, Taiwan, and Hong Kong clearly have helped promote and shape Chinese migration patterns between East Asia and the United States. In addition, Chinese American communities have played vital support roles in the immigration and resettlement processes for Chinese newcomers (Wong, 2006). There were a total of 2.5 million immigrants who came to the U.S. from China (including Hong Kong), as of 2019, making up about almost 18 percent of all immigrants from Asia, and about 372,000 immigrants (or 3 percent) were from Taiwan (Hanna & Batalova, 2021). Chinese immigrants were the largest group of international students in the United States in 2019 (Hanna & Batalova, 2021).

South Asians A substantial number of Asian Indians have also come to the United States since 1965. According to USCIS statistics, from 1961 to 2011, about 1,856,777 Asian Indian immigrants came to the United States (Migration Policy Institute, 2013). From 1980 to 2010, the population grew more than eleven-fold, roughly doubling every decade. As of 2019, almost 4.3 million immigrants came from South Asia, equating to over 30 percent of all immigrants from Asia in the United States (Hanna & Batalova, 2021). The largest share of South Asian immigrants come from India (2.7 million or 19 percent of all immigrants from Asia), followed by 398,000 immigrants from Pakistan (3 percent), 261,000 immigrants from Bangladesh (2 percent), and 167,000 immigrants from Nepal (1 percent) (Hanna & Batalova, 2021).

The earliest wave of South Asian immigrants to the United States were Punjabi Sikhs and Muslims, who arrived in the late 1800s and worked in the agriculture, lumber, and railroad industries (Dhingra, 2016). The largest waves of South Asian immigrants arrived post-1965 during the liberalized policy period. Viewed in the aggregate today, South Asians comprise an elite immigrant group, with high educational attainment and occupational status in fields including the sciences, engineering, and business (Kibria, 2006; Saran, 1985; Saran & Eames, 1980). From 1965 through the late 1970s, a majority immigrated to the United States via exclusive occupational categories in these fields. Subsequently, during the 1980s to mid-1990s, family reunification immigration complemented these professional channels.

In 2019, Asian Indians were the top recipients of high-skilled H-1B temporary visas and the second-largest group of international students in the United States (Hanna & Batalova, 2021). Given their fluency with the English language, one of the official languages of India, and history with British colonialism, Asian Indians tend to adjust quickly to the language and culture of the United States, similar to the Filipino immigrant experience. The American presence in India through economic and cultural exchanges in the post–World War II era facilitated transnational migration from India to the United States once immigration policies became more inclusive of Pacific migrations. However, the cultural networks and economic institutions that promoted and facilitated the migration currents were selective: only Asian Indians with exceptional socioeconomic status and social relations with American organizations had the necessary information and capacity to immigrate to the United States.

After 1965, South Asian immigrants to the United States from countries like Pakistan, Bangladesh, Sri Lanka, and Nepal came primarily on the basis of occupational skills. After 1980, South Asian immigrants to the United States from these same countries primarily entered through family reunification (Kibria, 2006). Like immigrants from India, other South Asian immigrants to the United States were comprised primarily of individuals who had attained high levels of occupational and educational status. However, with the increasing immigration flow from family reunification, the socioeconomic profile of South Asian immigrants has become more complex since 1980. For example, many South Asian immigrants settling in urban areas such as New York City (NYC) are employed in low-wage service positions, including taxi driving, restaurant work, or domestic work. Events in the home countries of South Asian Americans also impact the flow of migration and the profiles of who decides to immigrate to the United States. For example, in late 2020, the Indian government enacted agricultural acts (referred to as the Farm Bills) that were intended to modernize the farming industry by increasing privatization of the agricultural sector. However, opponents claimed that by providing fewer protections to farmers, the new laws posed threats to the national food supply and food security in India (Frayer, 2021). Predicting negative economic effects both on the domestic and global agricultural markets, Indian academics joined with farmers and others in vast demonstrations against the Farm Bills, with large-scale demonstrations also seen among the Asian Indian diaspora. The implementation of the Farm Bills was suspended by the Indian Supreme Court in January 2021 (Frayer, 2021). However, at the time of writing, the issue remains unresolved and provides an example of how political and economic developments in South Asian countries are impacting the socioeconomic profile of South Asian immigrant communities.

Today, South Asian immigrants are a much more diverse group, both ethnically and socioeconomically, than they were previously. Immigrants from India and Pakistan continue to account for a large proportion of the total South Asian American population. In the post-9/11 era and within the context of controlling terrorism, South Asian immigration has become a national security issue, especially for men from Muslim countries, such as Pakistan and Bangladesh, who may be subject to increasing U.S. government surveillance. This shift in national policy focus could lead to declining immigration from Muslim countries in the near future (Kibria, 2006). Islamophobia and hate violence persist in the Growing Restriction and Exclusion Period.

Filipinos Immigrants from the Philippines represent another major Asian group to migrate to the United States in the period since 1965. According to the USCIS, from 1961 to 2011, approximately 1,813,597 Filipino immigrants came to the U.S. (Migration Policy Institute, 2013). In 2019, about 2 million immigrants in the United States were from the Philippines, representing more than 14 percent of all Asian immigrants (Hanna & Batalova, 2021). Although the majority of Filipinos living abroad work as temporary contract laborers, most Filipino immigrants to the United States tend to be permanent settlers (Bankston, 2006; Cariño, 1987).

The strong political and economic relationships between the United States and the Philippines have served to facilitate the Pacific migration flow, initially through colonial and military relations and subsequently through labor recruitment and trade exchanges (Lee, 1986). At the end of the nineteenth century, the United States annexed the Philippines, ruling the country as a U.S. colony until recognizing its independence in 1946. Yet U.S. military and economic influences persisted long after independence, influencing the development of Filipino society and culture through post–World War II military, labor, and trade exchanges.

Because U.S. influences are pervasive and far-reaching in the lives of people from the Philippines, Filipino immigrants adjusted to living in the United States faster than most other Asian immigrant groups. Both the political and educational systems of the Philippines reflect U.S. systems. English is one of the official languages there, as well as the main medium of instruction in secondary schools and universities in the Philippines. In addition, Filipinos living or working near former U.S. military bases in the Philippines interact with U.S. military personnel on a routine basis. Some Filipinos qualified for U.S. citizenship after having served in the U.S. military. Some Filipinas married U.S. military men and moved to the U.S. along with their children and other family members, a phenomenon that contributed to the rise of the "mail-order bride" industry in the 1970s, wherein international matchmaking agencies connected Filipina women immigrating to the U.S. with men who were U.S. citizens or permanent residents (Demanarig & Acosta, 2016).

Many Filipinos seek opportunities outside of the Philippines (Bankston, 2006; Cariño, 1987; Chan, 1991). Economic prosperity in the United States and other parts of the world contrast greatly with the Philippines' large foreign debt, high unemployment rate, and distribution inequities. The economic challenges in the Philippines are exacerbated by its rising population growth. Many Filipino professionals, including physicians, nurses, and engineers, and Filipino labor workers come to the United States seeking better socioeconomic opportunities. Moreover, because the United States is the Philippines' largest international trade partner, U.S. corporations, financial institutions, and trade representatives have made major investments in promoting economic development and exchanges with the country. These political and economic influences, along with social and cultural exchanges between the Philippines and the United States have helped create transnational community networks and establish multiple migration streams over time. In addition, Filipino family and kinship networks in the United States facilitate the process of immigration and the social adjustment for new immigrants. Recent social and political shifts towards a more autocratic government under the Philippines President Rodrigo Duterte, such as the war on drugs, have led to human rights violations (Asis, 2017). These developments have increased tensions between the Philippines–United States transnational network and will have long-term implications on the labor migration and remittance (Asis, 2017).

Southeast Asians In the post-1965 era, mass refugee and immigrant flows from Vietnam, Cambodia, and Laos comprised another major source of Asian immigration. According to USCIS and Office of Refugee Resettlement data, from 1961 to 2011, approximately 1.6 million Southeast Asian immigrants (1,259,317 immigrants from Vietnam, 160,212 immigrants from Cambodia, and 183,768 immigrants from Laos) came to the United States (Migration Policy Institute, 2013), and most immigrants came after 1975 under refugee status (Barringer et al., 1993). Of the total Southeast Asian immigrant population in the United States, approximately 17 percent are ethnic Chinese and 100,000 are Amerasian (i.e., individuals of mixed Asian and American descent) (Rumbaut, 2006). During the conflicts of the Cold War and subsequent efforts to contain communism in Southeast Asia, the United States accepted its political responsibility to accommodate a large percentage of refugees from these countries. This acceptance was due in part to the political need to legitimate the status of the United States as an international superpower, demonstrate moral supremacy, and salvage the reputation of the United States after its military defeat in Southeast Asia (Chan, 1991; Hein, 1995).

The first major wave of refugees arrived in the United States in 1975, in the wake of the U.S. military withdrawal, when communist regimes assumed full power of Indochina (Rumbaut, 2006). These refugees were evacuated by air or escaped by land to Thailand and then were brought to the United States and other countries. Most of them were affiliated with the U.S. military and/or U.S.-supported regimes. Many were also well educated, wealthy, and of high social status. In addition, a significant percentage was Catholic.

The second major wave of Southeast Asian refugees arrived after 1978 from Vietnam, Cambodia, and Laos – a consequence both of dictatorial rule and war-ravaged socioeconomic systems (Chan, 1991; Rumbaut, 2006). From Vietnam, many Southeast Asians escaped by boat while the majority of Cambodian and Laotian refugees escaped by land to neighboring Thailand. In contrast to the first wave of immigrants, this second group came from less urbanized regions; was less educated, poorer, and more ethnically diverse; and included ethnic Chinese, Vietnamese, Cambodians, highland Hmong, and lowland Laotians. Southeast Asian refugee flows continued to come to the United States through the 1980s and 1990s. However, during the early to mid-1990s, due to new political alliances between Vietnam, Cambodia, and Laos and the United States as well as other Asian countries, Southeast Asian refugee flows slowed to a trickle (Robinson, 1999; Rumbaut, 2006). Immigration flow since then has been primarily through family reunification channels. In 2019, there were a total of 1.9 million Southeast Asian immigrants (14 percent of immigrants from Asia) in the United States, including 1.4 million immigrants from Vietnam (10 percent), 261,000 immigrants from Thailand (2 percent), 177,000 immigrants from Laos (1 percent), and 151,000 immigrants from Myanmar (1 percent) (Hanna & Batalova, 2021).

In 2020, United States and Vietnam commemorated 25 years of diplomatic relations and bilateral trade agreements. These agreements strengthened economic developments between the two countries, increasing trade from $451 million in 1995 to over $90 billion in 2020 (Bureau of East Asian and Pacific Affairs, 2021). In recent years, as an intensifying trade war between the United States and China has raised tariffs for imported Chinese goods, Vietnam has emerged as an alternative regional business partner for the United States (Bureau of East Asian and Pacific Affairs, 2021). A number of highly skilled Vietnamese Americans concerned about developments in their home country have been serving as middlemen, leveraging their professional networks on both sides and contributing actively to these U.S.–Vietnam bilateral economic developments.

Koreans In the post-1965 period, Korean immigrants have also arrived in the United States in significant numbers. According to USCIS statistics, from 1961 to 2011, approximately 1,082,613 Korean immigrants arrived in the United States (Migration Policy Institute, 2013). Korean immigrants consider the United States as their primary destination. Similar to the migration of Filipina women, there was a steady migration of Korean military brides, or marriages between Korean women and U.S. soldiers, in the 1970s that also resulted in the immigration of Korean family members to the United States thereafter (Yuh, 2005). In addition, many Korean professionals and entrepreneurs immigrated to U.S. urban centers seeking to build wealth and prosperity beyond what they perceive as possible in Korea (Kim, 2014; Light & Bonacich, 1991; Min, 2006b). By contrast, in other parts of the world, Korean immigrants work mainly in temporary contract positions and return to their country once their labor contract is completed. South Korea's competitive, cheap, skilled, non-unionized labor workers are especially attractive to international corporations seeking labor recruitment.

Similar to the Philippines, Korea's political and economic relations with the United States facilitated emigration (Chan, 1991; Koo & Yu, 1981). Although Korea was never a U.S. colony, American involvement in the

Korean War and the continued U.S. military alliance and international trade relations with South Korea have served to shape the social landscape and established and sustained Pacific migration streams between Korea and the United States. In addition, since 1962, as one of the world's most densely populated countries, South Korea promoted emigration as a means of population control to maintain the country's economic stability (Light & Bonacich, 1991). Growing Koreans American communities served as important networks for providing social support and economic opportunities to Korean immigrants, offering a means to better adapt to their new lives in the United States.

Recent Korean immigrants tend to be highly educated and of high socioeconomic status. Korean immigrants were the third-largest group of international students in the United States in 2019 (Hanna & Batalova, 2021). In 2019, there were 1 million Korean immigrants in the United States, representing 7 percent of all immigrants from Asia (Hanna & Batalova, 2021). This number represents a decrease from a high of 1.1 million Korean immigrants in 2010 and reflects a decline in incentives for Koreans to emigrate. Contemporary political and economic conditions in South Korea have improved and the South Korean government has attempted to increase return migration of the Korean diaspora through the expansion of economic and business opportunities. Despite this decline, the United States is still home to the largest South Korean diaspora in the world (O'Connor & Batalova, 2019).

Koreans have strong transnational networks that may be explained partially by the adoption of Korean children by American parents toward the end of the Korean War in 1953 – a trend that continued through the 1980s (Park Nelson, 2016). Korean adoptees make up approximately 10 percent of the total Korean American population, with the largest percent of Korean adoptees residing in Minnesota, where they comprise 50 percent of the Korean American population (Park Nelson, 2016). Over the last decade, numerous members of the large diaspora of Korean adoptees have returned to South Korea for myriad reasons, including searching for their Korean birth families or residing permanently in South Korea through special visas established to allow permanent residence status and pathways to dual South Korean–U.S. citizenship (Park Nelson, 2016).

The influence and rise of Korean pop culture (K-pop) that started in 1997 and exploded in the late 2000s has also facilitated the growth of transnational networks (Jin, 2018). Social networking platforms have served as a key driver of the expansion of K-pop's cultural influence within the United States. K-pop's popularity has become a global sensation that has penetrated numerous international markets, including the film, television, and music industries of the United States and the European Union.

Japanese In the last century, Japanese immigrants have migrated to the United States in smaller numbers than other major Asian groups. According to USCIS statistics, from 1961 to 2011, 318,225 Japanese immigrants arrived in the United States (Migration Policy Institute, 2013). Japanese political and economic systems were strong and prosperous in relation to Western powers during this period. Given the stability and abundance of opportunities in their homeland, relatively few Japanese have felt compelled to emigrate, with the exception of those employed by Japanese multinational corporations that are expanding their activities in the United States (Akiba, 2006; Takaki, 1998). Over the past few decades, more Japanese entrepreneurs have migrated to the United States than in earlier years, pushed by the persistent Japanese economic decline. As of 2019, there were a total of 333,000 Japanese immigrants in the United States (2 percent) (Hanna & Batalova, 2021). In recent years, to offset the loss of these migrants, Japan has expanded its visa programs for foreign workers and updated legislation to increase migration flows to Japan and address labor shortages related to caring for the aging Japanese population (Milly, 2020).

These different political periods and immigration flows have given rise to distinct generations of Japanese Americans. The Issei generation are Japanese immigrants who came to the United States before 1924 (Akiba, 2006; Takaki, 1998). The Nisei generation are the children of the Issei generation, born outside of Japan, followed by the Sansei (third), Yonsei (fourth), and Gosei (fifth) generations of Japanese Americans. There are distinct generational differences among Japanese Americans due to the internment experiences of the Issei and Nisei during World War II, as well as the subsequent redress campaigns carried out to acknowledge the harms and injustices they endured (Takahashi, 1997). Japanese immigrants have the highest interracial marriage rate (21 percent) compared to other Asian ethnic groups (range of 4 percent among Vietnamese immigrants to 11 percent among Filipino immigrants), and almost 19 percent of these marriages are with White spouses (Yang & Bohm-Jordan, 2018). Modern waves of Japanese immigrants are smaller and continue to decline compared to prior waves arriving to the United States.

Expanding Asian Populations

As the Asian immigrant population in the United States grew in the post-1965 liberalized immigration era, immigrants also brought their families (Chan, 1991; Espiritu, 2007). Immigrants with ethnic communities already established in the United States were able to gain entry more easily and adjust more quickly to life here. The economic recession in the 1970s resulted in the 1976 revision of the 1965 Immigration Act, which severely restricted the number of occupational immigrants, especially medical professionals (Yochum & Agarwal, 1988). However, the number of new immigrants qualifying under the family reunification criteria increased dramatically, leading to a substantial rise in the number of Asian Americans (Min, 1995b).

The Immigration Act of 1990 further revised the 1965 Immigration Act and intended to increase the number of occupational immigrants, with special preferences toward underrepresented European populations (Kim, 1994). However, contemporary Asian immigrants have adapted and found ways to negotiate the legal and political changes of the past four decades to ensure continued migration flows to the United States.

Asian immigrants continue to arrive in significant numbers today, and Asian American communities have expanded across the country beyond densely populated immigrant and ethnic enclaves (Min, 1995b, 2006c). The residential settlement patterns of Asian immigrants by state reflect the channels through which immigrants have arrived. For example, recent immigration of South Asians has occurred largely via work and student visas, leading these immigrants to settle in areas where companies and universities have drawn them, outside of traditional urban ethnic enclaves; by contrast, Southeast Asians have immigrated as refugees and resettled by the U.S. government in gateway communities across the United States (Budiman & Ruiz, 2021).

Indian Americans are the largest Asian origin group in the Southeast and Midwest, while Chinese Americans have the greatest concentrations in the West and Northeast (Budiman & Ruiz, 2021). Filipino Americans are the largest Asian origin group in nine states (Idaho, Montana, New Mexico, Nevada, North Dakota, and South Dakota); Vietnamese Americans comprise the largest Asian ethnic group in Louisiana, Mississippi, Oklahoma, and Nebraska; Korean Americans are the largest Asian ethnic group in Alabama; and Hmong Americans are the largest Asian ethnic group in Minnesota and Wisconsin (Budiman & Ruiz, 2021).

MAJOR ASIAN AMERICAN ISSUES

Contemporary Asian Americans are confronted by multiple social and racial/ethnic health disparities (Esperat et al., 2004; Institute of Medicine (US) Committee on Understanding and Eliminating Racial and Ethnic Disparities in Health Care, 2003). Social determinants, which include one's socioeconomic status, race/ethnicity, and gender, can either facilitate or restrict one's access and/or utilization of quality health care. These factors intersect and play a critical role in impacting health and well-being across Asian American communities. Intersectionality is a framework that may be used to demonstrate how individual social categorizations, including race, class, and gender, overlap and intersect to perpetuate systems of disadvantage and discrimination – a process that, in turn, impacts health outcomes (Crenshaw, 1990). This section provides insights and a structural context through which to view issues affecting Asian American health.

Socioeconomic Status, Social Welfare, and Inequality

Socioeconomic adjustment has been a critical measure of success for Asian Americans in U.S. society (Lai & Arguelles, 2003; Min, 1995b, 2006b; Ong et al., 1994). When comparing family income and educational status relative to other racial/ethnic groups, Asian Americans, on average, earn more than Whites, Blacks, Hispanic, and other racial/ethnic groups. However, a deeper examination of the data calls this conclusion into question. For example, Asian Americans earn less than Whites with the same educational status (Cabezas & Kawaguchi, 1988). This racial/ethnic inequality of income, like gender inequality of income, means that Asian Americans must work harder and longer to achieve the same socioeconomic status as Whites. Scholars have proposed that income inequality among Asian Americans results from the dual labor market phenomenon combined with the persistence of racial inequality (Cabezas & Kawaguchi, 1988; De Jong & Steinmetz, 2004; Piore, 1980). Some studies suggest that within the primary labor market, where jobs are characterized by relatively high status, high salaries, and good working conditions, Asian Americans are marginalized and limited to the periphery of power and social status (Shin & Chang, 1988; Taylor & Kim, 1980). Other Asian Americans are trapped in the secondary labor market, where their work status and income are not necessarily reflective of their educational status. Jobs in the secondary labor market pay lower wages, are less likely to be unionized, more likely to be insecure, and provide fewer opportunities for advancement than in the primary labor market. Examples include service industry jobs, such as retail and nail salons.

Additional factors impact Asian Americans differently than other racial/ethnic groups (Min, 1995b, 2006c). In Asian American families, more family members work outside the home as compared to White families. Thus, for an Asian American household to achieve the same income as a White household, more Asian American family members participate in the workforce than in a White household. Also, measuring the median family income of Asian Americans in a vacuum does not take into account the basic living expenses of the areas in which most Asian Americans reside. The majority of Asian Americans are concentrated in major metropolitan regions, such as New York City, San Francisco, and Los Angeles, where the standard of living is much higher than the national average. Furthermore, the Asian American population is not homogenous. When comparing between ethnic groups, the socioeconomic status of Asian populations can differ dramatically (see Table 1.4).

The positive depiction of socioeconomic success, sometimes referred to as the model minority myth, has negatively impacted Asian American communities (Hurh & Kim, 1989; Zhou & Xiong, 2005). Many Asian Americans have come to assume falsely that they have achieved socioeconomic parity with other ethnic/racial groups. In reality, Asian Americans are underrepresented in high-status jobs within the U.S. workforce and social hierarchy, as well as under-rewarded and overexerted in their jobs. In addition, the successful and problem-free images of Asian Americans have sometimes fostered anti-Asian sentiment as well as anti-Asian violence in

TABLE 1.4   **Median Annual Household Income and Percent Living in a Multigenerational Household Size, 2019**

	Median Annual Household Income	Percent Living in a Multigenerational Household
Total U.S.	$62,843	
Total Asian	$88,204	27
Asian Indian	$119,000	22
Bangladeshi	$59,500	36
Bhutanese	***	56
Burmese	$44,400	24
Cambodian	$67,000	42
Chinese, including Taiwanese	$81,600	25
Filipino	$90,400	34
Hmong	$68,000	36

Indonesian	$80,000	20
Japanese	$82,980	19
Korean	$72,200	20
Laotian	$61,000	40
Malaysian	***	16
Mongolian	***	13
Nepalese	$55,000	28
Pakistani	$78,000	35
Sri Lankan	$85,000	23
Thai	$63,000	25
Vietnamese	$69,800	34

Note: '***' means insufficient number of observations to provide a reliable estimate. Multigenerational households are households with two or more adult generations or one that includes grandparents and grandchildren. Abby Budiman and Neil G. Ruiz, "Key Facts about Asian Americans, a Diverse and Growing Population," Pew Research Center, April 29, 2021, https://www.pewresearch.org/fact-tank/2021/04/29/key-facts-about-asian-americans/

communities and universities (Gotanda, 1995; Osajima, 1988; Takaki, 1998). Furthermore, Asian American successes play into the "American dream" ideology and further stigmatize other racial/ethnic minority groups who have not achieved the same levels of success in their cultural and socioeconomic adjustments (Crystal, 1989). There are also some positive benefits to the model minority image for Asian Americans, including preferential treatment in regards to educational, employment, housing, and other opportunities (Min, 1995a).

The "glass ceiling" phenomenon, or the underrepresentation of Asian Americans workers in high-ranking and leadership positions within both public and private sectors, has been a major occupational mobility concern for the group (Chan, 1989; Der, 1993; Tang, 1993). For example, Asian American professors represent a significant percentage of professors nationwide, but few serve as presidents of major colleges and universities (Chan, 1989). In addition, in comparing career advancement between Asian and White engineers, White engineers clearly outpace their Asian colleagues in career mobility to managerial and other high-ranking positions (Tang, 1993). Furthermore, few Asian Americans are represented in government at local and federal levels (Der, 1993).

Similar to the glass ceiling phenomenon, Asian Americans face the "bamboo ceiling," which refers to the intersectionality of racial and other sociocultural barriers. Confronting the bamboo ceiling means that despite having higher educational attainment than their White colleagues, Asian Americans experience an invisible barrier to advancement in the workforce that results in underrepresentation of Asian Americans in executive/management positions. Stereotypes like the model minority myth contribute to the perpetuation of the bamboo ceiling. For example, one study found that within five large Silicon Valley companies (Google, Hewlett-Packard, Intel, LinkedIn, and Yahoo), Asian Americans were well-represented in nonmanagement positions and were the racial group least likely to be promoted to executive/management positions (Gee et al., 2015). The concept of intersectionality is discussed further in Chapter 12.

In addition to the search for better occupational opportunities and higher wages, many Asian immigrants come to the United States seeking educational advancement and opportunities for themselves and/or their children. Education is a major priority for Asian American families of all ethnic backgrounds (Takaki, 1998; Wang, 1993). Nationally, over the last four decades, the percentage of Asian Americans at major public and private universities has increased dramatically. For example, on several University of California campuses, Asian American students now represent the largest student group by race (Wang, 1993). Due to these changes in the racial/ethnic composition of the student population, many universities have established unequal policies to control admission of Asian Americans. These institutions discriminate against Asian Americans by applying stricter academic and supplemental guidelines to their applications for admission that go far beyond the standard grade point average and test scores requirements that are used to evaluate the fitness of candidates more broadly. The advent of these policies has been a point of contention between Asian American organizations and their allies who question the fairness of these policies and university authorities who claim to promote diversity yet develop policies against affirmative action (Takagi, 1990). Given the dominant ethnocentric policies that remain in place and are influenced by the model minority myth, as well as anti-Asian sentiment felt by other minority groups, these restrictive measures that discriminate against Asian Americans are unlikely to be removed in the near term.

Studies also indicate that the socioeconomic status of Asian Americans has a bipolar distribution (Min, 1995a, 2006a; Zhou & Xiong, 2005). Asian Americans as a whole can be found on both the very low and the very high ends of the socioeconomic scale. Proportionally, more Asian American households remain in poverty than White households, yet large numbers of Asian American individuals earn higher income than Whites (see Tables 1.4 and 1.5). Similarly, with respect to educational achievement, proportionally there are more Asian Americans than Whites who are considered excellent students and poor students. For example, Asian American students receive the highest and also the lowest SAT test scores, proportionally, as compared to other major ethnic/racial groups (Hu, 1989). The dichotomy that exists in these findings points toward the polarization by class of the Asian American population.

Within the Asian American population, considerable differences in socioeconomic status exist by ethnic group and income inequality is increasing more rapidly among Asian Americans than among any other racial/ethnic group (Kochhar & Cilluffo, 2018). When comparing different groups of Asian Americans, some populations are far above the average U.S. income level, while others fall far below average. Southeast Asian and mainland Chinese have far lower socioeconomic status than other Asian groups (Min, 1995a, 2006a). Within the Chinese American population, immigrants from Hong Kong and Taiwan have much higher socioeconomic status than immigrants from mainland China (Wong, 2006).

In sum, many challenges lie ahead for this diverse community. Priorities must include raising awareness in the national policy arena about the diverse socioeconomic realities facing Asian Americans and achieving parity for Asian Americans and other underrepresented groups in occupational, educational, and other socioeconomic indicators. The variation observed in socioeconomic attainment by ethnic group warrants further examination, particularly given the increasing diversity within the Asian American population. For example, future research must examine not only the impact of ethnic group on socioeconomic status but also the influence of diverse factors such as nativity, multiracial/multiethnic status, generational status, neighborhood characteristics, familial networks, and household structure (Sakamoto et al., 2009).

Racialization, Identity, and Cultural Politics

There are several images or social constructs of Asians that exist within U.S. national culture, history, and politics. These social constructs serve to marginalize both Asian immigrants and Asian Americans and classify them as the "other" (Lowe, 1991; Said, 1979). The racially biased label of the other is based on essentialist notions of "Asia" as the orient, exotic and alien, founded on the cultural ideology of the yellow peril (Hamamoto, 1994; Wu, 1982), within which Asian immigrants would steal jobs that would otherwise be given to U.S.-born Whites and – more broadly – threaten the dominance of White European power within U.S. society. This racialized construct is also perpetuated by the model minority myth (Hurh & Kim, 1989; Osajima, 1988; Zhou &

TABLE 1.5   **Asian American Percentage Below the Federal Poverty Line, 2019**

	Percentage Below the Federal Poverty Line
Total U.S.	13
Total Asian	10
Asian Indian	6
Bangladeshi	19
Bhutanese	13
Burmese	25
Cambodian	13
Chinese, including Taiwanese	13
Filipino	7
Hmong	17
Indonesian	11
Japanese	8
Korean	11
Laotian	13
Malaysian	16
Mongolian	25
Nepalese	17
Pakistani	15
Sri Lankan	8
Thai	14
Vietnamese	12

Source: U.S. Census Bureau, 2017–2019 American Community Survey 3-Year Estimates.

Xiong, 2005) wherein Asian Americans are presumed to be educated, professionally successful, and dominant in the upper socioeconomic strata of U.S. society.

Even though Asian immigrants have historically played important roles in projects of nation-building and development, they have been restricted from becoming U.S. citizens through legal, economic, and cultural exclusion policies and practices (Lowe, 1996). In addition, the social constructions of national culture and citizenship continue to be rooted in the exclusive racial ideologies of the founding fathers where White European traditions and practices dominate the core constructions of what makes up "America" and what it means to be "American." Asians in the United States continue to be perceived as being poised on the periphery of society, viewed as the other, immigrant, alien, and foreign. Full inclusion for Asian Americans has not yet been realized, even for ethnic Asians born in the United States and those whose backgrounds stem from several generations of predecessors living in America (Okihiro, 1994).

As a nation of immigrants, the United States is founded on values and ideological constructs including full integration of and equal opportunities for all immigrant populations and the availability of equal educational and socioeconomic opportunities for all. These ideals are in sharp contrast to the fragmented, silenced, and disenfranchised experiences that characterize the social history of Asian immigrants in the United States (Espiritu, 2007; Lowe, 1996). U.S. immigration policies and laws, with their selective inclusion and exclusion, have controlled and promoted labor migration flows based on the needs of the industrial sector. However, economic drivers cannot account for the institutional racism encountered by many Asian Americans and Asian immigrants. Asian "immigrant acts" or immigrant agency (Lowe, 1996) have been counter forces where resilience and resistance to dominant American cultural politics of nationhood and citizenship have often played out. Ethnic enclaves have been one of the arenas where ethnic formations and immigrant acts have served to lessen the impact of racialized economic and immigration policies and cultural practices found in American society (Portes & Rumbaut, 2014).

Fundamental contradictions exist between power politics, democracy, and capitalist development (J. O'Connor, 1979; Offe, 1984). In modern society, the economic development of Asian countries has come to represent both a political and an economic threat to U.S. global economic expansion and imperialism (Godement, 1996; Mahbubani, 1998). However, Asian immigrants continue to migrate to America and other parts of the world in significant flows, motivated both by transnational economic networks of labor recruitment across the Pacific and their desire to escape economic, political, and civil disruptions in their native lands (Sassen, 1998). In addition, the essentialist notion of "othering" Asians subordinates Asian identity within the United States, a country still rooted in a Western imperialist past (Lowe, 1991). Paradoxically, even as U.S. cultural and moral values, steeped in democratic ideology and Western capitalism, promote fair competition and equity for all, U.S. society continues to marginalize Asians at every level of social organization – regardless of whether they are Asian, Asian immigrants to the United States, or U.S.-born Asian Americans (Lowe, 1996).

Simultaneously, the shifting political and economic balance in the Pacific has reframed the cultural boundaries of nationhood and citizenship for Asian Americans and the Asian diaspora. Old divisive racial politics are being contested and replaced with new intercultural and transnational possibilities, which negotiate new forms and constructions of Asian and pan-Asian identities (Ong, 1996, 1999).

Despite progress toward racial inclusiveness within U.S. culture and society, racialized constructs of Asians as threatening U.S. values persist, merely disguised under new cultural terminology and political rhetoric (Espiritu, 2007; Lowe, 1996). Asian Americans continue to be excluded from the U.S. political arena due to lack of political volume, both in terms of the number of people of Asian descent who are politically active and who are elected. Historically, debates about race in politics and society have been framed as only a Black and White issue. More recently, these debates have expanded to include Hispanics as a third group deemed worthy of consideration and inclusion. Yet Asian Americans have remained peripheral to these conversations.

Fortunately, in the last decade, this scenario has shifted. During the 2008 U.S. presidential election, mainstream media started acknowledging the growing power of the Asian American electorate (Asian American Legal Defense and Education Fund, 2009). Continued high voter turnout and enthusiasm among Asian Americans was documented during the 2018 midterm and 2020 presidential elections (Ramakrishnan & Wong, 2020). In sum, three key issues that will impact socioeconomic mobility and political power for Asian Americans that merit future observation and research include: (1) the contradictions and contestations of race and identity politics; (2) the counter resistance of Pan-Asian American solidarity; and (3) the rise of Asia and its expansionism to dominant American political, economic and cultural forces.

Gender, Immigration, and Family

The central role of women in the history of Asian immigration to the United States has been minimized and neglected (Chan, 1991; Espiritu, 2007). Overall, more Asian women than men have emigrated to the United States, yet – for the most part – the voices of Asian Americans in political, economic, and educational settings have reflected issues viewed as important by Asian American men, such as racial discrimination and socioeconomic inequity. However, the last few decades have seen a shift toward the reconstruction, retelling, and rewriting of Asian American women's experiences in both the academic and policy arenas. As more Asian American women and their perspectives come to the forefront of contemporary Asian American movements, Asian American women's voices are transforming the priorities of social change and making new contributions to improving race, class and gender equity. As this section will show, Asian women's participation in the U.S. workforce has been a key avenue through which women have gained status and the ability to impact change.

Economics have always played a key role in Asian migration patterns, influencing family and social relationships throughout Asian American communities. During the early period of Asian immigration to the United States, in the nineteenth and early twentieth centuries, there was a large disparity in the proportion of Asian men as compared to women. This gender disparity decreased over time as Asian American communities grew in size. Many of the first Asian immigrant women to come to the United States were impoverished Chinese and Japanese women and girls sold into forced servitude and prostitution and Japanese and Korean women who immigrated as "picture brides," ordered by Asian immigrant men already residing in the United States, having been recruited as laborers for U.S. companies. Other women arrived in the United States with their husbands or joined them soon after, whether as wives of laborers or wealthy merchants. At this time, while Japanese and Chinese women made up the largest Asian immigrant groups, relatively more Japanese than Chinese women arrived in the United States because the Japanese government promoted Japanese family and community development among migrants overseas. Vastly fewer Korean, Filipina, and Asian Indian women arrived in the United States during this early period of Asian immigration.

Given that racialized, restrictive immigration laws allowed very few Asians to enter the United States before 1965 (Chan, 1991), it is not surprising that the majority of Asian immigrants were men recruited by U.S. agricultural and other corporations as temporary, low-wage, manual labor. Corporations generally preferred to select men without family attachments so that these new recruits would have no distractions from work and be more easily controlled by company management. At the same time, in the traditional communities from which these men were drawn, a woman's place was considered to be in the home. Few Asian women ventured beyond their local community and traveling to the American frontier – where conditions were quite difficult and unfamiliar – was rare. However, the few Asian women who did immigrate during this time played a vital role in the sustaining the material and social well-being of Asian immigrant families (Espiritu, 2007). Most of these Asian immigrant women took on dual roles, as agricultural or service industry workers as well as homemakers. While these demanding circumstances required the women to be especially tough and resilient to survive, an unintended positive consequence for the women was that their roles as income earners lifted their status in the family hierarchy.

The Immigration Act of 1965 facilitated an increase in immigration by Asian women through family reunification and occupation categories (Donato & Tyree, 1986), shifting the Asian immigration flow from one that was dominated by men filling temporary manual labor roles toward a majority of Asian immigrants arriving as families with long-term plans of settling in the United States (Chan, 1991). Indeed, Asian populations have comprised the largest source of immigration to the United States in the post-1965 era, with Asian women at the forefront of this contemporary migration stream (Espiritu, 2007). Once again, this shift was fueled by U.S. economic interests. The expansion of U.S. industries with jobs traditionally filled by women – such as service, health care, retail, and technology – opened the doors of the United States to many more Asian women of diverse ethnic, educational, and socioeconomic backgrounds. Not coincidentally, these sectors typically pay lower wages to women than men fulfilling the same responsibilities, in both skilled and unskilled jobs; nonetheless, these sectors opened doors through which Asian women were able to establish a foothold in the U.S. economy. Although prior to World War II, most Asian women immigrants came from poor backgrounds and worked primarily in lower status, labor-intensive industries, contemporary Asian women immigrants are a substantially more diverse group, filling positions in both professional and nonprofessional sectors.

The changing economic role of women has challenged traditional, gendered customs within Asian communities, particularly in situations where Asian women have found themselves working full-time jobs and contributing substantially to household income, eclipsing the contributions of husbands that struggle with persistent long-term unemployment (Kibria, 1993). Participation of Asian American women in the U.S. workforce has continued to increase throughout the last two decades, perpetuating and intensifying this gender role reversal. Employment among Asian American women increased from 2.5 million in 2000 to 4.3 million in 2021, with a peak of 4.8 million employed Asian American women in September 2019. There are significant occupational differences between Asian American men and women, in fields of all skill levels. For example, women with lower educational attainment may seek employment as nail technicians, while women with higher educational attainment may enter the nursing profession – neither of which are occupations that attract substantial numbers of men (Bleiweis, 2021). Asian American women have participated in the labor force at similar rates as women overall in the United States, fluctuating between 60 percent in January 2000 and 57 percent in January 2021 (Bleiweis, 2021). These rates remain lower than those of Asian American men, whose labor force participation rate changed from 79 percent in January 2000 to 74 percent in January 2021 (Bleiweis, 2021). Asian American women also experience large wage gaps as compared to White men across all job titles, and there is marked heterogeneity in annual earnings by Asian ethnic group, ranging from a median annual income of $30,000 among Burmese women to $70,000 among Taiwanese and Asian Indian women (Bleiweis, 2021). The evolution of economic opportunities and increased social power for Asian American women post-1965 is complicated by the intersections of race, gender, and sexuality, as Asian women continue to be hypersexualized and made vulnerable to violence. The mass shooting of eight people, including six Asian women, in three massage business in Atlanta, Georgia on March 16, 2021, brought to light the history and continued reality of racialized and gendered violence against Asian American women.

In sum, recognizing the historical context within which Asian women and their families have immigrated to the United States is critical to understanding contemporary migration patterns between Asian countries and the United States. The Immigration Act of 1965 was a key milestone in liberalizing immigration policy and allowing for increased migration from Asian countries, providing a stepping stone to a vastly larger flow of Asian women into the United States. The workplace provided an important environment for Asian immigrant women. The growing reliance on women's work for wage labor increased their overall workload dramatically, but also has reshaped the dynamics of traditional patriarchal systems and given more visible power to Asian women's lives in the family and beyond.

Social Determinants of Asian American Health

The complexities of the Asian American diaspora, including migration history, cultural and linguistic diversity, and intergenerational differences, contribute to unique social vulnerabilities and health issues across the life course for Asian Americans. Throughout this textbook, a *social determinants of health* approach is used as a lens through which to view the health issues impacting Asian American communities. The role of the social determinants of health for understanding the health status and health disparities of Asian Americans populations is further detailed in Chapter 2, while Chapter 3 describes key health issues impacting these communities. Understanding the intersectional and varied life experiences of Asian Americans provides the narrative for examining how health inequities manifest and guides the identification of risk and protective factors for health and well-being. Advancing health equity for Asian American communities will require innovative solutions that address the multiple determinants of health that create and perpetuate social vulnerabilities and health disparities, as well as promote resilience, like the role of cultural capital and food environments on health. Novel methods of understanding health, such as community-partnered systems science, are described in Chapter 6. Approaches to improving implementation of interventions through cultural adaptations is detailed in Chapter 7, with case studies describing the different approaches taken to tailor interventions to Asian American communities.

Acts of racism against Asian Americans are not new in U.S. history but remain concerning. Racism, a known social determinant of health, may exacerbate health disparities already present in the Asian American population (Le et al., 2020). Research has produced clear results demonstrating the negative impacts of racism on physical and mental health, through pathways such as increased allostatic load (i.e., the ongoing wear and tear of stress on the body) and continuous trauma and hypervigilance. Several example of the impact of heightened anti-Asian xenophobia and COVID-19 pandemic include high rates of long-term unemployment (Khan & Shih, 2020; Le et al., 2020) and economic downturn and business closures of Chinatowns across many U.S. metropolitan cities (Mar & Ong, 2020). Thus, solutions to promote overall health and health equity must include engagement of Asian American communities and support for capacity and coalition building, including multilevel strategies to increase community-clinic linkages (Chapter 9), advancing health in all policies across multiple sectors (Chapter 10), and data disaggregation for health equity (Chapter 4).

CONCLUSION

Asian Americans have become an increasingly important minority group, making American ethnic/racial processes far more sophisticated than before and Asian American visibility in the national arena continues to grow (Min, 1995a; P. Q. Yang, 2006). Overall, Asian Americans are a richly diverse group, in contrast to the myth of Asian homogeneity (Chan, 1991; Takaki, 1998). Culturally and economically, Asian Americans represent diverse religions, customs, languages, values, and social class backgrounds. There are no common languages, religions, and traditions that unite these various groups. Their socioeconomic status is also diverse, with some groups with median incomes comparable to Whites while other groups live in poverty at disproportionate rates. Furthermore, a clear divide exists between foreign- and U.S.-born Asian Americans vis à vis their ability to integrate socially within U.S. society (Min, 1995a; Yang, 2006). This finding is especially significant, as foreign-born individuals comprise the majority (57 percent) of the Asian American population (Budiman & Ruiz, 2021).

Despite the cultural, economic, and social diversity that exists among different ethnic Asian groups, Asian Americans share common experiences. This common ground has led to an Asian American movement that transcends ethnic, cultural, and economic differences (Wei, 1993). The creation of a Pan-Asian American identity and unity (Espiritu, 2007; National Council of Asian Pacific Americans, 2004) is based on the common values Asian Americans share, the similar perception and treatment of Asian Americans by the general public and government agencies, and with the shared goal among diverse Asian ethnic groups to protect their political, economic, health care, and other interests. As this new ethnic-political identity evolves, Pan-Asian institutions will voice the political needs of its constituents and make significant contributions to the Asian American agenda, which includes equity within the larger American institutions of politics, economics, health, and culture.

One setback faced by Asian American advocacy groups is the collateral damage that comes from American political and economic crises. In post-9/11 America, several challenges include tightening of immigration and national security policies, the emerging U.S. economic recession, and changes in government priorities at the federal level. Asian American health advocacy and service organizations lack political clout and knowledge compared to American mainstream institutions, and often are perceived as serving populations with little or no voting influence. Consequently, Asian American community organizations are the first to lose political support and to face budget cuts from government (Tseng, 2005). Nevertheless, some of these organizations have become experienced players, adept at managing with limited resources and skillfully utilizing their cross-cultural networks and capital. This ability to negotiate and advance health and social priorities of Asian Americans can help to reduce the negative impact felt by Asian American communities during such crisis periods. The Asian & Pacific Islander American Health Forum (APIAHF) was established in direct response to the invisibility of Asian American and NH/PI communities in federal health policy (Ko Chin, 2020). Over the span of 35 years, related policy advocacy organizations were created, including Asian Pacific Partners for Empowerment, Advocacy & Leadership (APPEAL), Association of Asian Pacific Community Health Organizations (AAPCHO), National Council of Asian Pacific Islander Physicians (NCAPIP), and Asian Americans Advancing Justice (AAJC). These organizations are also member organizations of the National Council of Asian Pacific Americans (NCAPA), a coalition of 37 national Asian American and NH/PI organizations that represent a national voice for Asian American and NH/PI issues.

Finally, American domestic and international policies on immigration not only affect Asian Americans and other communities of color but also dramatically influence U.S. politics and economy (Tseng, 2005). Post-globalization trends create supply and demand for cheap immigrant labor and provide explanation for the constant influx of new workers and their families from Asia and other world regions. Asian Americans play an ever-increasing role in the U.S. economy, politics, culture, and health care systems. Today, Asian Americans are essential to the United States, providing invaluable human labor and intellectual capital. As trends to promote diversity continue, national programs developed by the federal government must also address those issues affecting communities of color. The future of the United States, including its ability to innovate and thrive, is critically linked to the welfare of its multicultural communities. Fostering multicultural communities has become a national imperative and part of the national agenda.

DISCUSSION QUESTIONS

1. Discuss the different legal acts enacted to exclude and/or discriminate against various Asian American groups. How did these acts shape the demographic profile of the Asian American population as a whole? How do they contribute to racism and stereotyping of Asian Americans that persists today?

2. What are the *glass ceiling* and *bamboo ceiling* phenomena, and how do they relate to the *model minority* stereotype? How do these constructs affect social and political participation for Asian Americans?

3. Describe the concept of *intersectionality*. How does it contribute to health inequities?

REFERENCES

1946 Indian and Filipino Immigration and Naturalization (aka Luce-Celler Act), no. Pub. L. No. 79-483, 60 Stat. 416, United States Congress (1946).

Akiba, D. (2006). Japanese Americans. In *Asian Americans: Contemporary Trends and Issues* (2nd ed., pp. 148–177). SAGE Publications, Inc. https://doi.org/10.4135/9781452233802

Arnold, F., Minocha, U., & Fawcett, J. T. (1987). The Changing Face of Asian Immigration to the United States. In *Pacific Bridges: The New Immigration from Asia and the Pacific Islands* (pp. 103–152). Center for Migration Studies.

Asian American Legal Defense and Education Fund. (2009). *New Report on the Asian American Vote in the 2008 Elections Shows Widespread Support for Obama and Growing Numbers of First-Time Voters* [Press Release]. https://www.aaldef.org/press-release/new-report-on-the-asian-american-vote-in-the-2008-elections-shows-widespread-support-for-obama-and-g/

Asis, M. M. B. (2017, July 12). *The Philippines: Beyond Labor Migration, Toward Development and (Possibly) Return.* Migration Policy Institute. https://www.migrationpolicy.org/article/philippines-beyond-labor-migration-toward-development-and-possibly-return

Bankston, C. L. (2006). Filipino Americans. In *Asian Americans: Contemporary Trends and Issues* (2nd ed., pp. 180–203). SAGE Publications, Inc. https://doi.org/10.4135/9781452233802

Barringer, H. R., Gardner, R. W., & Levin, M. J. (1993). *Asians and Pacific Islanders in the United States.* Russell Sage Foundation; JSTOR. http://www.jstor.org/stable/10.7758/9781610440264

Bleiweis, R. (2021). *The Economic Status of Asian American and Pacific Islander Women* [Issue Brief]. Center for American Progress. https://www.americanprogress.org/issues/women/reports/2021/03/04/496703/economic-status-asian-american-pacific-islander-women/#fnref-496703-7

Brindis, C. D., Hadler, M. W., Jacobs, K., Lucia, L., Pourat, N., Raymond-Flesch, M., Siemons, R., & Talamantes, E. (2014). *Realizing the Dream for Californians Eligible for Deferred Action for Childhood Arrivals (DACA): Demographics and Health Coverage.* National Adolescent and Young Adult Health Information Center. https://nahic.ucsf.edu/wp-content/uploads/2014/04/DACA_health_coverage.pdf

Budiman, A. (2020, August 20). *Key findings about U.S. immigrants.* Pew Research Center. https://www.pewresearch.org/?p=290738

Budiman, A., & Ruiz, N. G. (2021, April 29). *Key facts about Asian origin groups in the U.S.* Pew Research Center. https://www.pewresearch.org/fact-tank/2021/04/29/key-facts-about-asian-origin-groups-in-the-u-s/

Bureau of East Asian and Pacific Affairs. (2021). *U.S. Relations with Vietnam* [Bilateral Relations Fact Sheet]. https://www.state.gov/u-s-relations-with-vietnam/

Cabezas, A., & Kawaguchi, G. (1988). Empirical evidence for continuing Asian American income inequality: The human capital model and labor market segmentation. In G. Y. Okihiro, S. Hune, A. A. Hansen, & J. M. Liu (Eds.), *Reflections on Shattered Windows* (pp. 144–164). Washington State University Press.

Cariño, B. V. (1987). *The Philippines and Southeast Asia: Historical roots and contemporary linkages. In Pacific Bridges: The New Immigration from Asia and the Pacific Islands* (pp. 303–325). Center for Migration Studies.

Chan, S. (1989). Beyond Affirmative Action. *Change: The Magazine of Higher Learning, 21*(6), 48–52. https://doi.org/10.1080/00091383.1989.9937605

Chan, S. (1991). *Asian Americans: An Interpretive History* (1st edition). Twayne Publishers.

Crenshaw, K. (1990). Mapping the Margins: Intersectionality, Identity Politics, and Violence against Women of Color. *Stanford Law Review, 43*(6), 1241–1300. https://heinonline.org/HOL/P?h=hein.journals/stflr43&i=1257

Crystal, D. (1989). Asian Americans and the Myth of the Model Minority. *Social Casework, 70*(7), 405–413. https://doi.org/10.1177/104438948907000702

De Jong, G. F., & Steinmetz, M. (2004). Receptivity Attitudes and the Occupational Attainment of Male and Female Immigrant Workers. *Population Research and Policy Review, 23*(2), 91–116. https://doi.org/10.1023/B:POPU.0000019929.59033.70

Demanarig, D. L. L., & Acosta, J. (2016). Phenomenological Look at the Experiences of Filipina Correspondence or Internet Brides. *SAGE Open, 6*(2), 2158244016654949. https://doi.org/10.1177/2158244016654949

Der, H. (1993). *Asian Pacific Islanders and the "glass ceiling" – New era of civil rights activism* (pp. 215–232) [The State of Asian Pacific America: Policy Issues to the Year 2020]. LEAP Asian Pacific Islander Public Policy Institute and UCLA Asian American Studies Center. http://www.aasc.ucla.edu/resources/policyreports/Policy_Issues_Year_2020/Policy_Higher_Education.pdf

Dhingra, P. (2016). Just Getting a Job Is Not Enough: How Indian Americans Navigate the Workplace. In *Contemporary Asian America* (3rd ed., pp. 217–235). New York University Press.

Donato, K., & Tyree, A. (1986). Family reunification health professionals and the sex composition of immigrants to the United States. *Social Sciences Review*, *70*, 226–230.

Esperat, M. C., Inouye, J., Gonzalez, E. W., Owen, D. C., & Feng, D. (2004). Health disparities among Asian Americans and Pacific Islanders. *Annual Review of Nursing Research*, *22*, 135–159.

Espiritu, Y. L. (2007). *Asian American Women and Men: Labor, Laws, and Love (Second edition)*. Rowman & Littlefield Publishers.

Frayer, L. (2021). India's Farmer Protests: Why Are They So Angry? *NPR*. https://www.npr.org/sections/goatsandsoda/2021/03/02/971293844/indias-farmer-protests-why-are-they-so-angry

Fujiwara, L. H. (1998). The Impact of Welfare Reform on Asian Immigrant Communities. *Social Justice*, *25*(1 (71)), 82–104. https://www.jstor.org/stable/29767060

García, J., & Sharif, M. Z. (2015). Black Lives Matter: A Commentary on Racism and Public Health. *American Journal of Public Health*, *105*(8), e27–e30. https://doi.org/10.2105/AJPH.2015.302706

Gee, B., Peck, D., & Wong, J. (2015). *HIDDEN IN PLAIN SIGHT: Asian American Leaders in Silicon Valley*. The Ascend Foundation. https://asiasociety.org/sites/default/files/inline-files/HiddenInPlainSight_Paper_042.pdf

Godement, F. (1996). *The New Asian Renaissance: From Colonialism to the Post-cold War*. Routledge.

Gotanda, N. (1995). Re-producing the model minority stereotype: Judge Joyce Karlin's sentencing colloquy in *People v. Soon Ja Du*. In W. L. Ng, S. Chin, J. S. Moy, & G. Y. Okihiro (Eds.), *ReViewing Asian America: Locating Diversity* (pp. 87–106). Washington State University Press.

Hamamoto, D. (1994). *Monitored Peril* (1st edition). University of Minnesota Press.

Hanna, M., & Batalova, J. (2021, March 9). *Immigrants from Asia in the United States*. Migration Policy Institute. https://www.migrationpolicy.org/article/immigrants-asia-united-states-2020

Hein, J. (1995). *From Vietnam, Laos, and Cambodia: A Refugee Experience in the United States*. Twayne Publishers.

Hing, B. O. (1994). *Making and Remaking Asian America Through Immigration Policy, 1850-1990* (1st edition). Stanford University Press.

Hoeffel, E. M., Rastogi, S., & Kim, M. O. (2012). *The Asian Population: 2010* [2010 Census Briefs]. U.S. Census Bureau. https://www.census.gov/prod/cen2010/briefs/c2010br-11.pdf

Hu, A. (1989). Asian Americans: Model Minority or Double Minority? *Amerasia Journal*, *15*(1), 243–257. https://doi.org/10.17953/amer.15.1.e032240687706472

Hurh, W. M., & Kim, K. C. (1989). The 'success' image of Asian Americans: Its validity, and its practical and theoretical implications. *Ethnic and Racial Studies*, *12*(4), 512–538. https://doi.org/10.1080/01419870.1989.9993650

Immigrant Legal Resource Center. (2021). *Executive Action Proposals for the Biden Administration to Protect DACA Recipients and their Families*. https://www.ilrc.org/sites/default/files/resources/executive_action_proposals_for_the_biden_administration_to_protect_daca_recipients_and_their_families.pdf

Institute of Medicine (US) Committee on Understanding and Eliminating Racial and Ethnic Disparities in Health Care. (2003). *Unequal Treatment: Confronting Racial and Ethnic Disparities in Health Care* (B. D. Smedley, A. Y. Stith, & A. R. Nelson, Eds.). National Academies Press (US). http://www.ncbi.nlm.nih.gov/books/NBK220358/

Jin, D. Y. (2018). An Analysis of the Korean Wave as Transnational Popular Culture: North American Youth Engage Through Social Media as TV Becomes Obsolete. *International Journal of Communication*, *12*(0), 19. https://ijoc.org/index.php/ijoc/article/view/7973

Khan, R., & Shih, H. (2020). *Impact of COVID-19 on Asian Employment in New York City*. Asian American Federation.

Kibria, N. (1993). *Family Tightrope*. Princeton University Press; JSTOR. http://www.jstor.org/stable/j.ctt1r2drf

Kibria, N. (2006). South Asian Americans. In *Asian Americans: Contemporary Trends and Issues* (2nd ed., pp. 206–227). SAGE Publications, Inc. https://doi.org/10.4135/9781452233802

Kim, H. C. (1994). *A Legal History of Asian Americans, 1790-1990:* Praeger.

Kim, I. (2014). *New Urban Immigrants: The Korean Community in New York*. Princeton University Press.

Ko Chin, K. (2020). A History of Asian American, Native Hawaiian, Pacific Islander Health Policy Advocacy: From Invisibility to Forging Policy. *Asian American Policy Review*, *30*. https://aapr.hkspublications.org/2020/10/04/a-history-of-asian-american-native-hawaiian-pacific-islander-health-policy-advocacy-from-invisibility-to-forging-policy/

Kochhar, R., & Cilluffo, A. (2018, July 12). *Income Inequality in the U.S. Is Rising Most Rapidly Among Asians*. https://www.pewresearch.org/social-trends/2018/07/12/income-inequality-in-the-u-s-is-rising-most-rapidly-among-asians/

Koo, H., & Yu, E.-Y. (1981). *Korean immigration to the United States: Its demographic pattern and social implications for both societies*. East-West Population Institute.

Lai, E. Y. P., & Arguelles, D. (Eds.). (2003). *The New Face of Asian Pacific America: Numbers, Diversity and Change in the 21st Century*. AsianWeek.

Le, T. K., Cha, L., Han, H.-R., & Tseng, W. (2020). Anti-Asian Xenophobia and Asian American COVID-19 Disparities. *American Journal of Public Health*, *110*(9), 1371–1373. https://doi.org/10.2105/AJPH.2020.305846

Lee, E. (2016). *The Making of Asian America: A History*. Simon & Schuster.

Lee, S. (1986). *Why People Intend to Move: Individual and Community-Level Factors of Out-Migration in the Philippines*. Westview Press.

Light, I., & Bonacich, E. (1991). *Immigrant Entrepreneurs: Koreans in Los Angeles, 1965–1982*. University of California Press.

Lowe, L. (1991). *Critical Terrains: French and British Orientalisms*. Cornell University Press.

Lowe, L. (1996). *Immigrant Acts On Asian American Cultural Politics*. Duke University Press.

Mahbubani, K. (1998). *Can Asians Think?* (4th edition). Times Book International.

Mar, D., & Ong, P. (2020). *University of Califonia Los Angeles. Asian American Studies Center. COVID-19's Employment Disruptions to Asian Americans.* http://www.aasc.ucla.edu/resources/policyreports/COVID19_Employment_CNK-AASC_072020.pdf

Migration Policy Institute. (2013, June 23). *Foreign-Born Population by Country of Birth.* MPI Data Hub: Migration Facts, Stats, and Maps. https://www.migrationpolicy.org/sites/default/files/datahub/MPIDataHub-Region-birth-1960.xlsx

Milly, D. J. (2020, February 20). *Japan's Labor Migration Reforms: Breaking with the Past?* Migration Policy Institute. https://www.migrationpolicy.org/article/japan-labor-migration-reforms-breaking-past

Min, P. G. (1995a). An Overview of Asian Americans. In *Asian Americans: Contemporary trends and issues* (pp. 10–37). SAGE Publications, Inc.

Min, P. G. (1995b). Major issues relating to Asian American experiences. In *Asian Americans: Contemporary trends and issues* (pp. 38–57). SAGE Publications, Inc.

Min, P. G. (2006a). Asian immigration: History and contemporary trends. In *Asian Americans: Contemporary trends and issues* (Second, pp. 7–31). SAGE Publications, Inc.

Min, P. G. (2006b). Korean Americans. In *Asian Americans: Contemporary Trends and Issues* (2nd ed., pp. 230–259). SAGE Publications, Inc. https://doi.org/10.4135/9781452233802

Min, P. G. (2006c). Settlement Patterns and Diversity. In *Asian Americans: Contemporary Trends and Issues* (2nd ed., pp. 32–53). SAGE Publications, Inc. https://doi.org/10.4135/9781452233802

National Council of Asian Pacific Americans. (2004). *Call to Action: Platform for Asian Pacific Americans National Policy Priorities.* Nactional Council of Asian Pacific Americans.

Nguyen, T. (2005). *We Are All Suspects Now: Untold Stories from Immigrant Communities after 9/11* (1st edition). Beacon Press.

O'Connor, A., & Batalova, J. (2019, April 10). *Korean Immigrants in the United States.* Migration Policy Institute. https://www.migrationpolicy.org/article/korean-immigrants-united-states-2017

O'Connor, J. (1979). *The Fiscal Crisis of the State.* St. Martin's Press.

Offe, C. (1984). *Contradictions of the Welfare State* (J. Keane, Ed.). MIT Press.

Oh, T. K. (1977). *The Asian Brain Drain: A Factual and Casual Analysis.* R & E Research Associates.

Okihiro, G. Y. (1994). *Margins and Mainstreams: Asians in American History and Culture.* University of Washington Press.

Ong, A. (1996). Cultural Citizenship as Subject-Making: Immigrants Negotiate Racial and Cultural Boundaries in the United States. *Current Anthropology, 37*(5), 737–762. https://www.jstor.org/stable/2744412

Ong, A. (1999). *Flexible Citizenship: The Cultural Logics of Transnationality* (2nd printing, edition). Duke University Press Books.

Ong, P., Bonacich, E., & Cheng, L. (1994). *The New Asian Immigration in Los Angeles and Global Restructuring.* Temple University Press.

Osajima, K. (1988). Asian Americans as the model minority: An analysis of the popular press image in the 1960s and 1980s. In G. Y. Okihiro, S. Hune, A. A. Hansen, & J. M. Liu (Eds.), *Reflections on Shattered Windows* (pp. 165–174). Washington State University Press.

Park Nelson, K. (2016). *Invisible Asians: Korean American Adoptees, Asian American Experiences, and Racial Exceptionalism.* Rutgers University Press.

Pew Research Center, "How the Asian Population Changed in Every State and D.C. from 2000 to 2019," April 9, 2021, https://www.pewresearch.org/fact-tank/2021/04/09/asian-americans-are-the-fastest-growing-racial-or-ethnic-group-in-the-u-s/ft_2021-04-09_asianamericans_05/.

Pimienti, M., & Polkey, C. (2019, March 29). *Snapshot of U.S. Immigration 2019.* National Conference of State Legislatures. https://www.ncsl.org/research/immigration/snapshot-of-u-s-immigration-2017.aspx

Piore, M. J. (1980). *Birds of Passage: Migrant Labor and Industrial Societies (1st PAPERBACK edition).* Cambridge University Press.

Portes, A., & Rumbaut, R. G. (2014). *Immigrant America: A Portrait, Updated, and Expanded (Fourth edition).* University of California Press.

Ramakrishnan, K., & Wong, J. (2020, September 15). New Survey: Asian Americans Enthusiastic for 2020, Favor Biden. *Data Bits (AAPI Data Blog).* http://aapidata.com/blog/2020-aa-voter-survey-enthusiasm/

Reimers, D. M. (1992). *Still the Golden Door: The Third World Comes to America.* Columbia University Press.

Robinson, W. C. (1999). *Terms of Refuge: The Indochinese Exodus and the International Response.* Zed Books.

Rumbaut, R. G. (2006). Vietnamese, Laotian, and Cambodian Americans. In *Asian Americans: Contemporary Trends and Issues* (2nd ed., pp. 262–289). SAGE Publications, Inc. https://doi.org/10.4135/9781452233802

Said, E. (1979). *Orientalism.* Random House.

Sakamoto, A., Goyette, K. A., & Kim, C. (2009). Socioeconomic Attainments of Asian Americans. *Annual Review of Sociology, 35*(1), 255–276. https://doi.org/10.1146/annurev-soc-070308-115958.

Saran, P. (1985). *The Asian Indian Experience in the United States.* Schenkman Books.

Saran, P., & Eames, E. (Eds.). (1980). *The New Ethnics: Asian Indians in the United States.* Praeger.

Sassen, S. (1998). *Globalization and Its Discontents (First Edition).* The New Press.

Shin, E. H., & Chang, K.-S. (1988). Peripherization of Immigrant Professionals: Korean Physicians in the United States. *International Migration Review, 22*(4), 609–626. https://doi.org/10.1177/019791838802200404

Takagi, D. Y. (1990). From Discrimination to Affirmative Action: Facts in the Asian American Admissions Controversy*. *Social Problems, 37*(4), 578–592. https://doi.org/10.2307/800583

Takahashi, J. (1997). *Nisei Sansei: Shifting Japanese American Identities and Politics (First Edition).* Temple University Press.

Takaki, R. (1998). *Strangers from a Different Shore: A History of Asian Americans, Updated and Revised Edition.* Little, Brown and Company.

Tang, J. (1993). The Career Attainment of Caucasian and Asian Engineers. *The Sociological Quarterly, 34*(3), 467–496. https://www.jstor.org/stable/4121108

Taylor, P. A., & Kim, S. S. (1980). Asian-Americans in the Federal Civil Service, 1977. *California Sociologist, 3*, 1–16.

Tseng, W. (2005). Government dependence of Chinese and Vietnamese community organizations and fiscal politics of immigrant services. *Journal of Health & Social Policy, 20*(4), 51–74. https://doi.org/10.1300/j045v20n04_03

U.S. Census Bureau. (1993). *1990 Census of Population, Asians and Pacific Islanders in the United States (CP-3-5).* (Table 262). U.S. Government Printing Office.

U.S. Census Bureau. (1973). *US Census of the Population: 1970, Subject Reports: Japanese, Chinese, and Filipinos in the US (PC[2]-1-C)*. (Table 140).

U.S. Census Bureau. (2020). *2015–2019 American Community Survey 5-year estimates*. https://www.census.gov/data.html

U.S. Immigration and Naturalization Service. (1960). *Annual Reports 1960–1978*. U.S. Government Printing Office.

U.S. Immigration and Naturalization Service. (1979). *Statistical Yearbook 1979–1992*. U.S. Government Printing Office.

Vespa, J., Medina, L., & Armstrong, D. M. (2020). *Demographic Turning Points for the United States: Population Projections for 2020 to 2060* (Current Population Report). https://www.census.gov/content/dam/Census/library/publications/2020/demo/p25-1144.pdf

Wang, L. L. (1993). *Trends in Admissions for Asian Americans in Colleges and Universities: Higher Education Policy* (pp. 49–59) [The State of Asian Pacific America: Policy Issues to the Year 2020]. LEAP Asian Pacific Islander Public Policy Institute and UCLA Asian American Studies Center. http://www.aasc.ucla.edu/resources/policyreports/Policy_Issues_Year_2020/Policy_Higher_Education.pdf

Wei, W. (1993). *The Asian American Movement*. Temple University Press.

Wong, M. G. (2006). Chinese Americans. In *Asian Americans: Contemporary Trends and Issues* (2nd ed., pp. 110–145). SAGE Publications, Inc. https://doi.org/10.4135/9781452233802

Wu, W. F. (1982). *The Yellow Peril: Chinese-Americans in American Fiction 1850–1940*. Archon Books.

Yang, P., & Bohm-Jordan, M. (2018). Patterns of Interracial and Interethnic Marriages among Foreign-Born Asians in the United States. *Societies*, 8(3), 87. https://doi.org/10.3390/soc8030087

Yang, P. Q. (2006). Future prospects of Asian Americans. In P. G. Min (Ed.), *Asian Americans: Contemporary Trends and Issues* (2nd ed., pp. 292–316). SAGE Publications, Inc.

Yochum, G., & Agarwal, V. (1988). Permanent Labor Certifications for Alien Professionals, 1975–1982. *The International Migration Review*, 22(2), 265–281. https://doi.org/10.2307/2546650

Yuh, J. Y. (2005). Moved by War: Migration, Diaspora, and the Korean War. *Journal of Asian American Studies*, 8(3), 277–291. https://doi.org/10.1353/jaas.2005.0054

Zhou, M., & Xiong, Y. S. (2005). The multifaceted American experiences of the children of Asian immigrants: Lessons for segmented assimilation. *Ethnic and Racial Studies*, 28(6), 1119–1152. https://doi.org/10.1080/01419870500224455

CHAPTER

HEALTH FRAMEWORK FOR UNDERSTANDING THE HEALTH AND HEALTH DISPARITIES OF ASIAN AMERICAN POPULATIONS

CHAU TRINH-SHEVRIN, RACHEL SACKS, SIMONA C. KWON, MATTHEW LEE, DEBORAH K. MIN, NADIA S. ISLAM

LEARNING OBJECTIVES

By the end of this chapter, readers will be able to:

- Understand the rationale for shifting from a health disparities research perspective to a population health equity framework.

- Identify strategies essential to operationalizing the population health equity framework to design, implement, and evaluate community-engaged research among Asian American communities.

- Identify new research methodologies that are components of the population health equity framework, including community-based participatory research, innovative data collection and analysis methods, ethnic and pan-ethnic advisory councils, and systems thinking.

Applied Population Health Approaches for Asian American Communities, First Edition. Edited by Simona C. Kwon, Chau Trinh-Shevrin, Nadia S. Islam, and Stella S. Yi.
© 2023 John Wiley & Sons, Inc. Published 2023 by John Wiley & Sons, Inc.
Companion Website: www.wiley.com/go/kwon/asianamerican

INTRODUCTION

This chapter describes a framework to guide research, training, and practice toward advancing population health equity. We present and explore strategies to assist in focusing attention on the highest attainment of the health for all, valuing everyone equally with focused and ongoing societal efforts to address avoidable inequalities, historical and contemporary injustices, and the elimination of health and health care disparities (Srinavasan & Williams, 2014).

THE POPULATION HEALTH EQUITY FRAMEWORK

The population health equity framework prioritizes the elimination of health disparities within racial/ethnic minority populations in order to advance the health of all (Srinavasan & Williams, 2014; Trinh-Shevrin, Kwon, et al., 2015). Health disparities refer to inequities in health and health care between groups of people (Artiga et al., 2020). These inequities are associated with social, economic, and/or environmental disadvantage and impact racial/ethnic groups as well as groups defined by immigrant status, disability, sex, gender, and geography (National Institutes of Health NIMHD, 2020). Health disparities and inequities facing Asian Americans are complex, multilevel, and tightly entrenched within larger social, political, historical, and economic constructs (Trinh-Shevrin, Islam, et al., 2015). The population health equity framework engages a social justice lens to identify the need for a deeper focus on engaging Asian American communities, employing a life course perspective, and tackling the root causes of inequalities through transdisciplinary partnerships and collaborations (Bravemen & Barclay, 2009). This approach prioritizes consideration of the profound impact that societies and environments have on the health outcomes of the vastly diverse ethnic groups that comprise the Asian American population. It incorporates structural and political factors that are constantly evolving, such as globalization, immigration, and intergenerational relationships, allowing for a dynamic and nuanced response to emerging issues that impact health.

Importantly, the population health equity framework shifts language and emphasis away from a focus on identifying problems (e.g., "health inequities") to designing solutions (e.g., "health equity for all") (Srinavasan & Williams, 2014). The framework is integrative and transdisciplinary, moving away from a disease-focused biomedical approach and incorporating advocacy, translation of research findings through communication, and adaptation and meaningful implementation of culturally relevant strategies and policies for underserved, culturally diverse populations (Trinh-Shevrin, Islam, et al., 2015).

BOX 2.1   Health Equity For All: Shifting The Paradigm

A *health disparity* generally refers to a disproportionate disease burden in health status or access to care that is experienced by one group compared with another, which stems from an array of factors that include behavioral, environmental, and social determinants (Srinivasan & Williams, 2014).

A *health inequity* refers to systematic health differentials across population groups that are a result of unjust burdens placed on individuals and communities (Braveman & Gruskin, 2003).

A *population health equity framework* moves beyond merely identifying these health disparities and inequities to translating them through meaningful stakeholder engagement in an iterative "policy-to-action" process, focusing attention on the highest attainment of health for all (Public Health Agency of Canada & World Health Organization, 2008; Trinh-Shevrin, Kwon, et al., 2015).

STRATEGIES FOR OPERATIONALIZING A HEALTH EQUITY FRAMEWORK

Shifting the paradigm from reducing health disparities among different population groups to increasing health equity for all represents a significant challenge. Researchers, clinicians, public health professionals, social service agencies, and communities must develop a balance between their ongoing inequities-focused research,

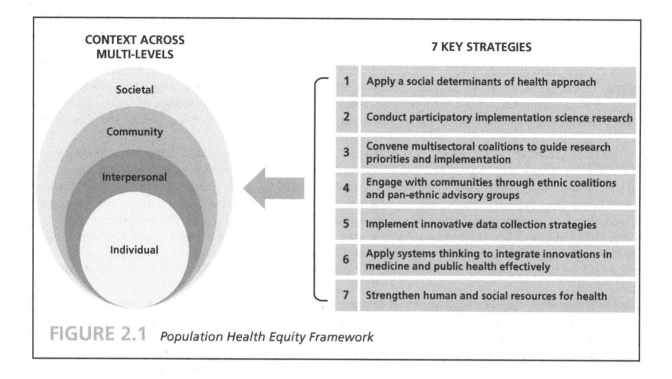

FIGURE 2.1   *Population Health Equity Framework*

policy efforts, and service provision and the development and implementation of innovative strategies to cultivate the necessary infrastructure to foster transdisciplinary progress toward health equity (Trinh-Shevrin, Kwon, et al., 2015).

Operationalizing a population health equity framework means integrating evidence-based practices into new community-engaged study designs to advance equity. Toward that end, we present seven strategies for operationalizing this framework. In our conceptualization, the population health equity framework (1) builds on the social determinants of health approach and (2) relies on participatory implementation science methodologies to ensure that health equity research is community-engaged, dynamic, and practical. We also (3) advocate for expanded implementation of innovative data collection and analysis methodologies to address well-documented inequities in current research methods. We (4) prioritize the engagement of multisectoral coalitions to ensure health equity research is guided by goals that resonate across policy and program domains and we (5) underscore the essential role of ethnic and pan-ethnic advisory groups in developing research agendas for their communities. We further (6) underscore the importance of cross-disciplinary systems thinking to integrate emerging technologies to address the goals and vision articulated by these communities. Finally, we (7) advocate for focused efforts to recruit, retain, and support additional human and social resources for health among racial/ethnic minority groups as a critical pathway sustainable development of internal community structures and self-reliance.

These seven strategies are depicted in Figure 2.1 and are described in detail below.

1. Apply a Social Determinants of Health Approach

The population health equity framework is founded on the social determinants of health approach, which prioritizes consideration of the impact of the conditions in which people are born, grow, work, live, and age along with the wider set of forces and systems shaping the conditions of daily life on their health and well-being (World Health Organization, 2020; Marmot et al., 2008). This wider set of forces and systems includes economic policies and systems, social norms, social policies, and political systems, all of which shape the distribution of money, power, and resources across U.S. regions, cities, and neighborhoods. Structural racism is a key concept within this approach, referring to the many ways in which racism is embedded in local, state, and federal laws, policies, and practices, oppressing communities of color while providing advantages to non-Hispanic Whites (Whites) (Bailey et al., 2017; Feagin & Bennefield, 2014; Williams et al., 2019). In addition to structural racism, social determinants of health include socioeconomic status, social structure, social position, and discrimination, as well as factors such as housing, transportation, political environment, and cultural beliefs and norms (Trinh-Shevrin, Islam, et al., 2015). An expansive view of this approach encompasses normative and cultural values as well as structural ones (Krieger, 2014; Brawner et al., 2015; Trinh-Shevrin, Islam, et al., 2015). Advocacy and policy change efforts to improve access to basic healthcare, education, housing, and other social programs for socially vulnerable and immigrant populations are integral components of a social determinants of health approach to increasing health equity. Additionally, this approach incorporates a life course perspective, identifying and integrating the effects of experiences from across the life span on health outcomes (Acevedo-Garcia et al., 2012).

These social and structural factors impact each racial/ethnic minority group in different ways. While efforts to address inequities across racial/ethnic groups are important to increasing health equity for all, tailored strategies are also needed that respond to the specific challenges faced by each racial/ethnic group. For example, migration factors comprise a critical variable within the life course perspective of Asian Americans, serving as an underlying cause of social and health disparities specific to this population. With high proportions of first- and second-generation immigrants throughout Asian American communities, a transnational approach that considers the impact of migration, immigration, and acculturative experiences on health is essential to elucidate the emergence and persistence of health inequities across generations and within family contexts (Trinh-Shevrin et al., 2018).

The *model minority* stereotype is another critical factor impacting social and health outcomes for Asian Americans. This "positive" stereotype paints a picture of Asian Americans as being educated, law-abiding, hardworking, and having high incomes, low crime rates, and close family ties (Yi et al., 2016). By extension, the model minority stereotype suggests that Asian Americans are an economically successful group that do not merit the consideration, resources, or attention that racial/ethnic minority groups are accorded in the United States. Not only does this myth deny Asian Americans consideration as a racial/ethnic minority group with a unique set of barriers and resource needs, but also the model minority stereotype has been used to drive a wedge between Asian Americans and other racial/ethnic groups, implying that other groups are lazy and unambitious (Kawai, 2005).

The model minority stereotype also ignores glaring socioeconomic disparities among the many different subcultures aggregated within the Asian American racial/ethnic category. For instance, South Asians – a diverse subgroup that includes Indians, Pakistanis, Bangladeshis, Sri Lankans, Nepalis, and Bhutanese – have a median household income of $72,000/year, substantially higher than the U.S. average of $53,000/year. Yet, within that group, Bangladeshi Americans have a median income of only $46,950/year, while Indian Americans have a median income of $95,000 (Trinh-Shevrin et al., 2018; Yi et al., 2016; Ramakrishnan & Ahmad, 2014). Furthermore, because South Asian households often support more members than the average U.S. household, direct comparisons between annual incomes for South Asian households with those of other nonwhite groups may be misleading.

The health consequences of the model minority stereotype are pervasive and persistent. Presuming that Asian Americans benefit from educational and economic advantages, health care professionals, policy makers, and the public at large assume that Asian Americans do not experience health-related disparities (Yi et al., 2016). This incorrect assumption leads to systemic barriers for Asian Americans seeking care. Due to the assumption that few Asian Americans will seek health care, health care practices and hospitals often lack culturally and linguistically tailored services for Asian Americans – yet it is the very lack of such services that contributes to lower health care utilization rates among Asian Americans (Cheng et al., 2017; Ihara et al., 2014). The fundamental lack of cultural competency in health issues affecting Asian populations across health care institutions extends to medical school training, which accords little time or attention to conditions that disproportionately impact Asian Americans or addressing the cultural contexts in which health issues emerge for different Asian populations.

As an example, obesity risk among Asian Americans has emerged as a topic of concern over the last decades as research has demonstrated higher prevalence of obesity-associated conditions, such as diabetes and hypertension, at lower body weights in this population (Kwon et al., 2017; Jih et al., 2014). The World Health Organization identified lower body mass index (BMI) cutoffs for obesity risk tailored to Asian Americans of 25 to 27 kg/ m^2 rather than the standard $\geq$ 30 kg/m^2 (Echeverria et al., 2017). Yet health care providers lack awareness about differences in the body composition of ethnic Asians as compared to whites. An attendant lack of cultural competency about Asian dietary practices may prevent clinicians from recommending dietary changes when indicated, leading to higher prevalence of preventable negative health outcomes for Asian Americans (Yi et al., 2016). Obesity risk among Asian Americans is discussed in more detail in Chapter 3.

2. Conduct Participatory Implementation Science Research

Effective and comprehensive implementation of the health equity framework requires innovative research that identifies and responds to emerging challenges in an efficient, practical manner. In recent years, evidence-based interventions developed in rigorously controlled clinical trials have increasingly faced challenges in uptake, practice, and adoption because the experimental conditions under which the interventions were tested were unable to account for the contextual factors that impact behavior, health status, and access to care (Kwon et al., 2018; Trinh-Shevrin, Islam et al., 2015). For this reason, researchers in the health equity space are shifting away from randomized controlled trials toward dissemination and implementation science research (hereafter referred to as *implementation science*) that fosters multidirectional, multidisciplinary integration of clinical research with patient-centered and population-based studies to improve health outcomes for all (Chambers et al., 2016; Kwon et al., 2018; Rubio et al., 2010).

Implementation science has been defined as "the scientific study of methods to promote the systematic uptake of research findings and other evidence-based practices into routine practice and, hence, to improve the quality and effectiveness of health services and care" (Eccles & Mttman, 2006). Implementation science is a dynamic field that offers frameworks, theories, and methods to support the movement of evidence-based practices – including programs, strategies, and policies supported by research findings – from the clinical and public health realms toward real-world settings, aiming to address the well-documented "research-to-practice" gap (Shelton et al., 2020; Ramanadhan et al. 2018; Colditz, 2012). For example, in a review, Shelton et al. (2020) highlighted striking evidence that among physicians, it takes an average of 17 years for 14% of research to be integrated into clinical practice (Balas, 1998), a timeframe that is likely to be even longer in community and low-resource settings (Green et al., 2009). Implementation science engages researchers across diverse disciplines including public health, social work, psychology, and medicine to identify and apply solutions to this challenge. Implementation science is further discussed in Chapter 8.

Stakeholder engagement is essential to designing and carrying out implementation research. Stakeholders include patients, practitioners, organizational leaders, community members, opinion leaders, and others in a community where research is being designed and implemented for the benefit of all (Ramanadhan et al. 2018). Equitably engaging stakeholders in designing and implementing research that is relevant to their needs, incorporates local resources, and encompasses cultural norms and expectations is critical and participatory research is a key methodology to achieve this engagement (Kwon et al., 2018). Participatory research may refer to any point along a spectrum of stakeholder engagement, with community-based participatory research (CBPR) representing the most fully engaged methodology (Ramanadhan et al., 2018). CBPR simultaneously contributes to scholarly discourse and social action by prioritizing community engagement in and ownership of research goals and outcomes, through partnership creation, coalition building, relationship development, planning and re-planning, co-learning, and coordinating action (Huffman, 2017; Kwon et al., 2018).

CBPR offers communities more control over the research process – a benefit that may be especially meaningful for Asian Americans and other racial/ethnic minority populations who are often treated as subjects of research rather than collaborators in its design, implementation, and evaluation (Zimmerman, 2008). While community participants acquire competencies through this process, such as problem-solving and data collection skills, they also contribute essential knowledge, expertise, and nuanced understanding of their own cultural, social, and environmental contexts to inform effective study design and intervention development. In this way, CBPR supports equitable implementation by placing communities on equal footing with researchers, explicitly addressing power dynamics in research-practice relationships (DuMont et al., 2019) CBPR channels community members' knowledge into rigorous research, promoting capacity building and change at the individual, systems, and community levels throughout the research process (Israel et al., 2008).

The full spectrum of community-based participatory research approaches is described in detail in Chapter 8. Examples of participatory research models can be found in Chapter 11.

3. Convene Multisectoral Coalitions to Guide Research Priorities and Implementation

Engaging a multisectoral coalition of stakeholders to work hand in hand with researchers to guide the research process is essential to shifting research meaningfully toward participatory implementation science. Recruiting and retaining individuals from diverse backgrounds to guide research helps to ensure that voices from multiple sectors and communities are integrated within in the design, implementation, and evaluation of research and also facilitates uptake of findings across sectors and policy areas (Trinh-Shevrin, Islam, et al., 2015; Rudolph et al., 2013). Often referred to as Health in All Policies (HiAP), this approach draws attention to the impact of social, economic, and environmental policies and programs on health, making the case for the integration of public health considerations and practice into all sectors. This integration fosters cross-sector connections, allowing for a focus on underlying social determinants of health to promote well-being in all sectors (Hahn, 2019). HiAP is further discussed in Chapter 10.

Representatives of local and state health departments, other government entities (e.g., education departments, criminal justice agencies), community-based organizations, and faith-based networks as well as community leaders, local opinion leaders, and other socially engaged leaders are important members to consider engaging in a multisectoral coalition to guide participatory implementation research (Trinh-Shevrin, Islam, et al., 2015).

4. Engage With Communities through Ethnic Coalitions and Pan-ethnic Advisory Groups

The success of CBPR and other community-engaged strategies depends on the integration of community-based cultural knowledge, expertise, and experience at the implementation level. Convening and supporting community advisory groups is essential to ensuring that studies are meaningful to communities and that all voices are heard throughout the design, implementation, and evaluation process (Trinh-Shevrin, Kwon, et al., 2015). Not only may these groups advise researchers and academic institutions, but also they may serve as mechanisms for community advocacy and self-reliance over the long term, designing and implementing their own projects in the community. See Chapter 5 for more details about engaging and working with community advisory boards (CABs) and other community-based groups.

To fulfill this purpose, pan-ethnic coalitions and advisory groups must include individuals from a wide range of backgrounds and life experiences, with potentially divergent viewpoints. Researchers have a key role to play in convening groups that include representatives of different age groups, with diverse immigration histories, national and regional backgrounds, and faiths. Failing to account for a variety of viewpoints and experiences risks reinforcing and replicating exclusionary methodologies that have plagued research to date. For example, to promote wellness and disease prevention at all stages of life, researchers must account for the lived social and cultural contexts of individuals at all points of the life course, from pregnancy and infancy to childhood and adolescence, through adulthood, and into old age. Each Asian ethnic group has its own expectations for individuals at each point along this spectrum, with intergenerational relationships featuring prominently within this paradigm. Including the perspectives of older adult Asian American women and men, many of whom may be first-generation immigrants, along with the voices of younger individuals is critical to ensuring that research is meaningful to the entire community. Furthermore, each Asian ethnic group is comprised of its own more vulnerable populations with unique needs and perspectives. Members of these vulnerable populations may not have opportunities to express themselves within traditional cultural structures or may find themselves completely excluded from community life. Lesbian, gay, bisexual, transgender, and queer (LGBTQ) people are an example. These individuals face multiple minority stressors, including racism toward people of color combined with heterosexism within their own Asian ethnic group and broader U.S. society (Sandil et al., 2015). Researchers must reach out to these individuals explicitly and establish safe and welcoming environments in which they may voice their ideas and concerns. See Chapter 12 for more information about considerations for working with LGBTQ Asian Americans.

Ensuring diverse membership in community advisory groups also creates the opportunity to identify and incorporate social and cultural themes that resonate across all groups. By identifying this common thread through multiple Asian ethnic groups, these studies illustrate a potential avenue for outreach and education to all Asian Americans. Diverse community advisory groups may provide a platform for multiple generations from different Asian ethnic groups to come together to discuss culturally appropriate messaging about this issue for the entire

Asian American population. Ultimately, pan-ethnic coalitions and advisory bodies may develop their own projects for community-based implementation. Researchers and academic institutions have an important role to play in providing training and technical assistance that not only supports coalitions to identify and address community needs as they arise but also to develop and implement culturally relevant and sustainable, high-impact policy-, systems-, and environmental-level strategies to improve health outcomes (Trinh-Shevrin et al., 2018). Examples include developing strategies for improving healthy eating options and increasing access to hypertension prevention and control opportunities in Asian American urban enclaves. See Case 1 in the Appendix for a detailed example.

5. *Implement Innovative Data Collection Strategies*

A critical and persistent challenge facing population health equity research is a basic lack of data for Asian Americans (Islam et al., 2010). Limitations include a lack of disaggregation of the Asian American category by ethnic group, inconsistent definitions of the term, "Asian American," small sample sizes and oversampling of Asian Americans as a composite group or of individual Asian populations, sampling techniques that may exclude Asian Americans, and a lack of or inconsistent reporting of race/ethnicity in disease registries, health plans, and hospitals. To overcome these limitations, innovative data collection strategies that bridge information gaps and promote equitable collection, reporting and analysis of data must be implemented, incorporating community-level data to inform city, state, and national efforts to identify population needs and inform health equity research (Alberti et al., 2013). In this section, we will introduce these issues. Refer to Chapter 4 for a more detailed discussion of strategies and approaches to address these challenges at the federal level.

The lack of disaggregated data for Asian Americans is an especially pernicious problem. National health surveys such as the National Health Interview Survey (NHIS), National Health and Nutrition Examination Survey, and the Behavior Risk Surveillance System Survey collect only limited information about Asian Americans (Islam et al., 2010). Until 2010, some national surveys, such as the National Immunization Survey, included only Asian, Native Hawaiian, and Pacific Islander categories (CDC, 2010). This classification system was expanded to include ethnicity data for six specific Asian American subgroups (Asian Indian, Chinese, Filipino, Japanese, Korean, and Vietnamese), with a seventh category for "Other Asian," in line with the Patient Protection and Affordable Care Act (2010). Yet limiting data collection to these six categories ignores the rapid growth of certain Asian American groups, such as the South Asian (e.g., Bangladeshi, Pakistani, or Sri Lankan) and Southeast Asian (e.g., Cambodian, Thai, Indonesian) American populations. Moreover, within the six existing categories, small sample sizes may pose obstacles to meaningful analyses. Because these large-scale surveys provide the population-based data that drive policy, program, and funding decisions, the lack of detail regarding Asian Americans is particularly troubling (Trinh-Shevrin, Islam, et al., 2015). Disaggregated data are essential to identify health issues disproportionately impacting Asian Americans, and to highlight which groups experience the most severe health disparities, why disparities exist and persist, and the best strategies to address them within each group.

Biases in data collection methods also contribute to inaccurate estimations of health status and disease risk for Asian Americans (Trinh-Shevrin, Islam, et al., 2015). For instance, national and regional surveys typically offer only a limited number of Asian languages for survey administration, if any. Because a high proportion of Asian Americans are first- or second-generation immigrants with low English proficiency, the lack of linguistic accessibility to these surveys leads to underrepresentation of Asian Americans in the data collected. Additionally, telephone sampling using random-digit dialing methods has been shown to exclude immigrant groups, including Asian Americans, and overrepresent older, white Americans. Survey data may also suffer from a lack of geographic representation or fail to account for the geographic distribution of Asian Americans across the United States. For example, one federal survey may include an Asian American sample that was largely drawn from Minnesota – a state in which the Asian American community is largely Hmong; another survey may have an Asian American sample largely sampled from Louisiana – a state in which the Asian American community is primarily Vietnamese. Survey administrators from the two surveys may claim to offer nationally representative samples of Asian Americans when, in fact, they represent very different Asian populations.

Researchers have identified creative and practical strategies to address these challenges. For instance, the National Academy of Medicine, formerly called the Institute of Medicine, recommends using indirect estimation strategies to assess ethnicity, including geocoding or surname analysis, in cases where directly collected race/

ethnicity data are not available or are insufficient for analytical purposes (Institute of Medicine, 2009). Data sets should be pooled across years in order to develop a sufficiently large dataset of Asian Americans for analysis, and innovative sampling strategies should be introduced, such as oversampling, targeted sampling, respondent-driven sampling, cumulations, and add-ons (Islam et al., 2010; Trinh-Shevrin, Islam, et al., 2015). One study showed that sampling of targets within households, oversampling selected macro-geographic units, and oversampling from an incomplete list frame effectively bolstered Chinese American representation within the NHIS (Elliot et al., 2008). Researchers should also engage health plans, disease registries, hospitals, and other health care providers to create community-based epidemiological data repositories. Collecting granular data, including country of birth and number of years in the United States, is another strategy that may facilitate detailed analysis of epidemiologic trends (Trinh-Shevrin, Islam et al., 2015).

At the community level, researchers have used CBPR and mixed-methods designs to supplement incomplete survey data with ethnicity-specific information. For example, The Population Study of Chinese Elderly in Chicago Study (The PINE Study) was a prospective study focused on health status and quality of life of Chinese American older adults in the greater Chicago area (Dong, 2017). This study has produced important new findings on diverse topics, such as cognitive decline (Li et al., 2017) and intergenerational relationships (Dong, Li, & Hua, 2017), to inform interventions for that community. Although the PINE Study's results cannot be generalized beyond the community of Chinese Americans in Chicago where the research was implemented, findings have suggested new directions for research. As the number and geographic diversity of smaller, community-based, ethnicity-specific studies like the PINE Study increase, cumulative findings from this research will create a more detailed national picture of Asian American health. An example of such research is detailed in Case 7, Forging Partnerships, in the Appendix.

6. Apply Systems Thinking to Integrate Innovations in Medicine and Public Health Effectively

Emerging technologies offer immense opportunities to reduce health disparities and inequities through new applications of artificial intelligence (AI), including precision medicine. In order to realize this promise, however, clinicians, researchers, public health practitioners, computer scientists, and communities must employ a systems science orientation to advance health equity. Systems science integrates diverse fields of study into a learning model that is dynamic and responsive to evolving needs, acknowledging that contemporary research challenges are interlinked, complex, and multidisciplinary (Hieronymi, 2013). To address these challenges, systems science highlights points of intersection between data science, analytics and medicine, and illuminates the larger system within which these fields operate. That larger system encompasses clinical and data-related systems as well as ethics, public health, sociology, and other fields. A systems science orientation facilitates cross-collaboration, bringing together diverse stakeholders to develop the tools and methodologies necessary to the realizing the opportunities of emerging technologies.

Precision medicine is a key platform for this work. By relying heavily on data and analytics, precision medicine aims to identify ways in which genetic, environmental, and lifestyle characteristics impact disease expression and develop tailored prevention strategies and clinical treatment for each individual (The White House, 2015). Yet precision medicine will only advance health equity if researchers, clinicians, and communities work hand in hand on a sustained basis to rapidly expand community-engaged strategies, including CBPR and implementation science, to recruit and retain diverse participants from traditionally marginalized communities into clinical research that informs precision medicine. The Precision Medicine Initiative (PMI), an ambitious initiative launched in 2015 by the National Institutes of Health (NIH), was designed to collect the data necessary to inform this field through the establishment of "All of Us" – a million-person cohort intended to be as diverse as the U.S. population itself (Collins & Varmus, 2015). To optimize its promise, All of Us must recruit and retain populations that typically are underrepresented in clinical research, including immigrant and racial/ethnic minority communities as well as populations with lower socioeconomic status and educational attainment (Caplan & Frisen, 2017). Ensuring a diverse study population will allow researchers to examine population-specific sequence variation linked to geographic ancestry, which may influence the presentation of the disease, accuracy of diagnosis, and response to medication and therapies (Fisher et al., 2020). Conversely, without this diversity in study populations, genetic researchers will not be able to accurately translate findings from majority-white study samples to other racial/ethnic groups, thereby deepening inequities in clinical medicine and health care rather than increasing health equity.

Asian Americans are a key population for inclusion in this cohort. However, recruiting and retaining more Asian Americans and other racial/ethnic minority groups in genetic studies requires researchers to address the multiple factors contributing to current low enrollment and retention rates of racial/ethnic minorities in clinical research more broadly. A recent review by Fisher et al. (2020) found high levels of interest among all racial/ethnic groups in undergoing genetic testing and participating in genetic research – a finding that undercuts traditional assumptions about medical mistrust figuring as a prominent obstacle to precision medicine research in racial/ethnic minority populations. Rather, Fisher et al. found that practical factors were more prominent in influencing the likelihood of individuals from racial/ethnic minority groups to participate in genetic research. A rapid scale-up of CBPR and other community-engaged strategies to encourage and sustain participation by racial/ethnic minorities in clinical research is an important way to identify such factors, including barriers as well as facilitators. For example, to increase participation by Asian American groups, researchers must engage with communities during the initial study design to develop clear culturally and linguistically tailored information about the purpose of the study, measures taken to ensure privacy, and when, how, and what types of biological samples would be used in future research. Supporting cross-collaboration among researchers, community and faith leaders, clinicians, and others to identify cultural facilitators and barriers to participation that are specific to each racial/ethnic population – and to the distinct cultural and linguistic groups that comprise the larger racial/ethnic population.

Precision medicine's reliance on the validity of big data analytics represents another area that must be addressed using a systems science orientation. To date, surprisingly little attention has been accorded to the methodological expertise and capacity needed to integrate and analyze large, complicated datasets. The massive computational resources used to manage the increasing volume and complexity of data derived from many sources, including the internet (e.g., Google, social media) and remote sensor networks, encompasses genetics, social media, environmental and lifestyle-related factors, as well as *omic* data, such as transcriptomics, epigenomics, proteomics, and metabolomics (Krittanawong et al., 2017; Benke & Benke, 2018). With the growing complexity of these datasets, increasingly sophisticated analytical tools will be needed to examine the integrative clinical, environmental, and -omics datasets to inform, educate and help with treatment and research (Low et al., 2018). Explicitly prioritizing health equity and declaring the intention to monitor and remove bias are essential to guarding against AI learning bias and prejudice that could lead to inaccurate conclusions and perpetuate bias toward historically disadvantaged populations (Ferryman & Winn, 2018; Rajkomar et al., 2018; Williams et al., 2018; Dankwa-Mullen, 2019). Toward this end, a systems science orientation offers a shared platform for health researchers, clinicians, and information technology specialists to contribute to the development of AI analytics used to develop the machine learning approaches that emulate what an intelligent human might decide (Bera et al., 2019).

The systems science orientation also allows for continuous evaluation of ethical concerns related to the collection of genetic data, including privacy, hacking, and data ownership (Benke & Benke, 2018). A particular concern is the rights to ownership of genetic information, control of its dissemination, and potential consumer use or abuse. There are particular privacy risks associated with gathering data from vulnerable populations, particularly given the history of malpractice, discrimination, and abuse that racial/ethnic minority populations have experienced in the U.S. health system (Nordling, 2019). For example, within precision medicine trials, a fear has been expressed that once genetic information is available for analysis, health insurance companies may add genetic testing information to their actuarial models to disadvantage racial/minority populations with multiple health risks, forcing them to pay higher premiums. (Stiles & Appelbaum, 2019). There is a need to be attentive to the tension between the push – no matter how benevolent – to gather data from historically marginalized and maligned populations and the need to protect those very populations from being exploited (Ferryman, 2018). A systems science orientation allows for consideration of ethics in conjunction with biomedical science, computer science, and community contexts, supporting the promise of precision medicine to advance health equity. Chapter 6 presents an in-depth discussion of systems science, including key systems science methodologies and applications within health equity research.

7. *Strengthen Human and Social Resources for Health*

Capacity building at multiple levels is critical to advance health equity. At the systems and institutional levels, there is a pressing need to diversify the biomedical and technology workforce. Increasing participation by members of racial/ethnic minority groups, women, and people with lower socioeconomic status will ensure that the workforce better reflects the U.S. population and that the interests of diverse subpopulations are represented within the biomedical and technological fields. According to the U.S. Department for Health and Human Services, Asian Americans are well represented within the physician workforce and other diagnostic and treatment fields (US DHHS, 2017). Yet they are underrepresented in certain categories, such as psychology, in which Asian Americans represent only 3.4 percent of the workforce. Increasing the number of Asian American mental health professionals, for example, is critical to increasing access to Asian ethnic- and language-concordant providers and expanding linguistically and culturally tailored services for different Asian ethnic groups. Increasing Korean American participation in the mental health workforce may be especially important, given the higher rates of depression and suicide documented in that population (Koh et al., 2018).

Similarly, as genomic studies move forward as part of the PMI, increasing the number and diversity of Asian American researchers working in this field is critical to advocating for and designing trials focusing on the genetic variations that impact disease expression in different Asian ethnic groups. Although Asian Americans as a whole appear to be well represented in the NIH-funded research workforce (Haggeness et al., 2019), disaggregated data describing participation by Asian ethnic group are unavailable. Attracting Asian Americans from less populous groups, such as Southeast Asian Americans, may be an important area for focus. Asian American researchers from diverse ethnic groups will be more adept at considering cultural, lifestyle, and environmental factors that impact the expression of cancers and other chronic diseases that disproportionately impact different Asian American groups, and more likely to be better able to engage with community-based organizations and providers to facilitate enrollment of Asian Americans in clinical trials.

With the increasing impact of big data on health and society, the lack of diversity in the computer sciences is particularly concerning. As already noted, avoiding the replication of historical biases against vulnerable populations in AI is a clear risk to the success of machine learning as a tool to contribute to the development of tailored treatments and preventions strategies for all Americans. Training datasets and analytic algorithms must be based on representative samples of the populations of interest; successfully developing this process depends on the ability of human researchers to recognize and correct the biases of their social milieu (Vaitla et al., 2020). Many forces complicate such awareness and action. For example, the original research question may not have been framed in terms that prioritize or are inclusive of vulnerable populations, including women; funding to collect larger training sets may not be available; and algorithmic procedures may be so complex that de-biasing depends on the attentiveness of a small set of programmers. There is also the issue of financial investment: many academic cancer centers and commercial testing laboratories have focused on a fraction of the frequently mutated genes that provide better cost-effectiveness, lower burden of data analysis, and rapid turnaround time for making clinical decisions (Low et al., 2017). Diversifying the technology workforce to include more women and racial/ethnic minorities is a critical means to avoid these pitfalls while also developing the capacity for advocacy and innovation within the workforce. As in the biomedical research field, Asian Americans as a whole are well represented within the computer sciences, but the internalization of the model minority stereotype in the technology field has constrained the industry from operationalizing an inclusive approach to addressing the needs of diverse Asian American populations within algorithms and programming efforts aimed to identify health challenges and solutions.

A multi-pronged approach is needed to increase representation of racial/ethnic minorities and women in these fields (Rodriguez et al., 2014; Rubio et al., 2018; Trinh-Shevrin, Islam, et al., 2015). As a foundational step, academic institutions must explicitly commit to diversifying their own workforce by increasing recruitment and retention of faculty from racial/ethnic minority groups. Providing these faculty with mentor training, peer support structures, grants, fellowships, and cross-institutional networking opportunities will be essential to sustaining this pipeline. In turn, these faculty may provide support to students through skills development combined with mentoring, seed funding, career advising, and opportunities for networking. Partnerships between academic institutions and organizations committed to workforce diversification are an important avenue to consider.

To strengthen resources at the community level, academic and research institutions have a role to play in providing skills-based training and technical assistance to community-based organizations, faith-based networks, and health care providers. As noted previously, this support will lead to sustainable development of internal community structures, such as the realization of community-driven projects to expand the evidence base to inform successful health interventions. In addition, providing internship opportunities to high school, undergraduate, and graduate students in community organizing, advocacy, and social change activities that improve access to care and other social resources that impact health is a key way that academic institutions and health agencies may encourage and support a pipeline for younger individuals to enter the health and social service professions.

Developing a cadre of community health workers (CHWs) is another way that communities may be strengthened for the long term (Trinh-Shevrin, Islam, et al., 2015). CHWs are frontline public health professionals that create a culture of health within their own neighborhoods, breaking down the barriers that typically separate the government and the health care system from socially disadvantaged, underserved communities. Recruiting and training CHWs, integrating CHWs within research and program design and implementation, and working with CHWs to develop interventions that build on existing community assets are all strategies that may promote sustainable resource development in the community. Importantly, CHWs may serve as key channels for fostering linkages between health care institutions and the community, including disseminating health information through community-based organizations and social service agencies.

SUMMARY AND RECOMMENDATIONS

The population health equity framework shifts language and emphasis away from a focus on identifying problems to designing solutions through an integrative, transdisciplinary approach that incorporates advocacy, translation of research findings through communication, and adaptation and meaningful implementation of culturally relevant strategies and policies for underserved, culturally diverse populations. Operationalizing the population health equity framework requires researchers to pursue multiple strategies simultaneously to ensure that studies balance ongoing health disparities work with novel studies to advance equity for all populations. Researchers working with Asian American communities have a unique opportunity both to operationalize the framework for the benefit of Asian American populations and to add their particular knowledge and experience to the integration of this framework in health research more broadly.

To increase uptake and adoption of the population health equity framework in Asian American health research, we recommend the following:

- *Build research questions and design studies based on a social determinants of health approach*, taking into account the unique effects of social, environmental, and cultural factors on Asian American communities, including structural racism.

- *Expand CBPR and engage implementation science methodologies* to ensure that research incorporates Asian American communities' priorities and integrates their ideas and feedback throughout the research and evaluation process.

- *Develop high quality datasets for Asian American ethnic groups,* utilizing innovative collection and analysis methodologies to bridge existing gaps.

- *Engage meaningfully with multisectoral coalitions* to facilitate the uptake of research findings across policies and programs, in line with a HiAP approach.

- *Consult and integrate recommendations from ethnic and pan-ethnic advisory groups* to ensure research responds to the diverse perspectives of Asian Americans, recognizing and incorporating different ethnic groups, generations, and immigration experiences.

- *Harness the power of systems thinking across disciplines* to ensure Asian Americans benefit from emerging research efforts, clinical practices, and technologies, such as precision medicine and AI.

- *Strengthen Asian American human and community resources* through grantmaking, training initiatives, and educational support.

DISCUSSION QUESTIONS

1. What is the rationale for the shift in perspective from health disparities to population health equity? What are some challenges that this change may present to researchers focused on identifying and reducing Asian American health disparities?

2. The authors emphasize the importance of community-engaged research. What are some ways that researchers may build sustainable partnerships with Asian American communities?

3. Developing research questions requires analysis of high quality data to identify issues of concern. When these data are not available for individual Asian American ethnic groups, either nationally or in communities, how can researchers identify key issues and design meaningful studies to address them?

REFERENCES

Abe-Kim, J., Takeuchi, D., Hong, S., Zane, N., Sue, S., & Spencer, M. S. (2007). Use of mental health-related services among immigrant and US-born Asian Americans: Results from the National Latino and Asian American Study. *American Journal of Public Health*, 97(1), 91–98. http://doi.org/10.2105/AJTH.2006.098541

Acevedo-Garcia, D., Sanchez-Vaznaugh, E. V., Viruell-Fuentes, E. A., & Almeida, J. (2012) Integrating social epidemiology into immigrant health research: a cross-national framework. *Social Science and Medicine, 75*(12), 2060–2068. http://doi.org/10.1016/j.socscimed.2012.04.040

Alberti, P. M., Bonham, A. C., & Kirch, D. G. (2013). Making equity a value in value-based health care. *Academic Medicine Journal of the Association of American Medical Colleges*, 88(11), 1619–1623. http://doi.org/10.1097/ACM.0b013e3182a7f76f

Artiga, S, Orgera, K, & Pham, O. (2020). Disparities in health and health care: Five key questions and answers. Issue Brief. Kaiser Family Foundation, March 2020. Available at: https://www.kff.org/disparities-policy/issue-brief/disparities-in-health-and-health-care-five-key-questions-and-answers/ Accessed June 4, 2020.

Bailey, Z. D., Krieger, N., Agénor, M., Graves, J., Linos, N., & Bassett, M. T. (2017). Structural racism and health inequities in the USA: evidence and interventions. *Lancet (London, England), 389*(10077), 1453–1463. https://doi.org/10.1016/S0140-6736(17)30569-X

Balas, E. A. (1998). From appropriate care to evidence-based medicine. *Pediatric Annals, 27*(9), 581–584.

Benke, K., & Benke, G. (2018). Artificial intelligence and big data in public health. *International Journal of Environmental Research and Public Health, 15*(12), pii: E2796. http://doi.org/10.3390/ijerph15122796

Bera, K., Schalper, K. A., Rimm, D. L., Velcheti, V., & Madabhushi, A. (2019). Artificial intelligence in digital pathology - new tools for diagnosis and precision oncology. *National Review of Clinical Oncology, 16*(11), 703–715. http://doi.org/10.1038/s41571-019-0252-y

Braveman, P., & Gruskin, S. (2003). Defining equity in health. *Journal of Epidemiology and Community Health, 57*(4), 254–258. http://doi.org/10.1136/jech.57.4.254

Braveman P, & Barclay C. (2009). Health disparities beginning in childhood: a life-course perspective. *Pediatrics, 124*(3), S163–S175. http://dx.doi.org/10.1542/peds.2009-1100D.

Brawner, B. M., Reason, J. L., Goodman, B. A., Schensul, J. J., & Guthrie, B. (2015). Multilevel drivers of HIV/AIDS among black Philadelphians: Exploration using community ethnography and geographic information systems. *Nursing Research, 64*(2), 100–110. http://dx.doi.org/10.1097/NNR.0000000000000076

Caplan, A., & Friesen, P. (2017). Health disparities and clinical trial recruitment: Is there a duty to tweet? *PLoS Biology, 15*(3), e2002040. https://doi.org/10.1371/journal.pbio.2002040

Centers for Disease Control and Prevention. (2010). National Immunization Survey Hard Copy Questionnaire, Q4/2010. Available at: https://www.cdc.gov/nchs/nis/data_files.htm Accessed April 7, 2020.

Cheng, A. W., Chang, J., O'Brien, J., Budgazad, M. S., & Tsai, J. (2017). Model minority stereotype: Influence on perceived mental health needs of Asian Americans. *Journal of Immigrant and Minority Health, 19*(3), 572–581. http://doi.org/10.1007/s10903-016-0440-0

Chau, V. Destigmatizing mental health in Asian American and Pacific Islander communities. Available at: https://blog.samhsa.gov/2019/05/22/destigmatizing-mental-health-in-asian-american-and-pacific-islander-communities. Accessed June 4, 2020.

Colditz, G. A. (2017). The promise and challenges of dissemination and implementation research. In R. C. Brownson, G. A. Colditz, E. K. Proctor (Eds.), *Dissemination and Implementation Research in Health: Translating Science to Practice (2ⁿᵈ edition)* (pp. 1–25).

Collins, F. S., & Varmus, H. (2015). A new initiative on precision medicine. *New England Journal of Medicine, 372*(9), 793–795. http://doi.org/10.1056/NEJMp1500523

Dankwa-Mullen, I. (2019). Examining health disparities in precision medicine. Available at: https://www.ibm.com/blogs/watson-health/examining-health-disparities-in-precision-medicine/# Published October 14, 2019. Accessed April 4, 2020.

Dong, X. (2017). Advancing Community and Health Equity: Health and Wellbeing of U.S. Chinese Populations. *The Journals of Gerontology Series A: Biological and Medical Sciences, 72* (S1), S1–S4, http://doi.org/10.1093/gerona/glx049

Dong, X., Li, M., & Hua, Y. (2017). The Association Between Filial Discrepancy and Depressive Symptoms: Findings From a Community-Dwelling Chinese Aging Population. *The journals of gerontology. Series A, Biological sciences and medical sciences, 72*(suppl_1), S63–S68. https://doi.org/10.1093/gerona/glx040

DuMont, K., Metz, A., & Woo, B. (2019). Five recommendations for how implementation science can better advance equity. Academy-Health. Available at: https://www.academyhealth.org/blog/2019-04/five-recommendations-how-implementation-science-can-better-advance-equity Accessed June 4, 2020.

Eccles, M. P, Mittman, B. S. (2006) Welcome to *Implementation Science. Implementation Sci. 1*(1):1. https://doi.org/10.1186/1748-5908-1-1

Elliott, M. N., Finch, B. K., Klein, D., Ma, S., Do, D. P., Beckett, M. K., Orr, N., & Lurie, N. (2008). Sample designs for measuring the health of small racial/ethnic subgroups. *Statistics in Medicine, 27*(20), 4016–4029. http://doi.org/10.1002/sim.3244

Feagin, J, & Bennefield, Z. (2014). Systemic racism and US health care. *Social Science & Medicine (1982), 103*, 7–14. https://doi.org/10.1016/j.socscimed.2013.09.006

Ferryman, K., & Winn, R. A. (2018) Artificial intelligence can entrench disparities – here's what we must do. *The Cancer Letter*. November 16, 2018. Available at: https://cancerletter.com/articles/20181116_1/ Accessed April 5, 2018.=

Fisher, E. R., Pratt, R., Esch, R., Kocher, M., Wilson, K., Lee, W., & Zierhut, H. A. (2020). The role of race and ethnicity in views toward and participation in genetic studies and precision medicine research in the United States: A systematic review of qualitative and quantitative studies. Molecular genetics & genomic medicine, 8(2), e1099. https://doi.org/10.1002/mgg3.1099

Green, L. W., Ottoson, J. M., García, C., & Hiatt, R. A. (2009). Diffusion theory and knowledge dissemination, utilization, and integration in public health. *Annual Review of Public Health, 30*(1), 151–174.

Heggeness, M. L., Evans, L., Pohlhaus, J. R., & Mills, S. L. (2016). Measuring diversity of the National Institutes of Health-funded workforce. *Academic Medicine: Journal of the Association of American Medical Colleges, 91*(8), 1164–1172. https://doi.org/10.1097/ACM.0000000000001209

Hahn, R. A. (2019). Two paths to health in all policies: The traditional public health path and the path of social determinants. *American Journal of Public Health, 109*(2), 253–254. http://doi.org/10.2105/AJPH.2018.304884

Hieronymi, A. (2013). Understanding systems science: A visual and integrative approach. *Systems Research and Behavioral Science, 30*, 580–595.

Huffman, T. (2017). Participatory/Action Research/CBPR. In The International Encyclopedia of Communication Research Methods (eds. J. Matthes, C.S. Davis and R.F. Potter).

Ihara, E. S., Chae, D. H., Cummings, J. R., & Lee, S. (2014). Correlates of mental health service use and type among Asian Americans. *Administration and Policy in Mental Health, 41*(4): 543–551. http://doi.org/10.1007/s10488-013-0493-5

Institute of Medicine. (2009). *Race, Ethnicity, and Language Data: Standardization for Health Care Quality Improvement*. Washington, DC: The National Academies Press.

Islam, N. S., Khan, S., Kwon, S., Jang, D., Ro, M., & Trinh-Shevrin, C. (2010). Methodological issues in the collection, analysis, and reporting of granular data in Asian American populations: historical challenges and potential solutions. *Journal of Health Care for the Poor and Underserved, 21*(4), 1354–1381. https://doi.org/10.1353/hpu.2010.0939

Israel, B. A., Schulz, A. J., Parker, E. A., Becker, A. B., Allen, A. J., III, & Guzman, J. R. (2008). Critical issues in developing and following community based participatory research principles. In M. Minkler & N. Wallerstein (eds.), *Community-Based Participatory Research for Health* (pp. 46–66). San Francisco: Jossey-Bass.

Kawai, Y. (2005). Stereotyping Asian Americans: The Dialectic of the Model Minority and the Yellow Peril. *Howard Journal of Communications, 16*(2), 109–130. doi:10.1080/10646170590948974.

Krieger, N. (2014). Discrimination and health inequities. *International Journal of Health Services, 44*(4), 643–710. http://dx.doi.org/10.2190/HS.44.4.b

Koh, E. (2018). Prevalence and predictors of depression and anxiety among Korean Americans. *Social Work in Public Health, 33*(1), 55–69. http://doi.org/10.1080/19371918.2017.1415178

Koh, S., Lee, M., Brotzman, L. E., & Shelton, R. C. (2020). An orientation for new researchers to key domains, processes, and resources in implementation science. *Translational Behavioral Medicine, 10*(1), 179–185. https://doi.org/10.1093/tbm/iby095

Krittanawong, C., Zhang, H., Wang, Z., Aydar, M., & Kitai, T. (2017) Artificial intelligence in precision cardiovascular medicine. *Journal of the American College of Cardiology, 69*(21), 2657–2664. http://doi.org/10.1016/j.jacc.2017.03.571

Low, S. K., Zembutsu, H., & Nakamura, Y. (2018). Breast cancer: The translation of big genomic data to cancer precision medicine. *Cancer Science, 109* (3), 497–506. http://doi.org/10.1111/cas.13463

Kwok, J. (2013). Factors that influence the diagnoses of Asian Americans in mental health: an exploration. *Perspectives in Psychiatric Care, 49*(4), 288–292. http://doi.org/10.1111/ppc.12017

Kwon, S. C., Tandon, S. D., Islam, N., Riley, L., & Trinh-Shevrin, C. (2018). Applying a community-based participatory research framework to patient and family engagement in the development of patient-centered outcomes research and practice. *Translational Behavioral Medicine, 8*(5), 683–691. https://doi.org/10.1093/tbm/ibx026

Leong, F. T. L., & Lau, A. S. L. (2001) Barriers to providing effective mental health services to Asian Americans. *Mental Health Services Research, 3*(4), 201–214. http://doi.org/10.1023/a:1013177014788

Li, L. W., Ding, D., Wu, B., & Dong, X. (2017). Change of cognitive function in U.S. Chinese older adults: A Population-Based Study. *The Journals of Gerontology, Series A: Biological Sciences and Medical Sciences, 72*(Suppl 1), S5–S10. https://doi.org/10.1093/gerona/glx004

Marmot M, Friel S, Bell R, Houweling, T. A., Taylor, S., & Commission on Social Determinants of Health (2008). Closing the gap in a generation: health equity through action on the social determinants of health. *Lancet, 372*(9650), 1661–1669. http://dx.doi.org/10.1016/S0140-6736(08)61690-6

National Institutes of Health. National Institute on Minority Health and Health Disparities: Overview. Available at: https://www.nimhd.nih.gov/about/overview/ Accessed June 4, 2020.

Nguyen, D. (2011). Acculturation and perceived mental health need among older Asian immigrants. *Journal of Health Behavioral Health Services and Research, 38*(4), 526–533. http://doi.org/10.1007/s11414-011-9245-z

Nordling, L. (2019). Mind the gap. *Nature. 573*, S103–S105.

Patient Protection and Affordable Care Act: PL-111-148, Section 3101, March 23, 2010. Available at: https://www.congress.gov/111/plaws/publ148/PLAW-111publ148.pdf Accessed April 7, 2020.

Public Health Agency of Canada, & World Health Organization. (2008), Health Equity Through Intersectoral Action: An Analysis of 18 Country Case Studies. Available at: https://www.who.int/social_determinants/resources/health_equity_isa_2008_en.pdf Accessed on April 6, 2020.

Rajkomar, A., Hardt, M., Howell, M. D., Corrado, G., & Chin, M. H. (2018). Ensuring Fairness in Machine Learning to Advance Health Equity. *Annals of Internal Medicine, 169*(12), 866–872. http://doi.org/10.7326/M18-1990

Ramanadhan, S., Davis, M. M., Armstrong, R., Baquero, B., Ko, L. K., Leng, J. C., Salloum, R. G., Vaughn, N. A., & Brownson, R. C. (2018). Participatory implementation science to increase the impact of evidence-based cancer prevention and control. *Cancer Causes & Control: CCC, 29*(3), 363–369. https://doi.org/10.1007/s10552-018-1008-1

Ramakrishnan K., & Ahmad, F. Z. (2014). State of Asian Americans and Pacific Islanders: Income and Poverty. Center for American Progress. Available from: https://cdn.americanprogress.org/wp-content/uploads/2014/08/AAPI-IncomePoverty.pdf Accessed April 6, 2020.

Rodríguez, J. E., Campbell, K. M., & Mouratidis, R. W. (2014). Where are the rest of us? Improving representation of minority faculty in academic medicine. *Southern Medical Journal, 107*, 739–744. http://doi.org/10.14423/SMJ.0000000000000204

Rubio, D. M., Mayowski, C. A., & Norman, M. K. (2018). A Multi-Pronged Approach to Diversifying the Workforce. *International Journal of Environmental Research and Public Health, 15*(10), 2219. https://doi.org/10.3390/ijerph15102219

Rubio, D. M., Schoenbaum, E. E., Lee, L. S., Schteingart, D. E., Marantz, P. R., Anderson, K. E., Platt, L. D., Baez, A., & Esposito, K. (2010). Defining translational research: implications for training. *Academic Medicine: Journal of the Association of American Medical Colleges, 85*(3), 470–475. https://doi.org/10.1097/ACM.0b013e3181ccd618

Rudolph L, Caplan J, Ben-Moshe K, & Dillon L. (2013). *Health in All Policies: A Guide for State and Local Governments*. Washington, DC, and Oakland, CA: American Public Health Association and Public Health Institute.

Shelton, R. C., Lee, M., Brotzman, L. E., Wolfenden, L., Nathan, N., & Wainberg, M. L. (2020). What is dissemination and implementation science? An introduction and opportunities to advance behavioral medicine and public health globally. *International Journal of Behavioral Medicine, 27*(1), 3–20. https://doi.org/10.1007/s12529-020-09848-x

Srinivasan, S., & Williams, S. D. (2014). Transitioning from health disparities to a health equity research agenda: the time is now. *Public Health Reports, 129*(Suppl 2), 71–76. https://doi.org/10.1177/00333549141291S213

Stiles, D., & Appelbaum, P. S. (2019). Cases in precision medicine: concerns about privacy and discrimination after genomic sequencing. *Annals of internal medicine, 170*(10), 717–721. https://doi.org/101.7326/M18-2666

Trinh-Shevrin, C., Islam, N. S., Nadkarni, S., Park, R., & Kwon, S. C. (2015). Defining an integrative approach for health promotion and disease prevention: A population health equity framework. *Journal of Health Care for the Poor and Underserved, 26*(2), 146–163. http://doi.org/10.1353/hpu.2015.0067

Trinh-Shevrin, C., Islam, N. S., Tandon, D., Abesamis N., & Ho-Asjoe, H. Rey, M. (2007). Using community-based participatory research as a guiding framework for health disparities research centers. *Progress in Community Health Partnerships: Research, Education, and Action, 1*(2), 195–205. http://doi.org/10.1353/cpr.2007.0007

Trinh-Shevrin, C., Kwon, S. C., Park, R., Nadkarni, S. K., & Islam, N. S. (2015). Moving the dial to advance population health equity in New York City Asian American populations. *American Journal of Public Health, 105*, e16–e25. http://doi.org/10.2105/AJPH.2015.302626

Trinh-Shevrin, C., Sacks, R., Ahn, J., & Yi, S. S. (2018). Opportunities and challenges in precision medicine: Improving cancer prevention and treatment for Asian Americans. *Journal of Racial and Ethnic Health Disparities. 5*, 1–6. http://doi.org/10.1007/s40615-016-0334-9.

U.S. Department of Health and Human Services, Health Resources and Services Administration, National Center for Health Workforce Analysis. (2017). Sex, Race, and Ethnic Diversity of U.S, Health Occupations (2011–2015), Rockville, Maryland. Available at https://bhw.hrsa.gov/sites/default/files/bhw/nchwa/diversityushealthoccupations.pdf Accessed on April 8, 2020.

Williams, A. M., Liu, Y., Regner, K. R., Jotterand, F., Liu, P., Liang, M. (2018). Artificial intelligence, physiological genomics, and precision medicine. *Physiological Genomics, 50*(4), 237–243. http://doi.org/10.1152/physiolgenomics.00119.2017

Williams, D. R., Lawrence, J. A., Davis, B. A. (2019). Racism and health: evidence and needed research. *Annual Review of Public Health, 40*, 105–125. https://doi.org/10.1146/annurev-publhealth-040218-043750

Woo, B. K. (2017). Comparison of mental health service utilization by Asian Americans and Non-Hispanic Whites versus their cardiovascular care utilization. *Cureus. 9*(8), e1595. http://doi.org/10.7759/cureus.1595.

World Health Organization. (2020). Social determinants of health. Available at: https://www.who.int/social_determinants/en/ Accessed June 4, 2020.

Zimmerman, M. A. (2000). Empowerment Theory. In J. Rappaport & E. Seidman E. (eds.), *Handbook of Community Psychology*. Boston, MA: Springer. https://doi.org/10.1007/978-1-4615-4193-6_2

CHAPTER

3

THE HEALTH OF ASIAN AMERICAN COMMUNITIES

SIMONA C. KWON, CHAU TRINH-SHEVRIN, YOUSRA YUSUF,
DEBORAH K. MIN, RACHEL SACKS

LEARNING OBJECTIVES

By the end of this chapter, readers will be able to:

- Describe current directions in health research among Asian Americans.
- Identify gaps in research and identify emerging issues.
- Examine the challenges and opportunities facing health researchers in this field.

Applied Population Health Approaches for Asian American Communities, First Edition. Edited by Simona C. Kwon,
Chau Trinh-Shevrin, Nadia S. Islam, and Stella S. Yi.
© 2023 John Wiley & Sons, Inc. Published 2023 by John Wiley & Sons, Inc.
Companion Website: www.wiley.com/go/kwon/asianamerican

INTRODUCTION

This chapter uses a health equity lens to review the current state of research exploring the health of Asian Americans, identify gaps in the literature, and highlight research opportunities for the years ahead. Epidemiological trends related to the major sources of mortality and morbidity among Asian Americans are presented, with health issues that disproportionately impact different ethnic groups highlighted.

Summarizing health data for Asian Americans is difficult due to the diversity of the ethnic groups that comprise this population. The term *Asian American* refers to someone with origins in East Asia, Southeast Asia, or South Asia and includes numerous populations that differ in language, geographic origin, immigration history, and acculturation status (Torre et al., 2016). Large population-based surveys aggregate data for the entire Asian American population, masking true differences among vastly diverse ethnic groups such that health trends seen in the largest Asian groups – i.e., Chinese (23%), Filipino (20%), Asian Indian (18%), Vietnamese (10%), and Korean (10%) – inform a limited picture of health and health disparities among Asian Americans. Many surveys also aggregate data for Asian Americans with the Native Hawaiian and Pacific Islander (NH/PI) populations, referring to this population as *AANHPI*. These aggregated data remain the key drivers of funding, research, and programming decisions.

In this chapter, we seek to expand this approach to draw a more detailed and nuanced picture of the health status of Asian Americans. We present data by Asian American ethnic group wherever possible. In many instances, disaggregated data are only available from regional surveys and community-based research. These studies have been instrumental in identifying health disparities and health issues of importance to Asian American populations. When analyzed in concert with national data describing broader trends, data from these smaller, focused studies highlight key areas for health research among the population as a whole.

THE STATE OF RESEARCH BY HEALTH TOPIC

Cancer

Cancer is the leading cause of death for Asian American men and women overall, accounting for 27% of all deaths in this population (ACS, 2016). Lung cancer is the leading cause of cancer among both Asian American men and women. Breast cancer is rising among Asian American women and is second only to lung cancer as the leading cause of cancer death among women. Among both men and women, colorectal cancers are on the rise and comprise the third leading cause of cancer death for both genders (Torre et al., 2016). Asian Americans also experience proportionally more cancers of infectious origin than other racial/ethnic groups, including viral hepatitis-associated liver cancer, *H. pylori*-associated stomach cancer, and human papillomavirus (HPV)-associated cervical and head and neck cancers (Chen, 2005; Trinh-Shevrin et al., 2018). Among men, liver cancer is second only to lung cancer as the leading cause of cancer death and among women, liver cancer is the fifth leading cause of cancer death (Torre et al., 2016). Although some of the leading cancer causes of death among Asian Americans are shared with the overall U.S. population (e.g., colorectal cancer and breast cancer for women), in this section, we will focus on the specific disparities Asian Americans experience for cancers of infectious origin.

Disaggregated data for cancer incidence among Asian Americans are severely limited, due in part to the ways in which data are collected and reported. The National Cancer Institute's (NCI's) Surveillance, Epidemiology, and End Results (SEER) program is the principal source of high-quality, population-based information on cancer incidence and survival in the United States. Regional SEER registries capture data for 28% of the U.S. population, including approximately 50% of Asians and 67% of NH/PIs. In SEER, Asian American and NH/PI populations are coded as Chinese, Filipino, Asian Indians/Pakistanis (grouped together in SEER), Vietnamese, Koreans, Japanese, Cambodians, Laotians, Native Hawaiians, Samoans, and non-Hispanic Whites (Whites) (Torre et al., 2016). One limitation of SEER data collection methods is that information on birthplace is often used as a proxy for immigrant status and ethnic identity. However, this practice may contribute to misclassification of ethnicity or a lack of nuanced data that, in turn, contributes to limited understanding of the role of ethnicity in incidence and survival statistics (Islam et al., 2010). For example, Chinese born in Vietnam or Asian Indians born in Malaysia do not align with a classification system that relies on birthplace (or parents' birthplace) to define ethnicity. An additional constraint is that SEER has only a limited number of registry sites in states that are home to higher numbers of Asian Americans, such as California and New York, representing a missed opportunity to capture more data for smaller Asian ethnic groups needed to enrich our understanding of disease incidence and progression in these populations. In addition to SEER data, state-level cancer registries capture data on disease incidence and mortality in each state (Torre et al., 2016). These registries cover nearly 96% of the U.S. population and 97% of the aggregate Asian American and NH/PI population. However, reporting requirements for race/ethnicity data vary from state to state, rendering aggregation of data across states difficult; moreover, the quality of the race/ethnicity data depends on the hospital reporting the data (Atekruse et al., 2017).

Despite these limitations, some trends are clear. Cancers of infectious origin disproportionately impact Asian Americans. To better understand the burden of disease in this population, disaggregated studies that capture ethnic group differences and nuances are urgently needed. For example, incidence of hepatitis-associated liver cancer is highest among Asian Americans as compared to all other racial/ethnic groups in the United States, with hepatitis B representing the predominant etiology (Ha et al., 2016). Yet Asian Americans also have the highest five-year survival rates of any ethnic group – a trend that is poorly understood and underresearched. The highest mortality rates from liver cancer have been documented among Chinese, Korean, and Vietnamese Americans (Thompson et al., 2016). There is an urgent need to identify effective clinical approaches and better treatment options for these ethnic groups. These high mortality rates also demand increased resource allocation to expand in-language, community-based prevention and education programs. Hepatitis B prevalence is especially high among the foreign-born, with as many as one in ten foreign-born Asian Americans chronically infected with hepatitis B, as compared 0.5% prevalence among the general U.S. population (Juon et al., 2014). Given the large proportion of the Asian American population that are immigrants, this finding is especially concerning. Disaggregated data from the California Health Interview Survey (CHIS) have shown that Southeast Asians (Vietnamese, Cambodians, and Laotians) have incidence rates twice as high as other Asian American groups and eight to nine times as high as Whites (Pham et al., 2018). That dataset also showed a decline in liver cancer incidence among Chinese Americans but rising rates among Filipino and Japanese men as well as Vietnamese and Laotian women. These divergent trends demand further research to develop meaningful multi-pronged strategies to prevent hepatitis B transmission and address the treatment needs of these populations. This critical need is further discussed in the Infectious Diseases subsection.

In the case of stomach cancer, incidence rates are declining overall. However, incidence rates among Asian Americans remain about twice as high as among Whites and disparities among ethnic groups persist (Torre et al., 2016; Gomez et al., 2013). *H. pylori* bacteria is the key risk factor for the noncardia gastric cancer that Asian Americans most often develop. Disaggregated data for stomach cancer, while limited, show that Korean Americans have the highest incidence and mortality rates of stomach cancer and that these rates have remained stable (Torre et al., 2016). Incidence and mortality rates for stomach cancer among Korean Americans are twice as high as those among Japanese Americans, who have the second highest rates of all Asian populations and for whom rates have declined in the last years. As with hepatitis-associated liver cancer, incidence is higher among the foreign-born, suggesting the need for more complex consideration of immigration experiences and the contextual factors in origin countries to better understand incidence and survival of stomach cancer within Asian ethnic groups. Stomach cancer is the second most common cancer in East Asia, accounting for approximately 50% of all cases of stomach cancer worldwide (McCracken et al., 2007). Despite declining rates, the Republic of Korea (Korea) continues to document the highest incidence of stomach cancer in the world while the incidence of stomach cancer in China has been documented as accounting for more than 40% of all new global cases. (Bray et al., 2013). Japan also continues to document a high burden of stomach cancer. These contextual factors contribute to differences in incidence among different Asian groups in the United States, including differences in rates between foreign- and U.S.-born Asian populations (Kim et al., 2015). Some data suggest that knowledge about *H. pylori* and stomach cancer remains particularly low in Korean American immigrant communities, indicating the need for more focused research and efforts on the factors preventing more widescale screening and treatment for *H. pylori* (Shah et al., 2020). As with liver cancer, Asian Americans have higher five-year survival rates than Whites – an advantage likely due in part to the earlier stage and younger age at diagnosis among Asian Americans as compared to Whites. Asian Americans may also have biological advantages that support survival, including mixed histological type and a higher prevalence of distal tumors, which are associated with better outcomes (Bautista et al., 2016). Genomic research could elucidate the mechanisms associated with this biologic advantage, with implications both for and beyond Asian American populations. Systemic factors may also impact survival. A retrospective review of a large health care system in California found that Asian American patients were more likely to undergo surgery and/or receive chemotherapy for stomach cancer than Whites (Bautitsta et al., 2016). These successful outcomes provide support for adapting tailored models of education, prevention, screening, and treatment for at-risk Asian American populations as a national priority (Kwon et al., 2019).

Finally, HPV causes nearly all cervical cancer in the United States, with Cambodian and Vietnamese women having disproportionately higher incidence as compared to Whites (ACS, 2016). Asian American women have among the lowest rates of cervical cancer screening as compared to other racial/ethnic groups, with considerable variation by Asian ethnic group, the result of complex system, provider, and patient factors (Hall et al., 2018; Shoemaker & White, 2016; Trinh et al., 2015). Screening rates have risen in recent years as culturally and linguistically tailored programs have been expanded, particularly among Cambodian, Vietnamese, and Laotian women (Fang et al., 2019; Fung et al., 2018). Yet screening rates remain low overall, with particularly low rates among Asian Indian, Chinese, and "Other Asian" groups (Shoemaker et al., 2016). HPV also causes oropharynx cancer, which affects the part of the throat behind the oral cavity and is more prevalent among men than women in the United States (ACS, 2020). While incidence of these cancers is lower among Asian Americans, research has yet to explore trends among Asian ethnic groups. Immigration and contextual factors play a role in these rates. Globally, 5% of women in North America are infected with any type of HPV, compared with 11% of women in Eastern Asia, 7% in Southern Asia, and 14% in Southeastern Asia (Bruni et al., 2010). The principal risk factor for HPV infection among men is sexual behavior, with higher risk associated with early age at sexual exposure, multiple sexual partners, and having partners who have had multiple partners, as well as frequency of oral sex (Berman & Schiller, 2017). HPV vaccination is recommended for both girls and boys at 11 or 12 years of age (Torre et al., 2016). Available data suggest that Asian American girls receive the vaccine at rates comparable to Whites, while Asian American boys are vaccinated at rates higher than Whites. However, disaggregated data are limited, contributing to an incomplete picture of health for Asian groups. In National Health Interview Survey (NHIS) data, foreign birth appears to be a barrier to uptake, but more research is needed (Budhwani & De, 2017). Nationally, Asian Indians had comparatively lower rates of HPV vaccine initiation than Whites (OR = 0.41; 95% CI = 0.207–0.832), and foreign-born Asian Indians had the lowest rate HPV vaccination of all subpopulations (2.3%). Yet Asian Indians also had high income, education, and health insurance coverage – all positive predictors of preventive health engagement and vaccine uptake. Acknowledging and addressing differences in Asian American care-seeking practices, access to culturally relevant and translated resources and information, and increasing access to preventive care and services among ethnic groups through the development of linguistically appropriate, conveniently located, and affordable services is imperative (Trinh-Shevrin et al., 2018).

Overall, incident cancer cases are expected to rise by 132% among Asian Americans by 2050 – an estimate that is especially concerning as Asian Americans have among the lowest cancer screening rates of all racial/ethnic groups (Kagawa-Singer et al., 2010). These low screening rates may reflect, in part, a lack of training for clinical providers and a lack of in-language, culturally tailored outreach to Asian American populations. For example, in a survey of New York and New Jersey health care providers, while liver cancer and stomach cancer were perceived as higher cancer risks among Asian Americans than among the general population, breast and prostate cancer were perceived as lower risks (Kwon et al., 2013) This lack of provider knowledge about cancer trends among Asian Americans contributes to lower rates of office-based screening for these types of cancer for Asian American patients. Clinical training programs to increase provider knowledge about the risk of all types of cancer among Asian Americans may help to reverse this trend. Provider recommendation has been consistently identified as a key facilitator in Asian Americans' decision to undergo all types of screening (Hall et al., 2018; Singh et al., 2017).

Providers' voices are necessary but not sufficient to increase cancer screening among Asian Americans. In clinical settings, language-appropriate services are also essential (Bodle et al., 2008). Even if the provider speaks the same language as the patient, the phlebotomist, radiologist, or other health care professional necessary to completing the screening process may not share the patient's language, presenting multiple points at which the process may break down. Community health workers (CHWs) and patient navigators may help to facilitate this process. A literature review examining interventions for breast, cervical, and colorectal cancer screening in the United States and abroad among Asian populations (including Vietnamese, Korean, Chinese and Taiwanese, Cambodians, Filipino, Mixed Asian Groups, Asians overseas) found that culturally tailored interventions utilizing

CHWs and delivering information through community-based channels (e.g., Asian grocery stores, churches) were effective in increasing screening rates (Hou et al., 2011). Still, these types of advances have improved screening rates among Cambodian, Vietnamese, and Laotian American women in the United States, even as rates remain low among Asian Americans overall (Hall et al., 2018) and particularly among the Asian Indian, Chinese, and "Other Asian" groups (Shoemaker et al., 2016). Continuing to research, develop, and implement multi-pronged strategies to facilitate access to cancer screening for all Asian Americans must be a priority, particularly as new, more effective screening technologies emerge in the coming years. Achieving this aim will require increased resource allocation to explore system-, provider-, and community-based strategies tailored to each ethnic group's risk profile and needs.

Heart Disease, Obesity, Diabetes

Cardiovascular disease (CVD), cerebrovascular disease (stroke) and other heart-related conditions are on the rise among Asian Americans, and proportionate mortality rates from these conditions are higher in every Asian American population, as compared with Whites (Jose et al., 2014). There is an urgent need to design and implement research that disaggregates data for ethnic groups and better quantifies and characterizes heart disease and stroke risk, incorporating consideration of potential geographic, cultural, and regional impacts as well as genetic predispositions. For example, stroke is higher in each of the largest Asian American populations as compared to Whites, yet lower rates of stroke among Asian Americans have been documented in the traditional "stroke belt" of the southeastern United States (Pu et al., 2017). Limited disaggregated data have shown that CVD-related morbidity and mortality is highest among Filipino and Indian Americans, followed by Japanese American men (Hastings et al., 2015), with approximately 80% of Filipino CVD deaths and 90% of Japanese CVD deaths occurring in the Pacific division of the United States (Pu et al., 2017). Indeed, the Pacific division has consistently documented the highest adjusted mortality rates of CVD and CVD subtypes among most Asian American ethnic groups.

Differences in health profiles have emerged in studies conducted among Chinese and South Asian populations both in the United States and overseas (Yi et al., 2016). Studies in China and Taiwan have shown a higher risk of hemorrhagic stroke in Chinese adults compared to Whites (Chen et al., 1992; Tsai et al., 2013). Similar results emerged from a community-based study of Chinese Americans in New York City (NYC), where Chinese American adults who had experienced stroke were more likely to have a history of hypertension and left ventricular hypertrophy than Whites (Fang et al., 2004). Yet Chinese Americans appear to be at a lower risk for coronary heart disease than Whites (Holland et al., 2011). By contrast, South Asians in both international and U.S.-based studies have been shown to be at higher risk for coronary heart disease and diabetes compared to other racial/ethnic groups and differences may exist across South Asian ethnic groups (Gupta et al., 2011; McKeigue et al., 1989; Rajpathak et al., 2010). Among Asian Indians in the United States, the leading cause of death is CVD and stroke mortality rates have been increasing over time (Hastings et al., 2015). Yet risk factors for CVD such as hypertension, smoking, elevated low density lipoprotein cholesterol, and coronary artery calcification have been documented at similar or lower rates in South Asian Americans compared to Whites (Gupta et al., 2006). Rates of diabetes are consistently higher among South Asian Americans than among Whites and rates of metabolic conditions including obesity, diabetes, hypercholesterolemia, and nonalcoholic fatty liver disease are rising among all Asian Americans (Virani et al., 2020; Wyatt et al., 2020).

These trends are poorly understood. Complex studies are needed to assess the interaction of the many demographic, contextual, and biologic factors that influence heart disease-related outcomes. For example, immigration has been shown to be a factor in CVD-related trends, as foreign-born individuals exhibit a different cardiometabolic risk profile compared with the U.S.-born, suggesting that assimilation into the American culture may be associated with important shifts in health behaviors across residence strata (Kalra et al., 2019). However, immigration status may interact with other sociodemographic variables that have been shown to contribute to these trends, including health insurance status, access to healthcare, treatment adherence rates, and access to in-language, culturally tailored disease prevention strategies. Identifying not only the relative burden of each of these factors but also the ways in which they interact is critical to understanding disparities in prevalence among ethnic groups. A better understanding of risk factors among ethnic groups is also needed, which will require focused studies examining dietary factors, physical activity levels, and smoking rates among individual Asian populations (Ancheta et al., 2015). For example, high smoking rates among Vietnamese and Korean Americans as compared to other groups may be a particular area for exploration and potential intervention.

Developing effective clinical treatments for the management of these conditions among Asian Americans also requires more research. Genetic differences in Asian Americans as compared to Whites and other racial/ethnic groups, as well as differences among Asian ethnic groups, may impact the effectiveness of pharmaceutical treatments (Trinh-Shevrin et al., 2018). For example, the presence of a unique loss-of-function point mutation in aldehyde hydrogenase 2 (ALDH2), referred to as ALDH2*2, affects 560 million people of East Asian descent globally (Gross et al., 2015) ALDH2*2 may compromise the effectiveness of nitroglycerin, rendering it less effective in reducing vasodilation among individuals with ALDH2*2 experiencing acute myocardial infarction, and acetaminophen, which may be detrimental to preserving tissue following ischemic injury among patients with ALDH2*2. Screening individuals of East Asian descent for ALDH2*2 using either a simple two-question screener or a rapid genotyping test could help health care providers to develop both personalized preventive care plans as well as treatment plans for their patients who test positive for the mutation. Additional research into the activation of ALDH2*2, leading to treatments based on this genotype, could substantially improve clinical care for Asian Americans.

Obesity has emerged as a key area of research. Whereas obesity prevalence was considered low among Asian Americans until recently, the World Health Organization (WHO) now recommends using lower body mass index (BMI) cutpoints for Asian Americans of 25 to 27 kg/m^2 rather than the standard ≥ 30 kg/m^2 (Echeverria et al., 2017). The rationale for lowering the BMI cutpoint from the standard ≥ 30 kg/m^2 to 25–27 kg/m^2 is that ethnic Asians tend to have a higher percent body fat for the same BMI as compared with Whites, possibly due to leg length relative to height and/or to smaller body frames (Yi et al., 2016). Some researchers have further suggested that waist circumference be used to evaluate obesity in Asian American groups rather than BMI cutpoints, since these cutpoints vary as a function of ethnicity (Ancheta et al., 2015). Using these lower cutpoints, obesity prevalence in U.S.-born Asian Americans (43%), foreign-born ≤ 20 years in the U.S. (38.6%) and those ≥ 20 years in the U.S. (45.1%) was higher than in Whites (36.2%) ($p = 0.0017$) (Echeverria et al., 2017). Filipino Americans, in particular, have been shown to have higher rates of obesity (Jih et al., 2014; Zhao et al., 2015; Ancheta et al., 2015). Recent studies, while limited, have demonstrated that Asian Americans identified as obese using the lower cutpoints have higher odds of having diabetes, high blood pressure and high cholesterol, providing support for this change (Kwon et al., 2017; Jih et al., 2014).

Diabetes is also a growing concern for Asian Americans (Cheng et al., 2019). Like WHO, the American Diabetes Association now recommends screening Asian Americans for diabetes at a BMI of 23 kg/m^2, a lower threshold than the standard 25 kg/m^2 (Echeverria et al., 2017). Asian Americans had higher diabetes prevalence at lower BMI than other ethnic groups, and their rates of combined undiagnosed and diagnosed diabetes exceeded Whites and Hispanics (Cheng et al., 2019). Disaggregated data for Asian ethnic groups are limited. One analysis of NHIS data showed that Asian Indians, followed by Filipino Americans, have the highest prevalence of diabetes as compared to Whites (Lee et al., 2011). More typically, however, studies have examined South Asians in aggregate, despite the substantial heterogeneity of this population, which includes individuals of Indian, Pakistani, Bangladeshi, Nepali, Sri Lankan, and Bhutanese descent. South Asians have been found to have particularly high co-morbidity of obesity and diabetes (Wyatt et al., 2020; Yi et al., 2016; Gupta et al., 2011). One perplexing and concerning aspect of this trend that merits further investigation is higher prevalence of cardiometabolic abnormalities, such as impaired glucose tolerance, documented at younger ages among South Asians than Whites (Volgman et al., 2018; Iyer et al., 2019).

Infectious Diseases

In 2020, the novel coronavirus pandemic upended the notion that rising rates of chronic disease prevalence dwarfed the threat to population health posed by infectious diseases. The virus that causes the novel coronavirus disease 2019 (COVID-19), known as severe acute respiratory syndrome coronavirus 2 (SARS-CoV-2), emerged in China in 2019, spread rapidly across the globe, and was declared a pandemic by WHO in March 2019 (Mayo Clinic, 2020). At the time of writing this chapter, there have been nearly 35 million COVID-19 cases in the United States and the disease has claimed more than 600,000 American lives, with disproportionate COVID-19-related morbidity and mortality in communities of color that is linked to structural racism (CDC, 2021; Millett et al., 2020; Yan et al., 2020). Asian Americans have experienced a 35% increase in deaths during the first seven months of 2020, second only to the Latino population (Flagg et al., 2020). This estimate includes a 44% increase in excess deaths this year, the majority of which have been attributed to COVID-19.

Disparities in COVID-19 testing, treatment, and outcomes have been documented. One study found that among 50 million patients in the Epic electronic health record system, Asian Americans were less likely than Whites to get tested for COVID-19 but twice as likely to have a positive test (Rubin-Miller et al., 2020). In some cities, COVID-19 case fatality rates have been shown to be higher or similar among Asian Americans and NH/PIs, as an aggregated group, as compared to other racial/ethnic groups (Yan et al., 2020). Drivers of these disparities may include high rates of virus transmission among frontline workers in industries such as health care, food service, farming, and food production – jobs held disproportionately by Asian American individuals (US Bureau of Labor Statistics, 2020). Additionally, higher rates of diabetes and hypertension among Filipino Americans, Native Hawaiians, Pacific Islanders, and South Asians, as these diseases are known to exacerbate the severity of COVID-19 (Wyatt et al., 2020).

Yet a lack of data continues to hamper assessment of the magnitude of the COVID-19-related burden on Asian American communities. Misclassification of Asian American patients, missing data, and a lack of disaggregated data by ethnic group has led to underestimation of the disease's impact. As a consequence, funding for Asian American-focused research has suffered. Two rounds of emergency federal funding totaling $283 million made available through the National Institutes of Health (NIH)'s Rapid Acceleration of Diagnostics for Underserved Populations (RADx-UP), an initiative dedicated to exploring the needs of vulnerable communities to ensure that COVID-19-related technologies and treatments are developed and disseminated in ways that accommodate cultural, ethnic, geographic, and community-based differences, included only two projects with outreach to Filipino Americans and one focused on Chinese, Vietnamese, and Hmong Americans (National Institutes of Health, 2021). Without increased resource allocation for research among Asian American communities, a true picture of the impact of COVID-19 in this population will not emerge.

Other infectious diseases also disproportionately impact Asian Americans. Viral hepatitis is a key example. Endemic throughout Southeast and East Asia, viral hepatitis contributes to a high burden of hepatitis B- and hepatitis C-related morbidity and among migrants from those countries to the United States (Ortiz et al., 2020). Hepatitis B, a factor in both liver cancer and cirrhosis, disproportionately impacts Cambodian, Chinese, Filipino, Hmong, Laotian, Korean and Vietnamese Americans, and particularly the foreign-born (Chen and Dang, 2015). Hepatitis B prevalence among Asian Americans ranges from 9 to 15%, with estimates reaching 25% in some groups of recent immigrants (Pollack et al., 2014). Yet vaccination rates remain suboptimal among Asian Americans, particularly adults (Chen & Dang, 2015), and in terms of treatment, differences in initiation (receipt) of antiviral therapy as compared to completion (full course) of therapy among Asian Americans are not known (Carabez et al., 2014).

In 2012, the Centers for Disease Control and Prevention (CDC) funded nine sites nationwide to increase hepatitis B screening and linkage of hepatitis B-positive individuals to care through the Racial and Ethnic Approaches to Community Health across the U.S. (REACH US) program, which uncovered even higher rates of infection and highlighted important areas for expansion of education, prevention, screening, and treatment. National studies have documented referral to care for hepatitis B-infected individuals at 40% (Cohen et al., 2011) and referrals among the communities of focus for REACH US at only 33% (Hu et al., 2013). REACH US demonstrated the importance of designing in-language, culturally appropriate messaging and programming for diverse immigrant communities. Referral to care was a key area of success. In aggregated data for three REACH US sites (San Diego, CA; Minneapolis, MN; New York, NY), one study documented referrals to care at 86% (Beckett et al., 2014).

In NYC, the disaggregation of data for Asian ethnic groups proved critical to success. The NYU Center for the Study of Asian American Health (CSAAH) at NYU Grossman School of Medicine's National Center of Excellence in the Elimination of Hepatitis B Disparities found that hepatitis B prevalence was highest among Chinese-born individuals, especially among those from Fujian province (23.2% and 33.1%, respectively) (Pollack et al., 2014) – community-based findings that emerged as essential to developing innovative, linguistically and culturally tailored prevention education, vaccination, and treatment programs (Trinh-Shevrin et al., 2015). Later broadened to serve multiple immigrant communities as "B Free NYC," CSAAH's work was recognized in a 2020 systematic review of the effectiveness of viral hepatitis interventions as a successful participatory multistrategy model, which prioritized reaching residents with limited English proficiency and immigrant communities by providing continual education, awareness, free screening, vaccination, and treatment and by collaborating with a wide range of stakeholders and thus facilitating access to care (Ortiz et al., 2020). The adaptation and expansion of such tailored and in-language approaches to education, vaccination, screening, and linkage to care programs will be critical to significantly reduce transmission of hepatitis B infection and rates of hepatitis B-associated liver cancer.

Hepatitis C, while not highly as prevalent as hepatitis B among Asian Americans overall, disproportionately impacts Vietnamese and Chinese Americans and contributes to higher liver cancer incidence and mortality in these groups (Lin et al., 2017; Lee et al., 2015). Prevalence in these groups is associated with older age, foreign birth, and exposure in health care settings (Lin et al., 2017). By contrast, in other racial/ethnic groups, hepatitis C transmission typically occurs through sexual exposure or shared injection drug use, underscoring the need for tailored outreach and treatment efforts among Asian American populations. Asian ethnicity must also be considered in treatment. Interferon-based therapies have been shown to be successful among Asian Americans, resulting in better sustained virologic response than in Whites (Chang et al., 2017; Su et al., 2017). Researchers have identified the favorable *IL28B* genetic polymorphism in Asians as a key contributor to this treatment success. Because newer, interferon-free therapies are not linked to *IL28B,* it is unclear whether these treatments will prove as successful for individuals of Asian descent. U.S.-based clinical trials conducted to date have failed to include sufficient numbers of ethnic Asians, a remarkable omission given the high prevalence of hepatitis C in this population. Engaging, recruiting, and retaining Asian Americans in research is critical to ensuring that these new therapies serve the needs of this disproportionately impacted population.

Other infectious diseases also disproportionately impact Asian Americans, including HIV/AIDS (discussed in detail in Chapter 12). Finally, tuberculosis remains a significant concern for the Asian American population. Although rates of infection are declining in the U.S. population overall, more cases have been detected among Asian Americans than other groups (CDC TB slides, 2018). Foreign birth is a key risk factor, with those born in the Philippines, India, Vietnam, and China together accounting for 36% of tuberculosis cases reported among foreign-born U.S. residents in 2018 (CDC TB slides, 2018). Yet a lack of more detailed, disaggregated data hampers the development of in-language, culturally tailored prevention and treatment efforts that will be critical to reducing the tuberculosis burden in the coming years. For example, in Michigan, researchers found that in new cases resulting from latent tuberculosis infection, Asian Americans, in aggregate, had an average incidence rate 24 times greater than Whites, after controlling for nativity, gender, and age. These findings underscore the need for disaggregated, community-based research that explores the social and environmental contexts that underlie this high incidence rate for the Asian American population as a whole (Noppert et al., 2017). Genotyping studies could also help to elucidate patterns of transmission and better inform focused prevention efforts (Stennis et al., 2016). More broadly, prevention and treatment programs must focus both on reducing transmission as well as reducing reactivation of latent tuberculosis. Routine contact tracing is an example of a program that has been seen as key to tuberculosis control. Culturally and linguistically appropriate strategies – along with staff and lay health workers to implement them – will be critical to the success of these programs.

Mental Health

National data describing the prevalence of mental disorders among Asian Americans are severely limited. Overall, Asian Americans have the lowest lifetime prevalence of mental disorders of any ethnic group in the United States (Alvarez et al., 2019). Because national surveys aggregate findings for Asian Americans, little is known about differences among ethnic groups, contributing to underestimation of the prevalence of mental health issues and insufficient allocation of resources to culturally relevant and language-appropriate mental health care and treatment services. This lack of services likely contributes to a lack of treatment-seeking among Asian Americans. Asian Americans been shown to have lower rates of mental health service utilization overall than the general population (in one study, 8.6% vs. 17.9%, respectively) (Abe-Kim et al., 2007). One national study found that among Asian Americans with severe, moderate, and mild need for mental health treatment, receipt of services was approximately 59.6%, 20.1%, and 9.2%, respectively, compared to 60.8%, 43%, and 28% in the general population (Ihara et al., 2014).

Because U.S.-born Asian Americans have been shown to have higher rates of service use than immigrant counterparts (6.2% vs 2.2%) and third or later generation have been shown to have higher rates of use of any services (19.3%) than first- or second-generation Asian Americans, some researchers have suggested that acculturation is the key factor impacting mental health service utilization (Abe-Kim et al., 2007). Feelings of shame, stigma, fear of "losing face," and an unwillingness to burden families or communities with individual problems have been identified as contributing factors to low utilization of mental health services by Asian Americans (Liu et al., 2017; Leong & Lau, 2001). Asian Americans are also more likely to somaticize psychological distress, presenting with physical symptoms in primary care rather than seeking mental health specialty treatment – a factor that contributes to under-reporting and undertreatment of mental disorders (Yang et al., 20). Researchers analyzing data from the National Latino and Asian American Survey found that Asian Americans who do present for mental health care do so at later stages than Latino individuals, with more serious disease (Ihara et al., 2014). Additionally, researchers have emphasized a low perceived need for mental health treatment services among Asian Americans as contributing to low service utilization overall and a need to improve cultural understandings of mental illness in order to increase demand for services (Breslau et al., 2017).

Yet cultural explanations for underutilization of mental health services by Asian Americans are insufficient to explain low service utilization rates. Not only does this perspective reflect the persistent impact of the model minority stereotype in assuming that Asian Americans do not have unmet mental health care needs, but also recent research has underscored the need to conduct studies designed to illuminate effective and efficient approaches to serving Asian American communities. For example, a recent analysis of five years of data from the National Survey on Drug Use and Health showed perceived need did not explain racial/ethnic differences in mental health care access between Asian Americans and Whites (Yang et al., 2020). To increase service utilization, there is a critical need to develop in-language, culturally appropriate clinical interventions, train health care providers to deliver those interventions, and implement community-based outreach and education for Asian American communities to raise awareness of service availability.

Limited disaggregated studies have explored specific mental health issues among Asian Americans. Small studies have shown that depression and suicide disproportionately impact Asian American adolescent girls and women, children of immigrants, and college students (Lau et al., 2013; Augsburger et al., 2015; Cheng et al., 2017). One literature review found that estimates of depression among Korean and Filipino Americans (33.3% and 34.4%, respectively) were twice as high as the estimates for Chinese Americans (15.7%; $p = .012$ for Korean, $p = .049$ for Filipino) (Kim et al, 2015). Among immigrants, discrimination and acculturative stress was strongly associated with lifetime prevalence of major depressive episode, even after controlling for demographics and other factors (odds ratio 2.27; 95% CI 1.44, 3.58) (Singh et al., 2017). Community-based studies have reflected these findings in studies conducted among individual ethnic groups. In a study conducted among older Chinese Americans in Chicago, self-reported discrimination was significantly associated with depressive symptoms, controlling for sociodemographic characteristics, migration-related variables, and personality factors (Li & Dong, 2017). CHIS data also suggest that treatment is also disproportionately low among Asian Americans. (Park et al., 2018). Moreover, some research suggests that Asian Americans may be more receptive to consulting a family doctor than a mental health specialist. In concert with the finding that many Asian Americans somaticize mental illness, these data suggest the need for increased resource allocation to increase access to needed mental health services in primary care (Kim, Park, et al., 2015; Kim-Mozeleski et al., 2018).

Substance use disorders remain understudied among Asian Americans. Limited data have shown low rates of substance use disorders, but these rates may be attributable to low prevalence among Chinese and South Asian Americans – the two most populous Asian American ethnic groups (Lee et al., 2013). Prevalence of alcohol and tobacco use disorders are higher among Korean, Japanese, and Filipino Americans than among Chinese or South Asian Americans (Wu & Blazer, 2015; Wu et al., 2013). A gender disparity has also been reported in the prevalence of substance use disorders, with Asian American women appearing to have lower rates than women of other racial/ethnic backgrounds. These analyses, however, do not consider ethnic group, acculturation, or generational status differences among Asian American women (Bersamira et al., 2017). In terms of treatment, although Asian Americans seek substance use disorder treatment at lower rates than other ethnic groups, treatment admissions increased at a faster rate for this population than other ethnic groups between 2000 and 2012

(Sahker et al., 2017). It is unclear whether this increase represents an increase in help-seeking or substance use disorder prevalence. Stimulants have been documented as the primary drug problem for a majority of first-time Asian American treatment clients, a significantly greater proportion than other ethnic groups (Wong & Bennett, 2010). In recent years, however, the most significant increase in treatment admissions has been found to be among Asian Americans using prescription opioids (Sahker et al., 2017). Taken together, these data indicate the urgent need for more research to examine substance use and treatment trends among Asian Americans.

Women's Health

Cancer is the leading cause of death among Asian American women, with lung, breast, and colorectal cancers responsible for the highest mortality rates (Torre et al., 2016). Rising rates of incident breast cancer are a particular concern, particularly in light of the fact that rates are declining among Whites. As compared to other racial/ ethnic groups, Asian American women have lower incidence and mortality rates associated with breast cancer but among younger Asian American women, rates are approaching those of Whites. Asian American women are diagnosed at younger ages than women of other racial/ethnic backgrounds (51.0 years, according to one study) (Warner et al., 2015) and with later stage disease (Gomez et al., 2013), highlighting the need for systemic improvements to increase screening paired with better public outreach and education. Overall, lower incidence and mortality rates are seen among recent immigrants, suggesting that changes to contextual factors impact pathogenesis. Rates and subtypes of breast cancer also differ significantly by ethnic group. A review of the SEER 18 registries database found that Asian Indian, Pakistani, and Korean American women may be at higher risk for triple negative breast cancer – the subtype that is most aggressive and difficult to treat – while Chinese and Filipina women may be at lower risk for this type (Iqbal et al., 2015). On the national level, in aggregate, among women aged 50–74 years, Asian American women have mammography screening rates (71%) comparable to White women (73%) (ACS, 2019). Yet analyses of multiple years of CHIS data showed pronounced disparities in mammography screening rates among Asian populations in California (Chawla et al., 2015; Ryu et al., 2013). In 2009, among Asian American women aged 50–74 residing in California, Korean (64.7%), and South Asian (69.7%) women had the lowest screening rates (Chawla et al., 2015). In contrast, during that same year, Japanese (93.8%) and Vietnamese (92.9%) women had the highest rates of mammography receipt among all Asian American women. A study of insured Korean American women in the Chicago area showed that only 53% had a mammogram in the past two years, suggesting that factors other than cost need to be considered to support screening in this population (Hong et al., 2018). A systematic review also found that women receiving care from Korean American providers had lower rates of breast cancer screening, highlighting a potential area for intervention by developing and implementing tailored provider education for this group (Oh et al., 2017). The same review found that spousal support for screening and incorporation of Korean American women's health beliefs within screening interventions were potential areas for improvement. Successful interventions in other Asian groups might also inform improvements. In CHIS data, Filipina and Vietnamese American women had the highest rates of mammography among all Asian American ethnic groups (Ryu et al., 2013). Differences in uptake among these communities likely indicate availability of in-language information, resources, access to culturally relevant navigation, and accessible health care, but more research is needed to understand and respond to these contextual factors.

There is an urgent need to explore the genetic and biologic factors that impact breast cancer tumorigenesis, and how these factors may interact with environmental factors to increase breast cancer risk and pathogenesis (Shi et al., 2017). Despite evidence showing Indian and Pakistani American women being diagnosed at a later stage and younger age than White women, this population has been shown to have better survival rates than other racial/ethnic groups (Iqbal et al., 2015). Reasons for this disparity are unknown. Research on racial differences has been hampered by insufficient numbers of Asian American women and Latinas included in studies, as well as a lack of information on human epidermal growth factor receptor 2 (HER2) status, and inconsistent assessment of other important factors affecting survival, including treatment, socioeconomic status, BMI, and comorbid conditions (Warner et al., 2015). Precision medicine trials, which focus on developing tailored treatments based on each individual's unique genetic and environmental profile, offer opportunities to address these issues, but only if sufficient numbers of Asian American women from diverse ethnic groups are successfully recruited and retained in cancer research.

Cervical cancer is declining among Asian Americans women, indicating an area of public health success (Gomez et al., 2013). Screening with a Papinacolaou (Pap) test, which may be combined with screening for HPV, is highly effective in identifying pre-cancerous lesions, which have a survival rate of nearly 100% (Nguyen-Truong et al., 2018). Yet cervical cancer remains a key concern for some Asian ethnic groups. Among Vietnamese American women, incidence and mortality rates are twice as high as among White women (Miller et al., 2008), and among the smaller population of Hmong women, cervical cancer incidence has been reported as three times higher than other Asian American women, and more than four times higher than Whites (Yang et al., 2004). Asian American women overall are diagnosed at later ages as compared to White women, suggesting the need for improved screening (Nghiem et al., 2016). Uptake of HPV vaccine also remains significantly lower among Asian American women than the general population (36.3% versus 44.7%) (US Department of HHS OMH, 2015). Foreign-born Asian American women having lower rates than foreign-born White women (Agénor et al., 2018), and lower rates of HPV vaccination have been linked to low health literacy, limited English proficiency, and immigration status (Becerra et al., 2020; Nguyen et al., 2012; Yi et al., 2013), highlighting the need for linguistically and culturally tailored messaging and programming to improve HPV vaccination rates.

Qualitative research studies have underscored the need for sensitivity to privacy issues related to women's health issues for Asian American women and the role that cultural norms and low health literacy may play in impacting care seeking among this population (Seo et al., 2018; Nguyen-Truong et al., 2018; Frost et al., 2016; Hahm et al., 2017). Interpersonal violence (IPV), including childhood, elder and intimate partner abuse, is severely underresearched (See Chapter 12).

Child and Adolescent Health

In areas impacting the health of very young children, such as completion of childhood immunizations, neonatal and infant mortality rates, and breastfeeding rates, data has shown that Asian American children fare as well or better than White children (Yu & Vyas, 2009). However, health issues emerging in later childhood and adolescence disproportionately impact certain Asian ethnic groups and contribute to health disparities seen among the adult population overall. Obesity is one such issue. Although obesity rates are generally lower among Asian American children than among other racial/ethnic groups in early childhood (Isong et al., 2018), the BMI cutpoints used to identify overweight and obesity among children do not differentiate among racial/ethnic groups. Interestingly, in a phenomenon not observed within other racial/ethnic groups, there is a sex difference in obesity prevalence, with Asian American boys having nearly twice the prevalence of overweight/obesity compared to girls (Ogden et al., 2016). Yet, like adults, Asian American children tend to have different body compositions as compared to Whites and other racial/ethnic groups, and reconsideration of current cutpoints is an area for future research (Cook & Tseng, 2019). Even at current cutpoints, children from certain ethnic groups experience disproportionate rates of overweight and obesity, including Filipino Americans and Southeast Asians (including Burmese, Cambodian, Hmong, Indonesian, Laotian, Malaysian, Thai and Vietnamese) (Diep et al., 2017; Braden et al., 2016; Cook & Tseng, 2019; Jain et al., 2012). Yet because Chinese Americans are the largest Asian American group, and because Chinese American children and adolescents are less likely than other groups to be overweight or obese throughout childhood and adolescence (Cook & Tseng, 2019), the low prevalence of overweight/obesity in this population masks the higher rates experienced by other ethnic groups when data are aggregated for the overall Asian American population. Moreover, a recent analysis comparing obesity cutpoints in the United States versus China found that using Chinese-specific measures was more effective at identifying overweight and obesity in Chinese American girls, negating the sex difference detected between Chinese American boys and girls that the CDC measures identified (Lau et al., 2020). Limited community-based studies have explored potential associations, linking poor diet quality and insufficient physical activity levels to higher BMI in the ethnic groups experiencing higher prevalence of overweight and obesity (Guerrero et al., 2015). Yet the social determinants of health, diet, and physical activity behaviors that underlie these pathways in specific populations remain understudied. While most research has found that less acculturated families with more traditional dietary practices have children with healthier weights, at least one study using national data found that mother's English proficiency was predictive of healthier weight (Diep et al., 2017). This finding illustrates the complexity of acculturation and its impact on the health of immigrant, first-generation, and second-generation children. Perhaps English-proficient mothers in the study were more adept at navigating nutritional information in mainstream U.S. society or that they engaged with the health care system more effectively and at higher rates. Alternatively, whereas lower levels of acculturation may be protective against higher BMI for populations with lower socioeconomic status, for groups with higher socioeconomic status, English proficiency, as a marker of higher acculturation, may be associated with healthier food intake patterns, acceptance of mainstream social norms, and greater social support. Refugee experiences also contribute to this complex array of acculturation factors. Prolonged food insecurity has been shown to contribute to excessive food consumption among refugee families in the United States, leading to higher prevalence of overweight and obesity in some Southeast Asian ethnic groups (Cook et al., 2019).

English proficiency has emerged as a predictor in other areas of child and adolescent health, further indicating the need for more research to better understand the complexity of its role as a determinant of health status. Mothers' limited English proficiency has been linked to low HPV vaccination rates among adolescents, and while increasing HPV vaccine uptake has been identified as a priority public health issue for all young people, improving vaccination rates among Asian Americans boys and girls is particularly urgent due to the high rates of cervical cancer among adult Asian American women in some ethnic groups, including among Cambodian, Vietnamese, and Hmong American women (Lee et al., 2016). Limited studies suggest that focusing on facilitators of vaccine uptake, including increasing provider recommendation, the sharing of HPV-related information through trustworthy sources (e.g., churches, community-based leaders), and school-based administration of the vaccine, may accelerate increases in rates among Asian American adolescents (Zhu et al., 2019; Hopfer et al., 2017; Lee et al., 2016; Kim, Kim, et al., 2015). Qualitative data has proven essential to developing effective interventions. For example, one study demonstrated that Vietnamese American women did not object to their daughters receiving the HPV vaccine, but they simply did not know about its benefits or that the vaccine could be obtained free of charge (Hopfer et al., 2017). The women's discomfort in discussing sexual health issues prevented them from raising the topic of HPV vaccination with their daughters, and they deferred decision-making to their health care providers.

Similarly, rich qualitative data are needed to inform interventions tailored to the health education needs of Asian American adolescents. Although, in aggregate, Asian American teens have lower rates of health risk behaviors overall (Lowry et al., 2011), some groups have shown higher rates of risk-taking and more research is needed to explore and address emerging trends. For example, Asian American adolescents have lower rates of cigarette use than other racial/ethnic groups nationally, but a California survey found that Asian American girls had the highest prevalence of e-cigarette use than any other group (Wong & Fan, 2018). A gender disparity was also found in rates of sexual initiation and behaviors in a national study, with more acculturated Asian American adolescent girls having earlier onset of sexual intercourse and a higher number of partners than boys (Tong, 2013). Reasons for these gender disparities are not known. Similarly, even as national data show that Asian American adolescents have lower rates of sexual activity as compared other racial/ethnic groups (Tong, 2013), they comprise the only group for which teen pregnancy has not declined in recent years nationally, a trend that is paired with rising rates of sexually transmitted infections (STIs), including HIV (Lee, Florez, et al., 2015). Alcohol use is increasing among Asian Americans in undergraduate university settings (Le & Iwamoto, 2019) and although prevalence of lifetime illicit drug use is markedly lower among Asian American adolescents than Whites nationally (17.9% versus 30.3%, respectively), use of the club drug ecstasy was similar to Whites and higher than Blacks and Hispanics (Wu et al., 2011). These findings are concerning not only because they are linked to negative health outcomes such as depression and suicide (Subica & Wu, 2018; Durand et al., 2016; Wyatt et al., 2015) but also because so little research has explored the underlying causes for these disparities. Factors such as bicultural socialization, acculturation, and acculturative stress among adolescents exert a complex influence on risk-taking and health but remain understudied (Wyatt et al., 2015).

Healthy Aging

National data describing the health status and needs of older Asian Americans are extremely limited, underscoring a critical need for population-based research regarding the unmet needs, sociocultural contexts, and health trajectories of the aging Asian American population. Smaller, community-based studies have begun to highlight directions for future research, including such issues as functional decline (Dallo et al., 2015; Fuller-Thomson et al., 2011), dementia (Jang et al., 2018; Li et al., 2017; Zheng & Woo, 2016), elder abuse (Dong & Wong, 2017), end-of-life planning (Chi et al., 2018; Kwak & Salmon, 2007), and intergenerational relationships (Dong, Li & Hua, 2017; Xu et al., 2017). These topics are discussed in detail in Chapter 11.

LGBTQ Health

Lesbian, gay, bisexual, transgender, and queer (LGBTQ) Asian Americans comprise a diverse population encompassing people with many different sexual orientations, sexual behaviors, and gender identities. Collectively, the term *LGBTQ* is commonly used, with the understanding that the term may not be exhaustive. Despite experiencing multiple minority stressors that likely contribute to disproportionate health disparities among this population, LGBTQ Asian Americans are underrepresented in health research (Barnett et al., 2019). Limited data indicate that LGBTQ Asian Americans are at risk for adverse health outcomes (e.g., substance use, sexual risk behaviors) compared to the general Asian American population. See Chapter 12 for a more detailed description about the stressors and health outcomes in this population.

SUMMARY AND RECOMMENDATIONS

Summarizing health data for Asian Americans is difficult due to the diversity of the ethnic groups that comprise this population and because large population-based surveys aggregate data for all of them, masking true differences among these vastly diverse populations. Despite these challenges, data show that cancers of infectious origin, heart-related conditions, and metabolic disorders are on the rise among Asian Americans, with nuanced differences by Asian ethnic group. Infectious diseases remain a uniquely important issue for Asian Americans, particularly for the foreign-born, and emerging data from the COVID-19 crisis increasingly demonstrate a high toll on Asian American communities, both in terms of morbidity and mortality.

Any research must make efforts to understand the nuanced social and structural determinants of health among Asian American ethnic groups. Health status and health issues in Asian American communities are informed and impacted by diverse genetic, socio-political, demographic, cultural, and economic factors that must be acknowledged in research. In terms of data collection and reporting, improved measures and methods to capture these determinants are necessary. Low health service utilization, often linked to limited availability of linguistically or culturally relevant services, is a key area for future research and action across all disease areas. Other measures that accurately capture immigration status and ethnic identity need to be developed and tested. Increasing the number and quality of disaggregated studies at the national, regional, and local levels to explore ethnic-specific health experiences will be critical to inform the development of appropriate and effective services for Asian Americans of all ethnic backgrounds, genders, ages, and sexual orientations in the years to come.

Clinical teams should aim to consist of diverse professionals from various trainings and backgrounds to provide holistic health care services to patients. Health care teams must employ culturally competent CHWs and patient navigators who are trained and comfortable in providing tailored services within Asian American communities. In addition, clinical training programs for health care providers must emphasize the importance of the role played by health care professionals in supporting early screening and disease prevention among patients. Clinical training should also address sources of bias against Asian American groups, which impacts disease screening and identification.

For research, engaging the community throughout the research process – from conceptualization to implementation to dissemination – is important to increase reach and acceptability of subsequent prevention and education programs. In-language and culturally competent materials are needed to provide community members with resources to address health concerns. Programs created and adapted for Asian American populations must be tailored to fit the cultural, ethnic, social, linguistic, and religious diversity of each community.

Tackling the dual burdens of chronic and infectious diseases on Asian American populations requires detailed, disaggregated data to be collected from and reported back to the communities of concern. Research developed through community-engaged processes must take into consideration the nuanced demographic, cultural, social, and economic diversity that exists among Asian ethnic groups to successfully build programs and services.

DISCUSSION QUESTIONS

1. Which diseases or health issues impact the Asian American population as a whole?

2. The authors presented numerous examples illustrating the importance of disaggregating data by Asian ethnic group to better understand the health needs of Asian American communities. What are some examples of diseases or health issues that disproportionately impact one or more Asian ethnic groups?

3. In many areas, Asian Americans have lower rates of health service utilization than other racial/ethnic groups. How might researchers and health service providers contribute to improving service utilization rates among Asian Americans overall? Can you identify any specific strategies that might be worth exploring for implementation with different Asian populations with respect to any specific health conditions?

REFERENCES

Abe-Kim, J., Takeuchi, D., Hong, S., Zane, N., Sue, S., & Spencer, M. S. (2007). Use of mental health-related services among immigrant and US-born Asian Americans: Results from the National Latino and Asian American Study. *American Journal of Public Health, 97*(1), 91–98. https://doi.org/10.2105/AJTH.2006.098541

Agénor, M., Abboud, S., Delgadillo, J.G., Pérez, A.E., Peitzmeier, S.M., & Borrero, S. (2018). Intersectional nativity and racial/ethnic disparities in human papillomavirus vaccination among U.S. women: a national population-based study. *Cancer Causes Control, 29,* 927–936. https://doi.org/10.1007/s10552-018-1069-1

Agénor, M., Pérez, A. E., Koma, J. W., Abrams, J. A., McGregor, A. J., & Ojikutu, B. O. (2019). Sexual Orientation Identity, Race/Ethnicity, and Lifetime HIV Testing in a National Probability Sample of U.S. Women and Men: An Intersectional Approach. *LGBT Health, 6*(6), 306–318. https://doi.org/10.1089/lgbt.2019.0001

Alvarez, K. Fillbrunn, M., Green, J. G., Jackson, J. S., Kessler, R. C., McLaughlin, K. A., Sadikova, E., Sampson, N. A., & Alegria, M. (2019). Race/ethnicity, nativity, and lifetime risk of mental disorders in US adults. *Social Psychiatry and Psychiatric Epidemiology, 54*(5), 553–565. https://doi.org/10.1007/s00127-018-1644-5

American Cancer Society (ACS). (2019). *Breast Cancer Facts & Figures 2019–2020.* Atlanta: American Cancer Society.

American Cancer Society (ACS). (2020). *Cancer Facts & Figures, 2020.* Atlanta: American Cancer Society.

ACS. *Special section: Cancer in Asian Americans, Native Hawaiians, and Pacific Islanders.* https://www.cancer.org/content/dam/cancer-org/research/cancer-facts-and-statistics/annual-cancer-facts-and-figures/2016/special-section-cancer-in-asian-americans-native-hawaiians-and-pacific-islanders-cancer-facts-and-figures-2016.pdf. Retrieved February 29, 2020.

Ancheta, I. B., Carlson, J. M., Battie, C. A., Borja-Hart, N., Cobb, S., & Ancheta, C. V. (2015). One size does not fit all: cardiovascular health disparities as a function of ethnicity in Asian-American women. *Applied Nursing Research, 28,* 99–105. https://doi.org/10.1016/j.apnr.2014.06.001

Atekruse, S. F., Cosgrove, C., Cronin, K., & Yu, M. (2017). Comparing Cancer Registry abstracted and self-reported data on race and ethnicity. *Journal of Registry Management, 44*(1), 30–33.

Abstracted and Self-Reported Data on Race and Ethnicity. *Journal of Registry Management, 44*(1), 30–33.

Barnett, A. P., Del Río-González, A. M., Parchem, B., Pinho, V., Aguayo-Romero, R., Nakamura, N., Calabrese, S. K., Poppen, P. J., & Zea, M. C. (2019). Content analysis of psychological research with lesbian, gay, bisexual, and transgender people of color in the United States: 1969–2018. *The American Psychologist, 74*(8), 898–911. https://doi.org/10.1037/amp0000562

Bautista, M. C., Jiang, S. F., Armstrong, M. A., Kakar, S., Postlethwaite, D., & Li, D. (2015), Significant racial disparities exist in noncardia gastric cancer outcomes among Kaiser Permanente's patient population. *Digestive Diseases and Sciences, 60*(4), 984–985. https://doi.org/10.1007/s10620-014-3409-7

Becerra, M. B., Avina, R. M., Mshigeni, S., & Becerra, B. J. (2020). Low human papillomavirus literacy among Asian-American women in California: An analysis of the California health interview survey. *Journal of Racial and Ethnic Health Disparities, 7*(4), 678–686. https://doi.org/10.1007/s40615-020-00698-7

Beckett, G. A., Ramirez, G., Vanderhoff, A., Nichols, K., Chute, S. M., Wyles, D. L., Schoenbachler, B. T., Bedell, D. T., Cabral, R., Ward, J. W., & Centers for Disease Control and Prevention (CDC). (2014). Early identification and linkage to care of persons with chronic hepatitis B virus infection – three U.S. sites, 2012-2014. *MMWR. Morbidity and mortality weekly report, 63*(18), 399–401.

Bersamira, C. S., Lin, Y. A., Park, K., & Marsh, J. C. (2017). Drug use among Asian Americans: Differentiating use by acculturation status and gender. *Journal of Substance Abuse Treat ment, 79,* 76–81. https://doi.org/10.1016/j.jsat.2017.06.002

Berman, T. A., & Schiller, J. T. (2017). Human papillomavirus in cervical cancer and oropharyngeal cancer: One cause, two diseases. *Cancer, 123*(12), 2219–2229. https://doi.org/10.1002/cncr.30588

Bi, S., Gunter, K. E., & Lopez, F. Y. (2019). Improving Shared Decision Making For Asian American Pacific Islander Sexual and Gender Minorities. *Medical Care, 57*(12), 937–944. https://doi.org/10.1097/MLR.0000000000001212

Bodle, E. E., Islam, N., Kwon, S. C., Zojwalla, N., Ahsan, H., & Senie, R. T. (2008). Cancer screening practices of Asian American physicians in New York City. *Journal of Immigrant and Minority Health, 10*(3), 239–246. https://doi.org/10.1007/s10903-007-9077-3

Braden, K. W., & Nigg, C. R. (2016). Modifiable determinants of obesity in Native Hawaiian and Pacific Islander youth. *Hawai'i Journal of Medicine & Public Health: A Journal of Asia Pacific Medicine & Public Health, 75*(6), 162–171.

Bray, F., Ren, J. S., Masuyer, E., & Ferlay, J. (2013). Global estimates of cancer prevalence for 27 sites in the adult population in 2008. *International Journal of Cancer, 132*(5), 1133–1145. https://doi.org/10.1002/ijc.27711

Breslau, J., Cefalu, M., Wong, E. C., Burnam, M. A., Hunter, G. P., Florez, K. R., & Collins, R. L. (2017). Racial/ethnic differences in perception of need for mental health treatment in a US national sample. *Social Psychiatry and Psychiatric Epidemiology*, *52*(8), 929–937. https://doi.org/10.1007/s00127-017-1400-2

Bruni, L., Diaz, M., Castellsague, X., Ferrer, E., Bosch, F. X., de Sanjose, S. (2010). Cervical human papillomavirus prevalence in 5 continents: meta-analysis of 1 million women with normal cytological findings. *Journal of Infectious Diseases*, 202, 1789–1799.

Budhwani, H., & De, P. (2017). Human papillomavirus vaccine initiation in Asian Indians and Asian subpopulations: A case for examining disaggregated data in public health research. *Public Health, 153,* 111–117. https://doi.org/10.1016/j.puhe.2017.07.036

Carabez, R. M., Swanner, J. A., Yoo, G. J., & Ho, M. (2014). Knowledge and fears among Asian Americans chronically infected with hepatitis B. *Journal of Cancer Education, 29*(3), 522–528. https://doi.org/10.1007/s13187-013-0585-7

Cené, C. W., Dilworth-Anderson, P., Leng, I., Garcia, L., Benavente, V., Rosal, M., Vaughan, L., Coker, L. H., Corbie-Smith, G., Kim, M., Bell, C. L., Robinson, J. G., Manson, J. E., & Cochrane, B. (2016). Correlates of successful aging in racial and ethnic minority women age 80 years and older: findings from the women's health initiative, *The Journals of Gerontology, Series A: Biological Sciences and Medical Sciences*, *71*(Suppl 1), S87–S99. https://doi.org/10.1093/gerona/glv099

Centers for Disease Control and Prevention (CDC). (2019). CDC HIV Prevention Progress Report, 2019. https://www.cdc.gov/hiv/pdf/policies/progressreports/cdc-hiv-preventionprogressreport.pdf.

CDC. (2021). CDC COVID Data Tracker. Available at: https://covid.cdc.gov/covid-data-tracker/?CDC_AA_refVal=https://www.cdc.gov/coronavirus/2019-ncov/cases-updates/cases-in-us.html#cases_casesper100klast7days.

Chang, C. Y., Nguyen, P., Le, A., Zhao, C., Ahmed, A., Daugherty, T., Garcia, G., Lutchman, G., Kumari, R., & Nguyen, M. H. (2017). Real-world experience with interferon-free, direct acting antiviral therapies in Asian Americans with chronic hepatitis C and advanced liver disease. *Medicine (Baltimore)*, *96*(6), e6128. https://doi.org/10.1097/MD.0000000000006128

Chawla, N., Breen, N., Liu, B., Lee, R., & Kagawa-Singer, M. (2015). Asian American women in California: A pooled analysis of predictors for breast and cervical cancer screening. *American Journal of Public Health*, *105*(2), e98–e109. https://doi.org/10.2105/AJPH.2014.302250

Chen, D., Román, G. C., Wu, G. X., Wu, Z. S., Yao, C. H., Zhang, M., & Hirsch, R. P. (1992). Stroke in China (Sino-MONICA-Beijing study) 1984–1986. *Neuroepidemiology*, *11*(1), 15–23. https://doi.org/10.1159/000110902

Chen, I. Y., Joshi, S., & Ghassemi, M. (2020). Treating health disparities with artificial intelligence. *Nature Medicine, 26*(1), 16–17. https://doi.org/10.1038/s41591-019-0649-2

Chen, M. S. Jr. (2005). Cancer health disparities among Asian Americans: what we do and what we need to do. *Cancer, 104*(12 Suppl), 2895–2902.

Chen, M. S., Jr, & Dang, J. (2015). Hepatitis B among Asian Americans: Prevalence, progress, and prospects for control. *World Journal of Gastroenterology*, *21*(42), 11924–11930. https://doi.org/10.3748/wjg.v21.i42.11924

Chen, W. T., Guthrie, B., Shiu, C. S., Wang, L., Weng, Z., Li, C. S., Lee, T. S., Kamitani, E., Fukuda, Y., & Luu, B. V. (2015). Revising the American dream: How Asian immigrants adjust after an HIV diagnosis. *Journal of Advanced Nursing*, *71*(8), 1914–1925. https://doi.org/10.1111/jan.12645

Cheng, A. W., Chang, J., O'Brien, J., Budgazad, M.S., Tsai, J. (2017). Model minority stereotype: Influence on perceived mental health needs of Asian Americans. *Journal of Immigrant and Minority Health, 19*(3), 572–581. https://doi.org/10.1007/s10903-016-0440-0

Cheng, Y. J., Kanaya, A. M., Araneta, M. R. G., Saydah, S. H., Kahn, H. S., Gregg, E. W., Fujimoto, W. Y., & Imperatore, G. (2019) Prevalence of diabetes by race and ethnicity in the United States, 2011-2016. *Journal of the American Medical Association, 322*(24), 2389–2398. https://doi.org/10.1001/jama2019.19365

Chi, H. L., Cataldo, J., Ho, E. Y., & Rehm, R. S. (2018). Please ask gently: Using culturally targeted communication strategies to initiate end-of-life care discussions with older Chinese Americans. *American Journal of Hospice and Palliative Medicine*, *35*(10), 1265–1272. https://doi.org/10.1177/1049909118760310

Choi, K. H., Paul, J., Ayala, G., Boylan, R., & Gregorich, S. E. (2013). Experiences of discrimination and their impact on the mental health among African American, Asian and Pacific Islander, and Latino men who have sex with men. *American Journal of Public Health*, *103*(5), 868–874. https://doi.org/10.2105/AJPH.2012.301052

Cohen, C., Holmberg, S. D., McMahon, B. J., Block, J. M., Brosgart, C. L., Gish, R. G., London W. T., & Block, T. M. (2011). Is chronic hepatitis B being undertreated in the United States? *Journal of Viral Hepatitis*, *18*, 377–383. https://doi.org/10.1111/j.1365-2893.2010.01401.x

Cook, W. J., & Tseng, W. (2019). Associations of Asian Ethnicity and Parental Education with Overweight in Asian American Children and Adolescents: An Analysis of 2011–2016 National Health and Nutrition Examination Surveys. *Maternal and Child Health Journal, 23*(4), 504–511. https://doi.org/10.1007/s10995-018-2662-3

Crowne, S. S., Juon, H. S., Ensminger, M., Bair-Merritt, M. H., & Duggan, A. (2012). Risk factors for intimate partner violence initiation and persistence among high psychosocial risk Asian and Pacific Islander women in intact relationships. *Women's Health Issues: Official Publication of the Jacobs Institute of Women's Health*, *22*(2), e181–e188. https://doi.org/10.1016/j.whi.2011.08.006

Dallo, F. J., Booza, J., & Nguyen, N. D. (2015). Functional limitations and nativity status among older Arab, Asian, Black, Hispanic, and White Americans. *Journal of Immigrant and Minority Health*, *17*(2), 535–542. https://10.1007/s10903-013-9943-0

Diep, C. S., Baranowski, T., & Kimbro, R. T. (2017). Acculturation and weight change in Asian-American children: evidence from the ECLS-K:2011. *Preventive Medicine*, *99*, 286–292. https://doi.org/10.1016/j.ypmed.2017.03.019

Dong, X., Li, M., & Hua, Y. (2017). The association between filial discrepancy and depressive symptoms: Findings from a community-dwelling Chinese aging population. *The Journals of Gerontology: Series A, 72*(suppl_1), S63–S68. https://doi.org/10.1093/gerona/glx040

Dong, X., Wang, B. (2017). Incidence of elder abuse in a U.S. Chinese Population: Findings from the longitudinal cohort PINE study. *The Journals of Gerontology: Series A, Biological Sciences and Medical Sciences*, *72*(Suppl_1), S95–S101. https://doi.org/10.1093/gerona/glx005

Durand, Z., Cook, A., Konishi, M., & Nigg, C. (2016). Alcohol and substance use prevention programs for youth in Hawaii and Pacific Islands: A literature review. *Journal of Ethnicity in Substance Abuse, 15*(3), 240–251. Epub 2015 Dec 7.

Echeverria, S. E., Mustafa, M., Pentakota, S. R., Kim, S., Hastings, K. G., Amadi, C., & Palaniappan, L. (2017). Social and clinically-relevant cardiovascular risk factors in Asian Americans adults: NHANES 2011–2014. *Preventive Medicine*, *99*, 222–227. https://doi.org/10.1016/j.ypmed.2017.02.016

Fang, C. Y., Lee, M., Feng, Z., Tan, Y., Levine, F., Nguyen, C., & Ma, G. X. (2019). Community-based cervical cancer education: Changes in knowledge and beliefs among Vietnamese American women. *Journal of Community Health, 44*(3), 525–533. https://10.1007/s10900-019-00645-6

Fang, J., Foo, S. H., Jeng, J. S., Yip, P. K., & Alderman, M. H. (2004). Clinical characteristics of stroke among Chinese in New York City. *Ethnicity & Disease, 14*(3), 378–383.

Flagg A., Sharma D., Fenn L., & Stobbe M. (2020). COVID-19's toll on people of color is worse than we knew. *The Marshall Project. August* 21, 2020. https://www.themarshallproject.org/2020/08/21/covid-19-s-toll-on-people-of-color-is-worse-than-we-knew.

Frost, M., Cares, A., Gelman, K., & Beam, R. (2016). Accessing sexual and reproductive health care and information: Perspectives and recommendations from young Asian American women. *Sexual and Reproductive Healthcare, 10,* 9–13. https://doi.org/10.1016/j.srhc.2016.09.007

Fuller-Thomson, E., Brennenstuhl, S., & Hurd, M. (2011). Comparison of disability rates among older adults in aggregated and separate Asian American/Pacific Islander subpopulations. *American Journal of Public Health, 101*(1), 94–100. https://doi.org/10.2105/AJPH.2009.176784

Fung, L. C., Nguyen, K. H., Stewart, S. L., Chen, M. S., Jr., & Tong, E. K. (2018). Impact of a cancer education seminar on knowledge and screening intent among Chinese Americans: Results from a randomized, controlled, community-based trial. *Cancer, 124* (Suppl. 7), 1622–1630. https://doi.org/10.1002/cncr.31111

Gomez, S. L., Noone, A. M., Lichtensztajn, D. Y., Scoppa, S., Gibson, J. T., Liu, L., Morris, C., Kwong, S., Fish, K., Wilkens, L. R., Goodman, M. T., Deapen, D., & Miller, B. A. (2013). Cancer incidence trends among Asian American populations in the United States, 1990-2008. *Journal of the National Cancer Institute, 105*(15), 1096–1110. https://doi.org/10.1093/jnci/djt157

Gross, E. R., Zambelli, V. O., Small, B. A., Ferreira, J. C., Chen, C. H., & Mochly-Rosen, D. (2015). A personalized medicine approach for Asian Americans with the aldehyde dehydrogenase 2*2 variant. *Annual Review of Pharmacology and Toxicology, 55,* 107–127. https://doi.org/10.1146/annurev-pharmtox-010814-124915

Guerrero, A. D., Ponce, N. A., & Chung, P. J. (2015). Obesogenic Dietary Practices of Latino and Asian Subgroups of Children in California: An Analysis of the California Health Interview Survey, 2007–2012. *American Journal of Public Health, 105*(8), e105–e112. https://doi.org/10.2105/AJPH.2015.302618

Gupta L. S., Wu, C. C., Young, S., & Perlman S. E. (2011). Prevalence of diabetes in New York City, 2002-2008: comparing foreign-born South Asians and other Asians with U.S.-born Whites, Blacks, and Hispanics. *Diabetes Care, 34*(8), 1791–1793. http://dx.doi.org/10.2337/dc11-0088

Gupta, M., Singh, N., & Verma, S. (2006). South Asians and cardiovascular risk: what clinicians should know. *Circulation, 113*(25), e924–e929. https://doi.org/10.1161/CIRCULATIONAHA.105.583815

Ha, J., Yan, M., Aguilar, M., Bhuket, T., Tana M. M., Liu, B., Gish, R. G., & Wong, R. J. (2016). Race/ethnicity-specific disparities in cancer incidence, burden of disease, and overall survival among patients with hepatocellular carcinoma in the United States. *Cancer, 122*(16), 2512–2523. https://doi.org/10.1002/cncr.30103.

Hahm, H. C., Augsberger, A., Feranil, M., Jang, J., & Tagerman, M. (2017). The Associations Between Forced Sex and Severe Mental Health, Substance Use, and HIV Risk Behaviors Among Asian American Women. *Violence Against Women, 23*(6), 671–691. https://doi.org/10.1177/1077801216647797

Hahm, H. C., Chang, S. T., Lee, G. Y., Tagerman, M. D., Lee, C. S., Trentadue, M. P., & Hien, D. A. (2017). Asian Women's Action for Resilience and Empowerment Intervention: Stage I Pilot Study. *Journal of Cross-cultural Psychology, 48*(10), 1537–1553. https://doi.org/10.1177/0022022117730815

Hahm, H. C., Lee, J., Chiao, C., Valentine, A., & Lê Cook, B. (2016). Use of Mental Health Care and Unmet Needs for Health Care Among Lesbian and Bisexual Chinese-, Korean-, and Vietnamese-American Women. *Psychiatric Services (Washington, D.C.), 67*(12), 1380–1383. https://doi.org/10.1176/appi.ps.201500356

Hall, I. J., Tangka, F. K. L., Sabatino, S. A., Thompson, T. D., Graubard, B. I., & Breen, N. (2018). Patterns and trends in cancer screening in the United States. *Preventing Chronic Disease, 15,* 170465. https://doi.org/10.5888/pcd15.170465

Hastings, K. G., Jose, P. O., Kapphahn, K. I., Frank, A. T. H., Goldstein, B. A., Thompson, C. A., Eggleston, K., Cullen, M. R., & Palaniappan, L. P. (2015). Leading causes of death among asian american subgroups (2003–2011). *PLoS One, 10*(4), e0124341. https://doi.org/10.1371/journal.pone.0124341

Holland, A. T., Wong, E. C., Lauderdale, D. S., & Palaniappan, L. P. (2011). Spectrum of cardiovascular diseases in Asian-American racial/ethnic subgroups. *Annals of Epidemiology, 21*(8), 608–614. https://doi.org/10.1016/j.annepidem.2011.04.004

Hong, H. C., Ferrans, C. E., Park, C., Lee, H., Quinn, L., & Collins, E. G. (2018). Effects of Perceived Discrimination and Trust on Breast Cancer Screening among Korean American Women. *Women's Health Issues, 28*(2):188–196. https://doi.org/10.1016/j.whi.2017.11.001

Hopfer, S., Garcia, S., Duong, H. T., Russo, J. A., & Tanjasiri, S. P. (2017). A Narrative Engagement Framework to Understand HPV Vaccination Among Latina and Vietnamese Women in a Planned Parenthood Setting. *Health Education & Behavior: The Official Publication of the Society for Public Health Education, 44*(5), 738–747. https://doi.org/10.1177/1090198117728761

Hou, S. I., Sealy, D. A., & Kabiru, C. W. (2011). Closing the disparity gap: cancer screening interventions among Asians – a systematic literature review. *Asian Pacific Journal of Cancer Prevention, 12*(11), 3133–3139.

Hu, D. J., Xing, J., Tohme, R. A., Liao, Y., Pollack, H., Ward, J. W., & Holmberg, S. D. (2013). Hepatitis B testing and access to care among racial and ethnic minorities in selected communities across the United States, 2009–2010. *Hepatology, 58,* 856–862. https://doi.org/10.1002/hep.26286

Ihara, E. S., Chae, D. H., Cummings, J. R., & Lee, S. (2014). Correlates of mental health service use and type among Asian Americans. *Administration and Policy in Mental Health, 41*(4), 543–551. https://doi.org/10.1007/s10488-013-0493-5

Iqbal, J., Ginsburg, O., Rochon, P. A., Sun, P., Narod, S. A. (2015). Differences in breast cancer stage at diagnosis and cancer-specific survival by race and ethnicity in the United States. *Journal of the American Medical Association, 313*(2), 165–173. https://doi.org/10.1186/s12879-019-4283-x

Isong, I. A., Rao, S. R., Bind, M. A., Avendaño, M., Kawachi, I., & Richmond, T. K. (2018). Racial and Ethnic Disparities in Early Childhood Obesity. *Pediatrics, 141*(1), e20170865. https://doi.org/10.1542/peds.2017-0865.

Iyer, D. G., Shah, N. S., Hastings, K. G., Hu, J., Rodriguez, F., Boothroyd, D. B., Krishnan, A. V., Falasinnu, T., & Palaniappan, L. (2019). Years of potential life lost because of cardiovascular disease in Asian-American subgroups, 2003–2012. *Journal of the American Heart Association, 8*(7), e010744. https://doi.org/10.1161/JAHA.118.010744

Jain, A., Mitchell, S., Chirumamilla, R., Zhang, J., & Horn, I. B. (2012). Prevalence of obesity among young Asian-American children. *Childhood Obesity, 8*(6), 518–525. https://doi.org/10.1089/chi.2011.0077

Jang, Y., Yoon, H., Park, N. S., Rhee, M. K., & Chiriboga, D. A. (2018). Asian Americans' concerns and plans about Alzheimer's disease: The role of exposure, literacy and cultural beliefs. *Health & Social Care in the Community, 26*(2), 199–206. https://10.1111/hsc.12509

Jih, J., Mukherjea, A., Vittinghoff, E., Nguyen, T. T., Tsoh, J. Y., Fukuoka, Y., Bender, M. S., Tseng, W., & Kanaya, A. M. (2014). Using appropriate body mass index cut points for overweight and obesity among Asian Americans. *Preventive Medicine, 65*, 1–6. https://doi.org/10.1016/j.ypmed.2014.04.010

Jose, P. O., Frank, A. T., Kapphahn, K. I., Goldstein, B. A., Eggleston, K., Hastings, K. G., Cullen, M. R., & Palaniappan, L. P. (2014). Cardiovascular disease mortality in Asian Americans. *Journal of the American College of Cardiology, 64*, 2486–2494. https://doi.org/10.1016/j.jacc.2014.08.048

Juon, H. S., Lee, S., Strong, C., Rimal, R., Kirk, G. D., & Bowie, J. (2014). Effect of a liver cancer education program on hepatitis B screening among Asian Americans in the Baltimore-Washington metropolitan area, 2009-2010. *Preventing Chronic Disease, 11*, 130258. https://doi.org/10.5888/pcd11.130258

Kagawa-Singer, M., Dadia, A. V., & Surbone , A. (2010). Cancer, culture, and health disparities: time to chart a new course? *CA: A Cancer Journal for Clinicians, 60*(1), 12–39. https://doi.org/10.3322/caac.20051

Kalra, R., Patel, N., Arora, P., Arora, G. (2019). Cardiovascular health and disease among Asian-Americans (from the National Health and Nutrition Examination Survey). *American Journal of Cardiology, 124*(2), 270–277. https://doi.org/10.1016/j.amjcard.2019.04.026

Kanuha, V. K. (2013). "Relationships so loving and so hurtful": the constructed duality of sexual and racial/ethnic intimacy in the context of violence in Asian and Pacific Islander lesbian and queer women's relationships. *Violence Against Women, 19*(9), 1175–1196. https://doi.org/10.1177/1077801213501897

Kim, B., & Aronowitz, T. (2019). Invisible Minority: HIV Prevention Health Policy for the Asian American Population. *Policy, Politics, & Nursing Practice, 20*(1), 41–49. https://doi.org/10.1177/1527154419828843

Kim, K., Kim, B., Choi, E., Song, Y., & Han, H. R. (2015). Knowledge, perceptions, and decision making about human papillomavirus vaccination among Korean American women: a focus group study. *Women's Health Issues: Official Publication of the Jacobs Institute of Women's Health, 25*(2), 112–119. https://doi.org/10.1016/j.whi.2014.11.005

Kim, G. H., Liang, P. S., Bang, S. J., & Hwang, J. H. (2016). Screening and surveillance for gastric cancer in the United States: Is it needed? *Gastrointestinal Endoscopy, 84*(1), 18–28. https://doi.org/10.1016/j.gie.2017.02.028

Kim, H. J., Park, E., Storr, C. L., Tran, K., Juon, H. S. (2015). Depression among Asian-American adults in the community: Systematic review and meta-analysis. *PLoS One. 10*(6):e0127760. https://doi.org/10.1371/journal.pone.0127760

Kim, Y., Park, J., Nam, B. H., & Ki, M. (2015c). Stomach cancer incidence rates among Americans, Asian Americans and Native Asians from 1988 to 2011. *Epidemiology and Health, 37*, e2015006. https://doi.org/10.4178/epih/e2015006

Kim-Mozeleski, J. E., Tsoh, J. Y., Gildengorin, G., Cao, L. H., Ho, T., Kohli, S., Lam, H., Wong, C., Stewart, S., McPhee, S. J., & Nguyen, T. T. (2018). Preferences for depression help-seeking among Vietnamese American adults. *Community Mental Health Journal, 54*(6), 748–756. https://doi.org/10.1007/s10597-017-0199-3

King, W. M., Restar, A., & Operario, D. (2019). Exploring multiple forms of intimate partner violence in a gender and racially/ethnically diverse sample of transgender adults. *Journal of Interpersonal Violence*, 088626051987602. https://doi.org/10.1177/0886260519876024

Kwak, J., & Salmon, J. R. (2007) Attitudes and preferences of Korean-American older adults and caregivers on end-of-life care. *Journal of the American Geriatric Society, 55*(11), 1867–72.

Kwon, H. T., Ma, G. X., Gold, R. S., Atkinson, N. L., & Wang, M. Q. (2013). Primary care physicians' cancer screening recommendation practices and perceptions of cancer risk of Asian Americans. *Asian Pacific Journal of Cancer Prevention, 14*(3), 1999–2004. https://doi.org/10.7314/apjcp.2013.14.3.1999

Kwon, S. C., Kranick, J. A., Bougrab, N., Pan, J., Williams, R., Perez-Perez, G. I., & Trinh-Shevrin, C. (2019). Development and assessment of a heliobacter pylori medication adherence and stomach cancer prevention curriculum for a Chinese American immigrant population. *Journal of Cancer Education, 34*(4), 519–525. https://doi.org/10.1007/s13187-018-1333-9

Kwon, S. C., Wyatt, L. C., Islam, N. S., Yi, S. S., & Trinh-Shevrin, C. (2017). Obesity and modifiable cardiovascular disease risk factors among Chinese Americans in New York City, 2009–2012. *Preventing Chronic Disease, 14*, E38. https://doi.org/10.5888/pcd14.160582

Lau, J. D., Elbaar, L., Chao, E., Zhong, O., Yu, C. R., Tse, R., & Au, L. (2020). Measuring overweight and obesity in Chinese American children using US, international and ethnic-specific growth charts. *Public Health Nutrition, 23*(15), 2663–2670. https://doi.org/10.1017/S1368980020000919

Lau, A. S., Tsai, W., Shih, J., Liu, L. L., Hwang, W. C., & Takeuchi, D. T. (2013). The immigrant paradox among Asian American women: are disparities in the burden of depression and anxiety paradoxical or explicable? *Journal of Consulting and Clinical Psychology, 81*(5), 901–911. https://doi.org/10.1037/a0032105

Le, T. P., & Iwamoto, D. K. (2019). A longitudinal investigation of racial discrimination, drinking to cope, and alcohol-related problems among underage Asian American college students. *Psychology of Addictive Behaviors, 33*(6), 520–528. https://doi.org/10.1037/adb0000501

Lee, J. W., Brancati, F. L., & Yeh, H. C. (2011). Trends in the prevalence of type 2 diabetes in Asians versus Whites: results from the United States National Health Interview Survey, 1997-2008. *Diabetes Care, 34*(2), 353–357. https://doi.org/10.2337/dc10-0746

Lee, Y. M., Florez, E., Tariman, J., McCarter, S., & Riesche, L. (2015a). Factors related to sexual behaviors and sexual education programs for Asian-American adolescents. *Applied Nursing Research, 28*(3), 222–228. https://doi.org/10.1016/j.apnr.2015.04.015

Lee., J., & Hahm, H. C. (2012). HIV risk, substance use, and suicidal behaviors among Asian American lesbian and bisexual women. *AIDS Education and Prevention, 24*(6), 549–563. https://doi.org/10.1521/aeap.2012.24.6.549.

Lee, H. K, Han, B., Gfoerer, J. C. (2013). Differences in the prevalence rates and correlates of alcohol use and binge alcohol use among five Asian American subpopulations. *Addictive Behaviors, 38*(3), 1816–1823. https://doi.org/10.1016/j.addbeh.2012.11.001

Lee, H., Kim, M., Kiang, P., Shi, L., Tan, K., Chea, P., Peou, S., & Grigg-Saito, D. C. (2016). Factors Associated with HPV Vaccination among Cambodian American Teenagers. *Public Health Nursing (Boston, Mass.), 33*(6), 493–501. https://doi.org/10.1111/phn.12294

Lee, S., Zhai, S., Zhang, G. (Yolanda), Ma, X. S., Lu, X., Tan, Y., Siu, P., Seals, B., & Ma, G. X. (2015b). Factors associated with hepatitis c knowledge before and after an educational intervention among Vietnamese Americans. *Clinical Medicine Insights: Gastroenterology, 8*, CGast. S24737. https://doi.org/10.4137/CGast.S24737

Leong, F. T. L., & Lau, A. S. L. (2001). Barriers to providing effective mental health services to Asian Americans. *Mental Health Services Research, 3*(4), 201–214. https://doi.org/10.1023/a:1013177014788

Lewis, N. M., & Wilson, K. (2017). HIV risk behaviours among immigrant and ethnic minority gay and bisexual men in North America and Europe: A systematic review. *Social Science and Medicine, 179*, 115–128. https://doi.org/10.1016/j.socscimed.2017.02.033

Li, L. W., Ding, D., Wu, B., & Dong, X. (2017). Change of cognitive function in U.S. Chinese older adults: A Population-Based Study. *The Journals of Gerontology, Series A: Biological Sciences and Medical Sciences, 72*(Suppl 1), S5–S10. https://doi.org/10.1093/gerona/glx004

Li, L. W., & Dong, X. (2017). Self-reported Discrimination and Depressive Symptoms Among Older Chinese Adults in Chicago. *The Journals of Gerontology, Series A: Biological Sciences and Medical Sciences, 72*(Suppl 1), S119–S124. https://doi.org/10.1093/gerona/glw174

Lin, O. N., Chang, C., Lee, J., Do, A., Martin, M., Martin, A., & Nguyen, M. H. (2017). *HCV Prevalence in Asian Americans in California Journal of Immigrant and Minority Health, 19*(1), 91–97. https://doi.org/10.1007/s10903-016-0342-1

Liu, H., Lieberman, L., Stevens, E. S., Auerbach, R. P., & Shankman, S. A. (2017). Using a cultural and RDoC framework to conceptualize anxiety in Asian Americans. *Journal of Anxiety Disorders, 48*, 63–69. https://doi.org/j.janxdis2016.09.006

Lowry, R., Eaton, D. K., Brener, N. D., & Kann, L. (2011). Prevalence of health-risk behaviors among Asian American and Pacific Islander high school students in the U.S., 2001–2007. *Public Health Reports, 126*(1), 39–49.

McCracken, M., Olsen, M., Chen, M. S., Jr, Jemal, A., Thun, M., Cokkinides, V., Deapen, D., & Ward, E. (2007). Cancer incidence, mortality, and associated risk factors among Asian Americans of Chinese, Filipino, Vietnamese, Korean, and Japanese ethnicities. *CA: A Cancer Journal for Clinicians, 57*(4), 190–205. https://doi.org/10.3322/canjclin.57.4.190

McKeigue, P. M., Miller, G. J., & Marmot, M. G. (1989). Coronary heart disease in south Asians overseas: a review. *Journal of Clinical Epidemiology, 42*(7), 597–609. https://doi.org/10.1016/0895-4356(89)90002-4

Mayo Clinic. (2020). *Coronavirus disease* 2019. https://www.mayoclinic.org/diseases-conditions/coronavirus/symptoms-causes/syc-20479963

Miller, B. A., Chu, K. C., Hankey, B. F., & Ries, L. A. G. (2008). Cancer incidence and mortality patterns among specific Asian and Pacific Islander populations in the U.S. *Cancer Causes & Control, 19*, 227–258. https://10.1007/s10552-007-9088-3.

Millett, G. A., Jones, A. T., Benkeser, D., Baral, S., Mercer, L., Beyrer, C., Honermann, B., Lankiewicz, E., Mena, L., Crowley, J. S., Sherwood, J., & Sullivan, P. S. (2020). Assessing differential impacts of COVID-19 on Black communities. *Annals of epidemiology, 47*, 37–44. https://doi.org/10.1016/j.annepidem.2020.05.003

National Institutes of Health. (2021, July 2). *Rapid Acceleration of Diagnostics (RADx)*. https://www.nih.gov/research-training/medical-research-initiatives/radx

Nghiem, V. T., Davies, K. R., Chan, W., Mulla, Z. D., & Cantor, S. B. (2016). Disparities in cervical cancer survival among Asian-American women. *Annals of Epidemiology, 26*(1), 28–35. https://doi.org/10.1016/j.annepidem.2015.10.004

Nguyen, G. T., Chen, B., & Chan, M. (2012). Pap testing, awareness, and acceptability of a human papillomavirus (HPV) vaccine among Chinese American women. *Journal of Immigrant and Minority Health, 14* (5), 803–808. https://doi.org/10.1007/s10903-012-9607-5

Nguyen-Truong, C. K. Y., Hassouneh, D., Lee-Lin, F., Hsiao, C. Y., Le, T. V., Tang, J. Vu, M., & Truong, A. M. (2018). Health care providers' perspectives on barriers and facilitators to cervical cancer screening in Vietnamese American women. *Journal of Transcultural Nursing, 29*(5), 441–448. https://doi.org/10.1177/1043659617745135

Nije-Carr, V. P. S., Sabri, B., Messing, J. T., Ward-Lasher, A., Johnson-Agbakwu, C. E., McKinley, C., Campion, N., Childress, S., Arscott, J., & Campbell, J. (2019). Methodological and ethical considerations in research with immigrant and refugee survivors of intimate partner violence. *Journal of Interpersonal Violence*, 886260519877951. https://doi.org/10.1177/0886260519877951

Noppert, G. A., Wilson, M. L., Clarke, P., Ye, W., Davidson, P., & Yang, Z. (2017). Race and nativity are major determinants of tuberculosis in the U.S.: evidence of health disparities in tuberculosis incidence in Michigan, 2004–2012. *BMC Public Health, 17*(1), 538. https://doi.org/10.1186/s12889-017-4461-y

Ogden, C. L., Carroll, M. D., Lawman, H. G., Fryar, C. D., Kruszon-Moran, D., Kit, B. K., & Flegal, K. M. (2016). Trends in Obesity Prevalence Among Children and Adolescents in the United States, 1988–1994 Through 2013–2014. *JAMA, 315*(21), 2292–2299. https://doi.org/10.1001/jama.2016.6361

Oh, K. M., Taylor, K. L., & Jacobsen, K. H. (2017). Breast Cancer Screening Among Korean Americans: A Systematic Review. *Journal of Community Health, 42*(2), 324–332. https://doi.org/10.1007/s10900-016-0258-7

Oliver, S. E., Hoots, B. E., Paz-Bailey, G., Paz-Bailey, G., Markowitz, L. E., Meites, E., & NHBS Study Group (2017). Increasing human papillomavirus vaccine coverage among men who have sex with men - national HIV Behavioral Surveillance, United States, 2014. *Journal of Acquired Immunodeficiency Syndrome, 75* Suppl 3, S370–S374. https://doi.org/10.1097/QAI.0000000000001413

Ortiz, E., Scanlon, B., Mullens, A., & Durham, J. (2020). Effectiveness of Interventions for Hepatitis B and C: A Systematic Review of Vaccination, Screening, Health Promotion and Linkage to Care Within Higher Income Countries. *Journal of Community Health, 45*(1), 201–218. https://doi.org/10.1007/s10900-019-00699-6

Park, H., Choi, E., Park, Y. S., & Wenzel, J. A. (2018). Racial and ethnic differences in mental health among Asian Americans and Non-Hispanic Whites: Based on California Health Interview Survey. *Issues in Mental Health Nursing, 39*(3), 208–214. https://doi.org/10.1080/01612840.2017.1379575

Pham, C., Fong, T.-L., Zhang, J., & Liu, L. (2018). Striking racial/ethnic disparities in liver cancer incidence rates and temporal trends in California, 1988–2012. *Journal of the National Cancer Institute, 110*(11), 1259–1269. https://doi.org/10.1093/jnci/djy051

Pollack, H. J., Kwon, S. C., Wang, S. H., Wyatt, L. C., Trinh-Shevrin, C., & on behalf of the AAHBP Coalition. (2014). Chronic hepatitis b and liver cancer risks among Asian immigrants in New York City: Results from a large, community-based screening, evaluation, and treatment program. *Cancer Epidemiology Biomarkers & Prevention, 23*(11), 2229–2239. https://doi.org/10.1158/1055-9965.EPI-14-0491

Pu, J., Hastings, K. G., Boothroyd, D., Jose, P. O., Chung, S., Shah, J. B., Cullen, M. R., Palaniappan, L. P., & Rehkopf, D. H. (2017). Geographic variations in cardiovascular disease mortality among asian american subgroups, 2003–2011. *Journal of the American Heart Association, 6*(7). https://doi.org/10.1161/JAHA.117.005597

Rajpathak, S. N., Gupta, L. S., Waddell, E. N., Upadhyay, U. D., Wildman, R. P., Kaplan, R., Wassertheil-Smoller, S., & Wylie-Rosett, J. (2010). Elevated risk of type 2 diabetes and metabolic syndrome among Asians and south Asians: results from the 2004 New York City HANES. *Ethnicity & Disease, 20*(3), 225–230.

Rubin-Miller L, Alban C, Artiga S, & Sullivan S. (2020, September 16). *COVID-19 Racial disparities in testing, infection, hospitalization, and death: analysis of Epic patient data.* Kaiser Family Foundation. https://www.kff.org/report-section/covid-19-racial-disparities-in-testing-infection-hospitalization-and-death-analysis-of-epic-patient-data-issue-brief/

Russ, L. W., Meyer, A. C., Takahashi, L. M., Ou, S., Tran, J., Cruz, P., Magalong, M., & Candelario, J. (2012). Examining barriers to care: provider and client perspectives on the stigmatization of HIV-positive Asian Americans with and without viral hepatitis co-infection. *AIDS Care, 24*(10), 1302–1307. https://doi.org/10.1080/09540121.2012.658756

Ryu, S. Y., Crespi, C. M., & Maxwell, A. E. (2013). What factors explain disparities in mammography rates among Asian-American immigrant women? A population-based study in California. *Women's Health Issues, 23*(6), e403–e410. https://doi.org/10.1016/j.whi.2013.08.005

Sahker, E., Yeung, C. W., Garrison, Y. L., Park, S., & Arndt, S. (2017). Asian American and Pacific Islander substance use treatment admission trends. *Drug and Alcohol Dependence, 171,* 1–8. https://doi.org/10.1016/j.drugalcdep.2016.11.022

Sandil, R., Robinson, M., Brewster, M. E., Wong, S., & Geiger, E. (2015). Negotiating multiple marginalizations: experiences of South Asian LGBQ individuals. *Cultural Diversity & Ethnic Minority Psychology, 21*(1), 76–88. https://doi.org/10.1037/a0037070

Seo, J. Y., Li, J., & Li, K. (2018). Cervical cancer screening experiences among Chinese American immigrant women in the United States. *Journal of Obstetric, Gynecologic, and Neonatal Nursing, 47*(1), 52–63. https://doi.org/10.1016/j.jogn.2017.10.003

Shah, S. C., Nunez, H., Chiu, S., Hazan, A., Chen, S., Wang, S., Itzkowitz, S., & Jandorf, L. (2020) Low baseline awareness of gastric cancer risk factors amongst at-risk multiracial/ ethnic populations in New York City: results of a targeted, culturally sensitive pilot gastric cancer community outreach program. *Ethnicity & Health, 25*(2), 189–205. https://doi.org/10.1080/13557858.2017.1398317

Shi, Y., Steppi, A., Cao, Y., Wang, J., He, M. M., Li, L., & Zhang, J. (2017). Integrative comparison of mRNA expression patterns in breast cancers from Caucasian and Asian Americans with implications for precision medicine. *Cancer Research, 77*(2), 423–433. https://doi.org/10.1158/0008-5472.CAN-16-1959

Shoemaker, M. L., & White, M. C. (2016). Breast and cervical cancer screening among Asian subgroups in the USA: estimates from the National Health Interview Survey, 2008, 2010, ad 2013. *Cancer Causes Control, 27*(6), 825–829. https://doi.org/10.1007/s10552-016-0750-5

Shover, C. L., Javanbakht, M., Shoptaw, S., Bolan, R. K., Lee, S. J., Parsons, J. T., Rendina, J., & Gorbach, P. M. (2018). HIV Preexposure prophylaxis initiation at a large community clinic: differences between eligibility, awareness, and uptake. *American Journal of Public Jealth, 108*(10), 1408–1417. https://doi.org/10.2105/AJPH.2018.304623

Singh, S., Schulz, A. J., Neighbors, H. W., Griffith, D. M. (2017). Interactive effect of immigration-related factors with legal and discrimination acculturative stress in predicting depression among Asian American immigrants. *Community Mental Health Journal, 53*(6), 638–646. https://doi.org/10.1007/s10597-016-0064-9

Stennis, N., Trieu, L., Perri, B., Anderson, J., Mushtaq, M., & Ahuja, S. (2015). Disparities in tuberculosis burden among South Asians living in New York City, 2001–2010. *American Journal of Public Health, 105*(5), 922–929. https://doi.org/10.2105/AJPH.2014.302056

Su, F., Green, P. K., Berry, K., & Ioannou, G. N. (2017). The association between race/ethnicity and the effectiveness of direct antiviral agents for hepatitis C virus infection. *Hepatology, 65*(2), 426–438. https://doi.org/10.1002/hep.28901

Subica, A. M., & Wu, L. T. (2018). Substance use and suicide in Pacific Islander, American Indian, and multiracial youth. *American Journal of Preventive Medicine, 54*(6):795–805. https://doi.org/10.1016/j.amepre.2018.02.003

Tan, J. Y., Xu, L. J., Lopez, F. Y., Jia, J. L., Pho, M. T., Kim, K. E., & Chin, M. H. (2016). Shared decision making among clinicians and Asian American and Pacific Islander sexual and gender minorities: An intersectional approach to address a critical care gap. *LGBT Health, 3*(5), 327–334. https://doi.org/10.1089/lgbt.2015.0143

Thompson, C. A., Gomez, S. L., Hastings, K. G., Kapphahn, K., Yu, P. Shariff-Marco, S., Bhatt, A. S., Wakelee, H. A., Patel, M. I., Cullen, M. R., & Palaniappan, L. P. (2016). The burden of cancer in Asian Americans: A report of national mortality trends by Asian ethnicity. *Cancer Epidemiology, Biomarkers and Prevention, 10,* 1371–1382. https://doi.org/0.1158/1055-9965.EPI-16-0167

Toleran, D. E., Friese, B., Battle, R. S., Gardiner, P. Tran, P. D., Lam, J., & Cabangun, B. (2013). Correlates of HIV and HCV risk and testing among Chinese, Filipino, and Vietnamese men who have sex with men and other at-risk men. *AIDS Education and Prevention, 25*(3), 244–254. https://doi.org/0.1521/aeap.2013.25.3.244

Torre, L. A., Sauer, A. M. G., Chen, M. S., Kagawa-Singer, M., Jemal, A., & Siegel, R. L. (2016). Cancer statistics for Asian Americans, Native Hawaiians, and Pacific Islanders, 2016: Converging incidence in males and females: Cancer statistics for Asian Americans, Native Hawaiians, and Pacific Islanders, 2016. *CA: A Cancer Journal for Clinicians, 66*(3), 182–202. https://doi.org/10.3322/caac.21335

Tong, Y. (2013). Acculturation, gender disparity, and the sexual behavior of Asian American youth. *Journal of Sex Research, 50*(6), 560–573. https://doi.org/10.1080/00224499.2012.668976

Trinh-Shevrin, C., Kwon, S. C., Park, R., Nadkarni, S. K., & Islam, N. S. (2015). Moving the dial to advance population health equity in New York City Asian American populations. *American Journal of Public Health, 105,* 216–e25. https://doi.org/10.2105/AJPH.2015.302626

Trinh-Shevrin, C., Sacks, R., Ahn, J., & Yi, S.S. (2018). Opportunities and challenges in precision medicine: improving cancer prevention and treatment for Asian Americans. *Journal of Racial and Ethnic Health Disparities, 5*(1), 1–6. https://doi.org/10.1007/s40615-016-0334-9

Tsai, C. F., Thomas, B., & Sudlow, C. L. (2013). Epidemiology of stroke and its subtypes in Chinese vs White populations: a systematic review. *Neurology, 81*(3), 264–272. https://doi.org/10.1212/WNL.0b013e31829bfde3

U. S. Bureau of Labor Statistics. (2020). *Labor Force Statistics from the Current Population Survey.* https://www.bls.gov/cps/cpsaat11.htm

U.S. Department of Health and Human Services-Office of Minority Health. (2018). *Immunizations and Asians and Pacific Islanders.* https://minorityhealth.hhs.gov/omh/browse.aspx?lvl=4&lvlid=52

Virani, S. S., Alonso, A., Benjamin, E. J., Bittencourt, M. S., Callaway, C. W., Carson, A. P., Chamberlain, A. M., Chang, A. R., Cheng, S., Delling, F. N., Djousse, L., Elkind, M. S. V., Ferguson, J. F., Fornage, M., Khan, S. S., Kissela, B. M., Knutson, K. L., Kwan, T. W., Lackland, D. T., . . . & Tsao, C. W. On behalf of the American Heart Association Council on Epidemiology and Prevention Statistics Committee and Stroke Statistics Subcommittee. (2020). Heart disease and stroke statistics—2020 update: A report from the American Heart Association. *Circulation, 141*(9). https://doi.org/10.1161/CIR.0000000000000757

Volgman, A. S., Palaniappan, L. S., Aggarwal, N. T., Gutpa, M., Khandelwal, A., Krishnan, A. V., Lichtman, J. H., Mehta, L. S., Patel, H. N., Shah, K. S., Shah, S. H., Watson, K. E., American Heart Association Council on Epidemiology and Prevention, Cardiovascular Disease and Stroke in Women and Special Populations Committee of the Council on Clinical Oncology, Council on Cardiovascular and Stroke Nursing, Council on Quality of Care and Outcomes Research, & Stroke Council. (2018). Atherosclerotic cardiovascular disease in South Asians in the United States: Epidemiology, risk factors, and treatments: A scientific statement from the American Heart Association. *Circulation, 138*(1), e1–e34. https://doi.org./10.1161/CIR.0000000000000580

Warner, E. T., Tamimi, R. M., Hughes, M. E., Ottesen, R. A., Wong, Y. N., Edge, S. B., Theriault, R. L., Blayney, D. W., Niland, J. C., Winer, E. P., Weeks, J. C., & Partridge, A. H. (2015). Racial and ethnic differences in breast cancer survival: Mediating effect of tumor characteristics and sociodemographic and treatment factors. *Journal of Clinical Oncology: Official Journal of the American Society of Clinical Oncology, 33*(20), 2254–2261. https://doi.org/10.1200/JCO.2014.57.1349

Wei, C., Raymond, H. F., Wong, F. Y., Silvestre, A. J., Friedman, M. S., Documet, P., McFarland, W., & Stall, R. (2011). Lower HIV prevalence among Asian/Pacific Islander men who have sex with men: a critical review for possible reasons. *AIDS and Behavior, 15*(3), 535–549. https://doi.org/10.1007/s10461-010-9855-0

Wong, D. N., & Fan, W. (2018). Ethnic and sex differences in E-cigarette use and relation to alcohol use in California adolescents: the California Health Interview Survey. *Public Health, 157*, 147–152. https://doi.org/10.1016/j.puhe.2018.01.019

Wu, L. T., Blazer, D. G. (2015). Substance use disorders and co-morbidities among Asian Americans and Native Hawaiians/Pacific Islanders. *Psychological Medicine, 45*(3), 481–494. https://doi.org/10.1017/S0033291714001330

Wu, L. T., Blazer, D. G., Swartz, M. S., Burchett, B., Brady, K. T., & NIDA AAPI Workgroup. (2013). Illicit and nonmedical drug use among Asian Americans, Native Hawaiians/Pacific Islanders, and mixed-race individuals. *Drug and Alcohol Dependence, 133*(2), 360–367. https://doi.org/10.1016/j.drugalcdep.2013.06.008

Wu, P., Liu, X., Kim, J., & Fan, B. (2011). Ecstasy use and associated risk factors among Asian-American youth: findings from a national survey. *Journal of Ethnicity in Substance Use, 10*(2), 112–125. https://doi.org/10.1080/15332640.2011.573304

Wyatt, L. C., Ung, T., Park, R., Kwon, S. C., & Trinh-Shevrin, C. (2015). Risk factors of suicide and depression among Asian American, Native Hawaiian, and Pacific Islander youth: A systematic literature review. *Journal of Health Care for the Poor and Underserved, 26*(2 Suppl), 191–237. https://doi.org/10.1353/hpu.2015.0059

Wyatt, L. C., Russo, R., Kranick, J., Elfassy, T., Kwon, S. C., Wong, J. A., Đoàn, L. N., Trinh-Shevrin, C., & Yi, S. S. 2012–2018 Health Atlas for Asian Americans, Native Hawaiians, and Pacific Islanders: A comprehensive look at AA and NH&PI health in the U.S. https://med.nyu.edu/departments-institutes/population-health/divisions-sections-centers/health-behavior/sites/default/files/pdf/csaah-health-atlas.pdf

Xu, L., Tang, F., Li, L. W., & Dong, X. Q. (2017). Grandparent caregiving and psychological well-being among Chinese American older adults – The roles of caregiving burden and pressure. *The Journals of Gerontology, Series A: Biological Sciences and Medical Sciences, 72*(Suppl 1), S56–S62. https://doi.org/10.1093/gerona/glw186

Yan, B. W., Ng, F., Chu, J., Tsoh, J., & Nguyen, T. (2020, July 13) *Asian Americans facing high COVID-19 case fatality. Health Affairs Blog.* https://www.healthaffairs.org/do/10.1377/hblog20200708.894552/full/

Yang, K. G., Rodgers, C., Lee, E., & Lê Cook, B. (2020). Disparities in Mental Health Care Utilization and Perceived Need Among Asian Americans: 2012–2016. *Psychiatric Services (Washington, D.C.), 71*(1), 21–27. https://doi.org/10.1176/appi.ps.201900126

Yang, R. C., Mills, P. K., & Riordan, D. G. (2004). Cervical cancer among Hmong women in California, 1988 to 2000. *American Journal of Preventive Medicine, 27*(2), 132–138. https://doi.org/10.1016/j.amepre.2004.04.003

Yi, J. K., Anderson, K. O., Le, Y. C., Escobar-Chaves, S. L., & Reyes-Gibby, C. C. (2013). English proficiency, knowledge, and receipt of HPV vaccine in Vietnamese-American women. *Journal of Community Health, 38*(5), 805–811. https://doi.org/10.1007/s10900-013-9680-2

Yi, S. S., Thorpe, L. E., Zanowiak, J. M., Trinh-Shevrin, C., & Islam, N. S. (2016). Clinical characteristics and lifestyle behaviors in a population-based sample of Chinese and South Asian immigrants with hypertension. *American Journal of Hypertension, 28*, 631–639. https://doi.org/10.1093/ajh/hpw014

Yoshihama, M., Blazevski, J., & Bybee, D. (2014). Enculturation and attitudes toward intimate partner violence and gender roles in an Asian Indian population: Umplications for community-based prevention. *American Journal of Community Psychology, 53*(3–4), 249–260. https://doi.org/10.1007/s10464-014-9627-5

Yu, S. M., & Vyas, A. N. (2009). The health of children and adolescents. In C. Trinh-Shevrin, N. S. Islam, & M. J. Rey (Eds.) *Asian American Communities and Health (pp. 107–131).* Jossey-Bass.

Zhao, B., Jose, P. O., Pu., J., Chung, S., & Ancheta, I. B. (2015). Racial/ethnic differences in hypertension prevalence, treatment, and control for outpatients in northern California 2010–2012. *American Journal of Hypertension, 28*, 631–639. https://doi.org/10.1093/ajh/hpu189

Zheng, X., & Woo, B. K. (2016). Association between recognizing dementia as a mental illness and dementia knowledge among elderly Chinese Americans. *World Journal of Psychiatry, 6*(2), 233–238. https://doi.org/10.5498/wjp.v6.i2.233

Zhu, L., Zhai, S., Siu, P. T., Xia, H. Y., Lai, S., Zambrano, C. N., & Ma, G. X. (2019). Factors Related to Chinese Parents' HPV Vaccination Intention for Children. *American Journal of Health Behavior, 43*(5), 994–1005. https://doi.org/10.5993/AJHB.43.5.10

PART

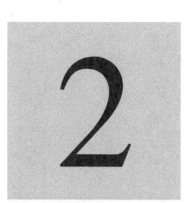

MEASURES

CHAPTER

4

OVERVIEW OF METHODOLOGIES USED TO GENERATE MEANINGFUL DATA FOR ASIAN AMERICAN POPULATIONS

RITI SHIMKHADA, NINEZ A. PONCE

LEARNING OBJECTIVES

By the end of this chapter, readers will be able to:

- Describe the federal data collection standards for gathering Asian American data in population-based studies.
- Identify strengths and challenges of different population-based study types for Asian American-focused health research.
- Describe data collection and study design best practices adapted from studies that have examined Asian American population health outcomes.

Applied Population Health Approaches for Asian American Communities, First Edition. Edited by Simona C. Kwon, Chau Trinh-Shevrin, Nadia S. Islam, and Stella S. Yi.
© 2023 John Wiley & Sons, Inc. Published 2023 by John Wiley & Sons, Inc.
Companion Website: www.wiley.com/go/kwon/asianamerican

INTRODUCTION

Collecting data about Asian Americans has improved remarkably since the early 1990s, when advocacy efforts began calling for the disaggregation of data for Asian American populations based on the diversity of their cultures, languages, and health needs (Ponce, 2011; Srinivasan & Guillermo, 2000). To date, disaggregated health data from large population-based surveys have shed light on disparities in morbidity and mortality between Asian American populations and provided insights on how health care providers and policymakers might better serve their Asian American patients (Choi, 2016; Mui et al., 2018; Ye et al., 2012; Zhang et al., 2020). Yet, to a surprising degree, studies using data from large population-based health surveys in the United States may not report disaggregated data for Asian American populations. Typically, this lack of disaggregated data is not the result of researchers disavowing the importance of disaggregation to better understand health trends for diverse groups of Asian Americans but rather because of the methodologic challenges that prevent them from studying a large enough sample of Asian Americans overall to allow for disaggregation and reporting of data for smaller Asian American groups (Ponce et al., 2015). In recent years, researchers and their community-based partners have intensified the demand to increase population-based survey data to better elucidate potentially dramatic health disparities between Asian American populations and address each population's specific health needs (Holland & Palaniappan, 2012; Islam, 2010; Ponce et al., 2015; Ro, 2002). The imperative to develop more robust health datasets for ethnic populations is particularly urgent for underserved Asian Americans with low socioeconomic status (Fuller-Thomson et al., 2011; Ghosh, 2010; Kuo, 1998; Lin-Fu, 1993; Nguyen, 2014; Quach et al., 2014; Srinivasan & Guillermo, 2000).

FEDERAL DATA COLLECTION STANDARDS FOR ASIAN AMERICANS

Developing and implementing supportive policies and guidance on collecting and reporting data for Asian Americans separately from Native Hawaiians and Pacific Islanders (NH/PIs) in federal population surveys was a critical step toward more complete disaggregation of Asian American and NH/PI populations (Holup et al., 2007). In 1997, the U.S. Office of Management and Budget (OMB) revised its Statistical Policy Directive No. 15, providing a common language for reporting data on race and ethnicity. The original 1977 directive defined only five distinct population groups by race and ethnicity (i.e., American Indian or Alaskan Native; Asian or Pacific Islander; Black; Hispanic; and White). The update defined the five groups by race only (i.e., American Indian or Alaska Native; Asian; Black or African American; Native Hawaiian or Other Pacific Islander; and White), while the Hispanic category was included as an ethnic categorization, complementary and potentially additional to any of the five racial categories. Subsequently, in 2011, the U.S. Department of Health and Human Services (HHS) issued data standards for race/ethnicity for all surveys conducted or sponsored by HHS per Section 4302 of the Affordable Care Act (ACA), insisting on further granularity for Asian Americans to distinguish between Asian Indian, Chinese, Filipino, Japanese, Korean, Vietnamese, and Other Asian subgroups. All of these subcategories aggregated to the five OMB standard categories. Similarly, the NH/PI category was disaggregated to four subgroups (Table 4.1).

POPULATION-BASED STUDIES

Population estimates from the U.S. Census Bureau, which administers the Census and the American Community Survey (ACS), suggest that Asian Americans comprise the fastest growing population in the United States. According to the 2000–2010 U.S. Census, the fastest-growing Asian American populations were Bhutanese (8,255% increase), Nepalese (561% increase), and Burmese Americans (500% increase). The U.S. Census is sent to every household in the United States every ten years to produce an accurate snapshot of the U.S. population.[1] Apart from being a key source of information for researchers across disciplines, the Census provides counts of people for the purposes of congressional apportionment and legislative redistricting.

In contrast to the U.S. Census, which collects data about each person in the population being surveyed, the ACS is a population-based survey. Population-based surveys collect data on a random sample of the population that is representative of the larger population of interest residing within defined geographic boundaries. To offer statistical reliability to researchers seeking to infer conclusions regarding key variables about the population of

TABLE 4.1 Federal Standards for the Collection of Data on Race and Ethnicity by HHS and OMB

Federal survey question and possible responses	Description
What is your race (one or more categories may be selected)? 1 White 2 Black 3 American Indian or Alaska Native	Three of the five OMB standards for reporting race in federal surveys
4 Asian Indian 5 Chinese 6 Filipino 7 Japanese 8 Korean 9 Vietnamese 10 Other Asian	These categories disaggregate Asian Americans into seven ethnic subgroups. All categories roll up to the OMB standard, "Asian"
11 Native Hawaiian 12 Guamanian or Chamorro 13 Samoan 14 Other Pacific Islander	These categories disaggregate NH/PI into four ethnic subgroups. All categories roll up to the OMB standard, "Native Hawaiian or Other Pacific Islander"

interest, the sample collected must be large enough to offer statistical reliability. Accordingly, the ACS is implemented on a continual basis and collects data on race/ethnicity, employment, education, transportation, and other demographic variables about populations residing within defined geographic boundaries. Each member of the population residing within the identified geographic zone has an equal and mutually exclusive chance of being selected for participation in the survey. ACS data is often the source of the Asian American control totals for comparison with data collected in other, more limited population-based health surveys.

The National Center for Health Statistics (NCHS), housed within HHS, collects data on health behaviors through a number of population-based health surveys. The two major federal health surveys include the National Health Interview Survey (NHIS) and the National Health and Nutrition Examination Survey (NHANES), which provide estimates of health and health care access and have been used extensively to track health status and progress toward achieving health objectives. NCHS datasets are the main sources of data used to describe health disparities and were among the first datasets used to examine the health of Asian American communities. Because of the large proportion of the total Asian American population residing in California, the California Health Interview Survey (CHIS), a statewide population-based health survey, was among the first datasets that brought to light the importance of examining Asian American health disparities. The CHIS is described in detail in a later section of this chapter.

Large population-based surveys are not appropriate for studies examining research questions specific to small groups, like individual Asian American ethnic groups. This is because pooled data from multiple survey years will not yield a large enough sample of the population of interest to allow for statistically stable results. Furthermore, while useful for studying disease prevalence, population-based surveys are not ideal for studying incidence or other, more granular aspects of diseases. Because of these and other limitations, researchers examining Asian American populations often turn to alternative data sources to examine health disparities and seek answers to detailed research questions about specific diseases or other health-related issues. Many researchers use data from epidemiologic studies or focused health surveys for Asian American groups of interest and for specific disease conditions. Increasingly, researchers are linking datasets, such as electronic health records (EHR), disease registries, and genomic data, across disparate systems. These linkages both facilitate more

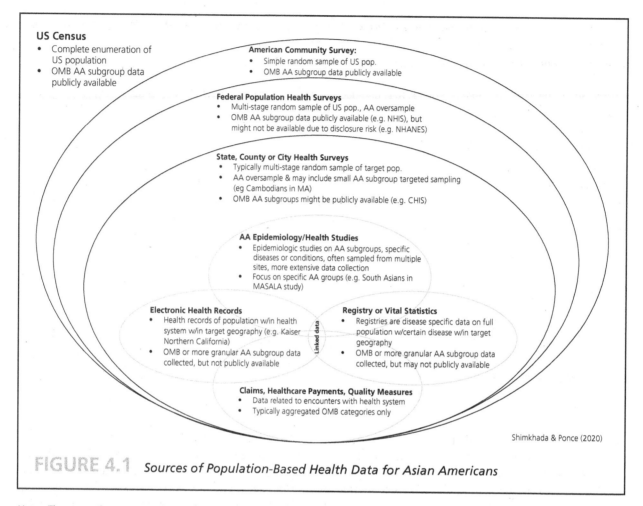

US Census
- Complete enumeration of US population
- OMB AA subgroup data publicly available

American Community Survey:
- Simple random sample of US pop.
- OMB AA subgroup data publicly available

Federal Population Health Surveys
- Multi-stage random sample of US pop., AA oversample
- OMB AA subgroup data publicly available (e.g. NHIS), but might not be available due to disclosure risk (e.g. NHANES)

State, County or City Health Surveys
- Typically multi-stage random sample of target pop.
- AA oversample & may include small AA subgroup targeted sampling (eg Cambodians in MA)
- OMB AA subgroups might be publicly available (e.g. CHIS)

AA Epidemiology/Health Studies
- Epidemiologic studies on AA subgroups, specific diseases or conditions, often sampled from multiple sites, more extensive data collection
- Focus on specific AA groups (e.g. South Asians in MASALA study)

Electronic Health Records
- Health records of population w/in health system w/in target geography (e.g. Kaiser Northern California)
- OMB or more granular AA subgroup data collected, but not publicly available

Registry or Vital Statistics
- Registries are disease specific data on full population w/certain disease w/in target geography
- OMB or more granular AA subgroup data collected, but may not publicly available

Linked data

Claims, Healthcare Payments, Quality Measures
- Data related to encounters with health system
- Typically aggregated OMB categories only

Shimkhada & Ponce (2020)

FIGURE 4.1 *Sources of Population-Based Health Data for Asian Americans*

Notes: The rectangle represents the entire United States. Ovals capture progressively smaller geographic boundaries and depict the major studies and sampling methods typically used in health research to obtain data about Asian American populations. OMB = Office of Management and Budget; NHIS = National Health Interview Survey; NHANES = National Health and Nutrition Examination Survey; CHIS = California Health Interview Survey; MASALA = Mediators of Atherosclerosis in South Asians Living in America.
Source: Adapted from Shimkhada & Ponce (2020).

detailed study of conditions and enrich the numbers of study subjects in particular populations to study, which is especially critical for studies of Asian American and NH/PI ethnic groups. Data related to encounters with the health system, such as health care quality measures, health care payments, and insurance claims, are also used in health disparities research among Asian American populations. Figure 4.1 summarizes these key sources of data. Case 2 in the Appendix provides an example of applying an integrative approach to studying lung cancer among Asian Americans.

DIVERSITY OF POPULATIONS AND POPULATION SIZES

Even though OMB Asian American data collection standards have largely been embraced by the research community, challenges persist. A key obstacle to conducting research on Asian American subpopulations is the lack of large enough samples to allow for sophisticated analyses of Asian ethnic groups. The Asian American population currently comprises about 6% of the total U.S. population (Lopez et al., 2017). Accordingly, in a survey sample of 10,000 U.S. households, we may expect to find only about 600 Asian Americans. Such a small number of Asian Americans within the total sample may preclude reliable multivariable analyses of Asian American

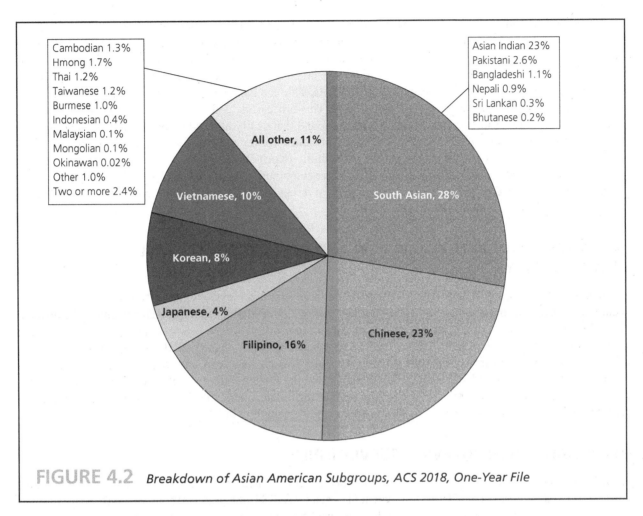

Cambodian 1.3%
Hmong 1.7%
Thai 1.2%
Taiwanese 1.2%
Burmese 1.0%
Indonesian 0.4%
Malaysian 0.1%
Mongolian 0.1%
Okinawan 0.02%
Other 1.0%
Two or more 2.4%

Asian Indian 23%
Pakistani 2.6%
Bangladeshi 1.1%
Nepali 0.9%
Sri Lankan 0.3%
Bhutanese 0.2%

All other, 11%
South Asian, 28%
Vietnamese, 10%
Korean, 8%
Japanese, 4%
Filipino, 16%
Chinese, 23%

FIGURE 4.2   *Breakdown of Asian American Subgroups, ACS 2018, One-Year File*

Source: American Community Survey 2018,1 year file; Asian alone, United States.

populations. This is particularly true for smaller Asian ethnic groups, such as Nepalis, Bhutanese, and Burmese – the very groups that have seen the largest population increases in the last U.S. Census but which still comprise small groups within the total U.S. population. Given the trade-offs in likelihood of selection of these smaller groups in a finite probability sample, Asian American populations are often aggregated into a single group.

Nationally, the largest Asian American subgroups – South Asian, Chinese, Filipino, Vietnamese, Korean, and Japanese Americans – make up nearly 90% of Asian Americans (Figure 4.2). In larger surveys that disaggregate Asian American subgroups, OMB standards identify and report data for these populations. The "Other Asian" subgroup includes a diverse mix of Asian Americans, many of whom are from groups with higher prevalence of lower socioeconomic status, such as Hmong and Cambodian Americans, as compared to larger Asian American subgroups, such as Chinese or Indian Asian Americans. For smaller subgroups, health surveys explicitly tailored to the unique needs of each group of interest must be developed and implemented. Because Asian American subgroup populations often cluster in particular counties, cities, or neighborhoods, examining health outcomes among Asian American groups residing in ethnic enclaves or larger areas with sizable proportions of the Asian American groups of interest can provide a wealth of information (see Case 3 in the Appendix).

As an example, due to the small size of the total Cambodian American population, federal and state-level population-based health surveys lack data for Cambodian Americans. Because the city of Lowell, Massachusetts, is home to the second largest Cambodian American community in the United States, the federal Centers for Disease Control (CDC) Racial and Ethnic Approaches to Community Health (REACH) initiative funded the Cambodian Community Health 2010 Project, a survey conducted by researchers in partnership with community-based organizations to identify health disparities among Cambodian Americans residing in Lowell.

Researchers conducted an area probability sample of Lowell focused on Cambodian American adults age 25 or older (Koch-Weser, 2006). To identify the geographic areas of Lowell most likely to include Cambodian American residents, investigators used data from the 2000 U.S. Census to focus on city blocks with a large proportion of respondents reporting Asian race and Khmer language. The blocks were stratified into groups based on high, medium, or low density of Cambodian residents. Thirteen blocks were selected from each stratum and participants were randomly selected from the stratum. This process yielded a sample of 381 Cambodian adults age 25 years or older. Within this sample, researchers found that nearly half (44%) of respondents reported fair or poor health. Those most likely to report fair or poor health were female, had fewer years living in the United States, were older, and were unable to work due to disability (Koch-Weser, 2006).

This example underscores the importance of collecting community-based data and working with community-based organizations to develop and implement surveys for Asian American populations in order to inform disease prevention and health promotion efforts.

ASIAN AMERICAN DATA COLLECTION AND REPORTING IN FEDERAL HEALTH SURVEYS

As mentioned previously, NCHS implements multiple large health surveys, including NHIS and NHANES, to generate statistical information to guide HHS policies and recommendations to improve the health of Americans. In 1990, the passage of the Disadvantaged Minority Health Improvement established subgroup classifications for racial/ethnic minority groups in NCHS surveys. In accordance with this change, NHIS began collecting data for Chinese, Japanese, Vietnamese, Filipino, Asian Indian, and Korean American subgroups, all of which rolled up to the Asian American standard category. Recognizing that the limited total population of Asian American prevented detailed analyses, in 2006, NHIS began oversampling Asian American to improve Asian American representation in the survey. NHANES began Asian American oversampling in 2011.

NATIONAL HEALTH INTERVIEW SURVEY (NHIS)

NHIS is the largest face-to-face health survey conducted in the United States (Centers for Disease Control and Prevention, n.d.; Parsons et al., 2014). Implemented annually, NHIS is the principal source of information for the non-institutionalized U.S. population on health status, health care access, and progress toward achieving national health objectives. To develop its sample population, NHIS uses multistage probability sampling of households to select clusters of households and non-institutional group quarters (e.g., homeless shelters) that are nested within primary sampling units (PSUs) that consist of a county, a small group of adjacent counties, or a metropolitan statistical area. Interviewers visit selected households and collect basic demographic information for each member of the household. Within each household, one adult and, if available, one child are randomly selected for a detailed health interview. Interviews are conducted only in English or Spanish, effectively excluding Asian American respondents who have low English proficiency. NHIS Public Use Files report data from the survey that serve as the key source of national health data for researchers.

From 2006–2015, the NHIS included an oversample of Asian Americans. Oversampling, which involves taking larger samples of certain populations than would otherwise be collected if random sampling were done, allowed for more Asian Americans to be interviewed than would have been possible if the NHIS sample was proportional to the U.S. population. This methodology was discontinued in 2016. From 2018 onward, instead of oversampling racial/ethnic minority groups at the household level, NHIS increased the probability of selection to be included in the survey if the sampled adult is a member of an underrepresented group that was oversampled in prior years. These groups included Asian Americans, as well as non-Hispanic Blacks (Blacks), Hispanics (Latino), and adults over age 65.

To determine race/ethnicity, interviewers ask respondents to identify the race and ethnicity, using OMB standard categories, for everyone living in the household. For Asian Americans, respondents may choose from the following ethnic subgroups: Asian Indian, Chinese, Filipino, Japanese, Korean, Vietnamese, or Other Asian. If a respondent reports more than one race for an individual in the household, the interviewer asks which one of the groups best represents the respondent's race. This response is then considered the individual's primary race.

Multiple race categories are not included in NHIS Public Use Files. When data from the interviews are imputed, respondents reporting more than one race are collapsed into a single multiracial category. For example, if a respondent reports her race as being both non-Hispanic White (White) and Asian American, those data are lost: the race is recorded only as "multiracial" – a category that includes all individuals reporting more than one race. Additionally, for respondents reporting that their race does not fall into one of the five OMB standards (American Indian or Alaska Native, Asian, Black or African American, Native Hawaiian or Pacific Islander, or White), the reported race is recoded or imputed into one of the five standard categories. For Asian Americans, only the largest subgroups – Chinese, Asian Indian, and Filipino – are reported in NHIS Public Use datasets. Due to small sample sizes, the OMB standard categories, Vietnamese, Japanese, Korean, and Other Asian, are not included in NHIS Public Use Files. Data for these smaller subgroups are made available to researchers only upon request to the NCHS Research Data Center.

NATIONAL HEALTH AND NUTRITION EXAMINATION SURVEY (NHANES)

NHANES assesses the health and nutritional status of noninstitutionalized adults and children in the United States on a continual basis. The survey is conducted in person and includes an interview, a physical examination, and laboratory tests. The interview component is conducted in the selected households, while the medical and laboratory components are conducted by physicians at Mobile Examination Centers (Centers for Disease Control and Prevention, n.d.; Chen et al., 2018).

As part of the in-person interview, demographic data are collected for each member of the selected household, including race and ethnicity data. For respondents who report more than one race, the interviewer does not ask the respondents with which race they most identify. When the selected respondent is a child, a parent is present for the interview and may respond on the child's behalf.

NHANES data describing the Asian American population are somewhat limited. For NHANES conducted during 2011–2018, oversampling of Asian Americans allowed NCHS to publish reliable estimates related to the health status of Asian Americans as a whole. However, despite oversampling, sample sizes for Asian American subgroups were small during each survey year and multiple survey cycles must be pooled to allow for analysis of those subgroups.

Due to the small sample sizes of Asian American subgroups and disclosure concerns associated with analyzing these data, disaggregated Asian American subgroup data are not publicly released. However, NHANES maintains restricted files that may be requested from the NCHS Research Data Center to allow for some subgroup analyses, provided that researchers use multiple years of pooled data for each Asian American subgroup of interest. These restricted files also contain more detailed data regarding race and ethnicity than are available publicly, including specific responses regarding race from respondents who reported more than one race.

GAPS AND OPPORTUNITIES

Although NHIS and NHANES are important sources of data on Asian American health, the lack of sufficient sample sizes to allow for rigorous data analyses limits the use of these datasets in health research focused on Asian American populations. Studies on diabetes using NHANES datasets, for example, have only presented Asian Americans in aggregate, masking ethnic differences that other studies have shown exist between Asian American subgroups (Menke et al., 2015).

To advance Asian American health research, building research and data capacity to contribute to a comprehensive study pipeline will allow for better monitoring and identification of Asian American health disparities. Regional, statewide, and county-based efforts are critical in building capacity. Typically, these sub-national initiatives are linked to local and community-based support, facilitating closer study of smaller Asian American ethnic groups. For example, the New York City (NYC) Department of Health and Mental Hygiene conducts the annual NYC Community Health Survey (CHS), through which the city has identified important health-related trends among Asian American subgroups (King & Deng, 2018). One such finding is that prevalence of diabetes among South Asians in NYC is higher than that of any other Asian American population – a worrying trend that warrants further study to inform the development of tailored interventions for that community. Investing additional financial resources in these types of local or regional studies over time will also contribute to building a more comprehensive database of health information for Asian Americans overall. Longitudinal studies on Asian American populations are expensive and, given the financial constraints inherent in funding large-scale follow-up studies, these studies must be limited to only a few Asian American populations. Yet the information gathered could accelerate our understanding of Asian American health behaviors, as prospectively collected data can mitigate biases associated with recall bias and exposure ascertainment and are particularly valuable for capturing exposures and outcomes over the life-course.

Community engagement is an essential piece of this process. Not only may community engagement help to identify areas where capacity building is most essential, but also community-based organizations and other community partners may assist in fundraising or advocacy efforts to develop new data collection efforts that build the datasets necessary for sophisticated analyses of health trends for each Asian American subgroup.

Over the last decade, several large studies have been conducted that offer models for study design and provide a foundation upon which future studies about Asian American populations may build. Several examples are described below.

EPIDEMIOLOGIC STUDIES ON ASIAN AMERICAN POPULATIONS

NLAAS

The National Latino and Asian American Study (NLAAS) was a groundbreaking cross-sectional study focused on mental health and mental health service utilization among Latino and Asian American adults age 18 and over. NLAAS was the first epidemiological study that prioritized data collection for Asian Americans (Takeuchi et al., 2012). To allow for subgroup analyses, respondents were stratified into the following ethnic subgroup categories: Puerto Rican, Cuban, Mexican, Other Latinos, Chinese, Vietnamese, Filipino, and Other Asians. Unlike other national studies, NLAAS engaged fully bilingual lay interviewers capable of administering the survey instrument in the respondent's choice of the following languages: English, Spanish, Chinese, Vietnamese, or Tagalog. The NLAAS included a multistage national area probability sample of the noninstitutionalized U.S. adult population. In order to obtain large enough samples of Latino and Asian Americans, NLAAS used supplemental samples focusing on regions with a high density of Latino and Asian American households (Heeringa et al., 2004).

MESA and MASALA

The Multi-Ethnic Study of Atherosclerosis (MESA) was a prospective cohort study conducted over two decades (2000–2020) that examined predictors of cardiovascular disease (CVD) in an ethnically diverse population (Bild et al., 2002). The sample was drawn from adults age 45–84 years residing in the catchment area of one of six field centers across the United States. Most Asian Americans in the sample were of Chinese descent. Consequently, results from MESA have proven instrumental to understanding CVD risk factors and outcomes among Chinese Americans. Modeled on MESA, the Mediators of Atherosclerosis in South Asians Living in America (MASALA), launched in 2010 and currently still underway, is a longitudinal cohort study of South Asian adults without known CVD (Kanaya et al., 2013). Study participants were drawn from two clinical sites in two different geographic locations in the United States: the San Francisco Bay Area and the greater Chicago area. To be eligible for participation, MASALA respondents had to identify with South Asian origin and have at least three grandparents born in one of the following countries: India, Pakistan, Bangladesh, Nepal, or Sri Lanka.

MEC

The Multiethnic Cohort (MEC) study, which recruited participants during 1993–1996 and remains ongoing, is a prospective cohort study designed to provide data on cancer and other chronic diseases for a diverse range of ethnic groups across various socioeconomic levels (Kolonel et al., 2000). The MEC sample included over 215,000 adults from the states of Hawaii and California (predominately Los Angeles County) who were between the ages of 45–75 years at the time of recruitment. Participants were coded as being from one of five racial/ethnic groups: African American, Japanese American, Latino, Native Hawaiian, and White. Because the MEC includes a specific category for Japanese Americans, with 56,921 enrolled at baseline, the MEC is a key source of cancer-related data for this Asian American group. Additionally, unlike NHANES and NHIS, participants could report identification with more than one ethnic group.

The cohort was assembled primarily through Department of Motor Vehicle files for the state of Hawaii and Los Angeles County, California. To identify incident cancers in the sample population, cohort data are linked to the Hawaii and California National Cancer Institute (NCI)-funded Surveillance, Epidemiology, and End Results (SEER) tumor registries. SEER data include information about cancer site, stage, histology, differentiation, grade, and disease-specific and overall survival. The MEC cohort also links to state and national vital statistics data, various claims databases, and neighborhood and environmental data.

EHRs

Due to the specific health care needs as well as the limitations in studying small Asian American populations using survey data, there has been much interest in exploring alternate data sources that can be used for research, such EHR data. In 2009, the Institute of Medicine (IOM) Subcommittee on Standardized Collection of Racial/Ethnicity Data for Healthcare Quality Improvement recommended that more granular race and ethnicity information be captured in EHRs (Institute of Medicine, 2009). Recent studies using EHR data have illuminated variations in clinical outcomes among different Asian American populations (Devers, 2013). For example, a large cohort study using EHR data conducted by a health system in Northern California that serves a large population of Asian Americans found that Filipino, South Asians, and PIs had a significantly higher risk of CVD as compared to other Asian American and NH/PI groups, to the extent that the authors recommended these particular populations never be combined with other Asian American ethnic groups in future CVD-related research (Gordon et al., 2019).

EHR data may also be used to identify patients from Asian American ethnic groups for recommended preventive screenings and for tailored interventions. These data may also be used to produce quality metrics for disease management and prevention specific to Asian American subgroups. Importantly, EHR data may allow clinicians and researchers to examine health outcomes for these groups, reducing the reliance on self-report data.

As noted earlier, to further examine associations among health-related and other variables for Asian American populations, EHRs may be linked with disease registries, genomics databases, insurance claims databases, and health care payment (payor) databases. To create deterministic linkages between these data sources, researchers typically use a combination of individual identifiers, such as social security numbers and date of birth, with health insurance claim numbers or medical record numbers. Hospital- or area-level identifiers may link EHR data to geographic- or facility-level data.

Disease Registries

Most health care institutions collect detailed information for chronic conditions such as cancer, diabetes, and asthma in disease registries. Disease registries are databases that contain information about patients who have been diagnosed with those particular conditions. These databases allow clinicians, administrators, and researchers to examine quality measures related to the disease of interest among their patient populations. Typically, these registries link to the institution's EHRs; and ideally, because health care institutions collect race/ethnicity data in their EHRs, these registries should allow for the exploration of disease-related outcomes and other variables in racial/ethnic groups of interest. For example, in a federally qualified health center that serves a racially diverse low-income population, the development of a diabetes registry linked to the EHR will allow clinicians to query the system to explore diabetes outcomes among South Asian patients – an Asian American population known to have higher rates of diabetes than the general population.

On a broader scale, national disease registries provide detailed information that may facilitate Asian American subgroup analyses. For example, NCI's SEER registries and the CDC's National Program of Cancer Registries (NPCR) collect detailed race/ethnicity data related to individuals with incident cancers. Although state cancer registries collect Asian American subgroup data with designated codes, statistics are often aggregated due to small sample sizes of distinct Asian American populations. In states with large Asian American populations, such as California, disaggregated Asian American data are available from population-based cancer registries and have been a key source of data for many studies, such as liver cancer (Pham et al., 2018), colorectal cancer (Ellis et al., 2018), breast cancer (Gomez et al., 2017), and lung cancer (see Case 2 in the Appendix). With pooling and other interpolation methods, cancer trends among specific Asian American ethnic groups have been examined across states and regions (Gomez, 2013).

METHODOLOGICAL CHALLENGES AND BEST PRACTICES

Population-based sampling aims to obtain a representative sample of the total population of interest; that is, members of the sample must have characteristics similar to those of the broader population. Developing a representative sample of any single Asian American ethnic group presents methodological challenges that must be resolved to ensure the resulting dataset allows for meaningful analyses. In this section, we describe the methodologies currently being adapted to overcome these challenges and build representative samples for Asian Americans.

Typically, in order to study specific Asian American populations, researchers employ regional sampling and oversampling from regions with high concentrations of Asian Americans. (Feinleib, 1993; Holland & Palaniappan, 2012; Islam et al., 2010; Ponce, 2009; Ponce, 2011; Srinivasan & Guillermo, 2000). However, within larger surveys, such as the NHIS, multistage sampling is used to build a representative sample of smaller populations, including Asian American ethnic groups. With this methodology, researchers first focus on a fixed number of census tracts known be home to a minimum level of the Asian American group of interest. This minimum level varies and is defined by the specific study protocol. At the second stage, researchers randomly select census blocks for further study. Lastly, researchers may use lists of phone numbers or addresses of households on those blocks and select residents with surnames that match the particular ethnic group of interest. These data may then be pooled across several survey cycles to build a larger Asian American sample to facilitate analyses. Yet, even when researchers employ these methodologies to bolster Asian American population size, the samples used in survey-based studies remain relatively small, leading to inconsistent findings across studies. Small Asian American group samples have also limited researchers' ability to examine variation by gender and age within each Asian American ethnic group.

According to the Pew Research Center, new methods of polling the population of interest may increase the number of Asian Americans included in research (Kennedy and Ruiz, 2020). An example of these new methods is switching the survey methodology from telephone random digit dialing (RDD) to internet-based selection to increase survey participation. In the new sampling method for Pew's American Trends Panel (ATP), a nationally representative panel of randomly selected U.S. adults, researchers identify a sample of individuals by their residential addresses and then mail a letter to the selected individuals detailing instructions for accessing and completing an online self-administered survey panel consisting of multiple cross-sectional surveys. Potential participants who do not have internet access at home are given a table and wireless connection. With this approach, Pew is able to increase the number of Asian American panel participants over time on an ongoing basis rather than needing to build new samples at the start of each survey. It should be noted, however, that the survey is administered only in English and Spanish, potentially limiting participation by Asian Americans with limited English proficiency.

It may also be useful to learn from non-random sampling methodologies that have been developed for surveying traditionally hard-to-reach populations to identify strategies for better capturing Asian American groups that are small or difficult to include using standard survey methods (Badowski et al., 2017; Galinsky et al., 2019). Quasi-probability sample designs are increasingly used to sample populations that may not be found with traditional oversampling methods due to their small sizes and lack of neighborhood clustering. These designs include respondent-driven sampling (RDS) and venue-based sampling. RDS is similar to what is known as "snowball sampling," in which researchers begin with a purposive selection of a few members of the hard-to-reach population of interest. These individuals are referred to as "seed participants." From among their acquaintances, each seed participant recruits a predetermined number of additional members of the population of interest. Venue-based sampling relies on the assumption that members of the hard-to-reach population may be sampled at locations they are likely to visit, such as special ethnic markets or festivals. Unlike traditional probability sampling designs, RDS and venue-based sampling do not employ random selection. Thus, the biggest drawback to the use of these methods is that the population of interest may not be adequately represented in the study sample, limiting the generalizability of results.

CALIFORNIA HEALTH INTERVIEW SURVEY

The California Health Interview Survey (CHIS) offers an excellent example of how researchers may adapt methodologies to effectively gather and analyze data about small racial/ethnic groups to inform policy and programming. Conducted since 2001, CHIS is the largest state-based population health survey in the United States and has facilitated the generation of population-based Asian American subgroup estimates used in studies nationwide (Ponce, 2009; Ponce, 2011). Researchers continue to develop innovative approaches to implementing the CHIS, focusing on improving cost-effective approaches to increasing the sample yield for NH/PI populations, including address-based sampling and respondent-driven sampling (UCLA Center for Health Policy Research, 2018b). The CHIS represents the forefront of data disaggregation for both Asian American and NH/PI for several reasons. First, CHIS collects detailed health and sociodemographic data by Asian American and NH/PI subgroup. These data roll up to the larger OMB category for Asian Americans, but CHIS also makes the disaggregated data for each ethnic group publicly available to researchers, community-based groups, and other interested parties. Second, CHIS uses oversampling to ensure sufficient numbers of Asian Americans are included in the data collection procedures to allow for meaningful analyses. Third, CHIS conducts interviews in six Asian languages (i.e., Cantonese, Mandarin, Korean, Vietnamese, Khmer, and Tagalog), in addition to English and Spanish, to facilitate participation by a diverse cross-section of Asian Americans with various immigration histories and socioeconomic and education levels.

CHIS uses a continuous data collection strategy that aims to reach 40,000 households during every two-year survey cycle. Data are collected from adults (age 18 and older), adolescents (age 12-17), and, for children age 0-11, the most knowledgeable adults able to answer on their behalf. Demographic information, including race/ethnicity, are self-reported directly by adult and adolescent respondents and by the most knowledgeable adult (usually a parent) for children age 0-11. CHIS collects information on race/ethnicity using several questions (see Table 4.2). Consistent with OMB race/ethnicity questions, interviewers first inquire about Latino ethnicity. Next, interviewers ask about race in a separate question with the following response categories: Native Hawaiian, Other Pacific Islander, American Indian, Alaska Native, Asian, Black/African American, White, or other. Respondents may select as many racial categories as applicable. For respondents who report Asian American race, interviewers ask a follow-up question about ethnicity, which includes eighteen possible population categories. Responses to these questions are coded into summary measures that are published in the Public Use File. To code race measures, CHIS combines responses from all of these subgroups into OMB's five standard categories for single race and offers an additional category for those who report more than one race. Another race variable categorizes respondents based on single race, and for those who report more than one race, the race with which they most identify. In addition to the Public Use Files, CHIS maintains restricted access data files that provide even more granular data for racial subpopulations.

To better understand associations between immigration status and race/ethnicity, CHIS gathers data on mother's and father's place of birth, English language proficiency, and other characteristics essential to understanding immigrant health. Since its inception, CHIS has also asked questions about citizenship and permanent resident status, using a consistent format. California has the nation's largest foreign-born population, both in terms of absolute size and percent of total population. Immigration status has been shown to impact access to health and other essential services and also to influence the lived experiences of immigrant communities (Ingram, 2020; Martinez, 2014; Park et al., 2019). However, questions related to immigration are not easy to ask, particularly within the current political climate, which is unfavorable to undocumented immigrants and even to those holding temporary or permanent resident status. To protect the data of respondents, CHIS has explicitly outlined privacy protections for individuals being surveyed which include clear language regarding the confidentiality of respondents' data and data security technology that is regularly updated and monitored to protect against data breaches. With these measures in place, CHIS has demonstrated that it is possible to include questions on citizenship and immigrant status in population health surveys to describe the health needs of immigrant populations and advance health equity for all Americans.

From 2001 until 2018, the CHIS sample design and data collection methodology used RDD computer-assisted telephone interviews (CATI) (UCLA Center for Health Policy Research, 2018a). Beginning in 2019, CHIS transitioned to a methodology more similar to that used by the Pew Research Center's ATP, described above. CHIS now uses a mixed-mode methodology (internet and telephone) to identify respondents (UCLA

TABLE 4.2 **CHIS Questions Relevant to Asian American Data Collection**

Are you Latino or Hispanic?

Yes/No

[You said you are Latino or Hispanic. Also,] please tell me which one or more of the following you would use to describe yourself. Would you describe yourself as Native Hawaiian, Other Pacific Islander, American Indian, Alaska Native, Asian, Black, African American, or White?

White/ Black or African American / Asian
American Indian or Alaska Native
Native Hawaiian/ Other Pacific Islander
Other (Specify:_____)

You said, Asian, and what specific ethnic group are you? Check all that apply
1. Bangladeshi
2. Burmese
3. Cambodian
4. Chinese
5. Filipino
6. Hmong
7. Indian (India)
8. Indonesian
9. Japanese
10. Korean
11. Laotian
12. Malaysian
13. Pakistani
14. Sri Lankan
15. Taiwanese
16. Thai
17. Vietnamese
Other Asian (specify:____)

You said you are [multiple responses from above]; do you identify with one race in particular?

Which race do you most identify with?

What languages do you speak at home? Check all that apply
1. English
2. Spanish
3. Cantonese
4. Vietnamese
5. Tagalog
6. Mandarin
7. Korean
8. Asian Indian languages
9. Russian
10. Japanese
11. French
12. German
13. Farsi
14. Armenian
15. Arabic

(Continued)

TABLE 4.2 (*Continued*)

[Since you speak a language other than English at home, we are interested in your own opinion of how well you speak English] Would you say you speak English. . .
1. Very well
2. Well
3. Not well
4. Not at all

In what country were you born
1. United States
2. American Samoa
3. Canada
4. China
5. Guam
6. Japan
7. Korea
8. Mexico
9. Philippines
10. Puerto Rico
11. Vietnam
12. Virgin Islands
13. Other (specify:____)

In what country was your mother born? (same categories as above)
In what country was your father born? (same categories as above)

Are you a citizen of the United States?
1. Yes
2. No
3. Application pending

Are you a permanent resident with a green card? Your answers are confidential and will not be recorded to Immigration Services.
1. Yes
2. No
3. Application pending

About how many years have you lived in the United States?
Year first came to live in the U.S.

Center for Health Policy Research, 2018b). Using a random sample of California addresses, CHIS randomly selects households for participation and mails a letter inviting one adult member of the household to complete the survey online. For households with eligible children age 0 to 11 years, a parent or other responsible adult is asked to respond to questions about one randomly selected child in the household, identified by CHIS. For households with adolescents age 12 to 17 years, the parent or responsible adult is asked for permission to allow one randomly selected adolescent complete the survey online or by telephone.

The mailed letter provides information in multiple languages about CHIS and instructions on how to securely access the study website. The online survey is currently available in five languages: English, Spanish, Chinese, Korean, and Vietnamese. Following the initial letter, CHIS sends a reminder postcard and, if needed, a second letter to the household to encourage participation. For households with a valid telephone number who do not complete the survey within about a five-week time frame, interviewers attempt to complete the interview over the telephone. Households are also be provided a telephone number that they can call if they prefer to complete the survey with a trained telephone interviewer. Trained interviewers are able to conduct the survey over the telephone in the same five languages as the online survey, as well as Tagalog.

SUMMARY AND RECOMMENDATIONS

Developing national policies to require the collection and reporting of data on Asian American populations has been a critical step in facilitating Asian American data disaggregation in health research (Ponce et al., 2016). State legislation can further help encourage disaggregation efforts. For example, under the auspices of Assembly Bill No. 1726 (AB-1726), which was passed in 2016 and will come into full effect in 2022, the State of California will track major disease and mortality trends, pregnancy rates, and housing-related data for additional Asian American populations including Bangladeshi, Hmong, Indonesian, Malaysian, Pakistani, Sri Lankan, Taiwanese, Thai, Fijian, and Tongan Americans. The bill also authorizes the collection of education-related data to track admission, enrollment, completion, and graduation rates for these populations.

Researchers have a key role to play in pushing these efforts forward. As detailed in this chapter, methodologies that prioritize data disaggregation may be woven into the fabric of study design at all levels – neighborhood/community, city, state, regional, and national. Looking toward the future, we highlight the following strategies and priorities:

- Community involvement should be considered a high priority in Asian American research not simply to improve Asian American participation but also to ensure that study results are disseminated to the community and used to improve the health of the populations of interest.

- Careful consideration of the needs of the populations of interest must drive decisions regarding which populations require oversampling, how data should be disaggregated, and how results should be disseminated. In general, population-based surveys should aim to oversample Asian Americans in the population of interest and ensure that Asian Americans from the largest ethnic groups residing within the geographic boundaries of the survey area are represented. However, when small Asian American populations in the area are known to have unique needs (e.g., Hmong, Bhutanese), researchers should prioritize these smaller populations.

- Sampling methodologies must encompass individuals representing the wide range of socioeconomic levels and demographic characteristics that may be found among Asian Americans.

- Surveys must be translated into multiple Asian languages to facilitate participation by smaller Asian American populations.

- Extant non-research datasets (e.g., claims, payor databases) offer great potential as reference populations for the exploration of potential associations between sociodemographic characteristics and chronic disease outcomes. Increasing the availability of disaggregated data for Asian American populations in these datasets through greater investment in data collection and more consistent reporting of disaggregated data must be a priority to facilitate use of these data for health disparities research.

DISCUSSION QUESTIONS

1. What are the main challenges of conducting population-based studies among Asian Americans?

2. What are the strengths and weaknesses of federally supported large national datasets in examining Asian American health outcomes?

3. Are there ways to better survey small Asian American populations?

NOTE

1. In statistics, a population is a group of people defined by boundaries of geography and any other restrictions, such as a particular ethnicity, age group, sex, or occupation, from which information is gathered.

REFERENCES

Badowski, G., Somera, L. P., Simsiman, B., Lee, H.-R., Cassel, K., Yamanaka, A., & Ren, J. (2017). The efficacy of respondent-driven sampling for the health assessment of minority populations. *Cancer Epidemiology, 50*, 214–220. https://doi.org/10.1016/j.canep.2017.07.006

Bild, D. E. (2002). Multi-ethnic study of atherosclerosis: Objectives and design. *American Journal of Epidemiology, 156*(9), 871–881. https://doi.org/10.1093/aje/kwf113

Centers for Disease Control and Prevention. (n.d.). *National Health and Nutrition Examination Survey.* https://www.cdc.gov/nchs/nhanes/

Centers for Disease Control and Prevention. (n.d.). *National Health Interview Survey.* https://www.cdc.gov/nchs/nhis

Chen, T. C., Parker, J. D., Clark, J., Shin, H. C., Rammon, J. R., & Burt, V. L. (2018). National health and nutrition examination survey: Estimation procedures, 2011–2014. *Vital and Health Statistics. Series 2, Data Evaluation and Methods Research, 177*, 1–26.

Choi, S. (2016). Sub-ethnic and geographic variations in out-of-pocket private health insurance premiums among mid-life Asians. *Journal of Aging and Health, 29*(2), 222–246. https://doi.org/10.1177/0898264316635563

Devers, K. (2013, September). *The Feasibility of Using Electronic Health Records (EHRs) and Other Electronic Health Data for Research on Small Populations. Urban Institute.*

Ellis, L., Abrahão, R., McKinley, M., Yang, J., Somsouk, M., Marchand, L. L., Cheng, I., Gomez, S. L., & Shariff-Marco, S. (2018). Colorectal cancer incidence trends by age, stage, and racial/ethnic group in California, 1990–2014. *Cancer Epidemiology Biomarkers & Prevention, 27*(9), 1011–1018. https://doi.org/10.1158/1055-9965.EPI-18-0030

Feinleib, M. (1993). Data needed for improving the health of minorities. *Annals of Epidemiology, 3*(2), 199–202. https://doi.org/10.1016/1047-2797(93)90138-T

Fuller-Thomson, E., Brennenstuhl, S., & Hurd, M. (2011). Comparison of disability rates among older adults in aggregated and separate Asian American/Pacific Islander subpopulations. *American Journal of Public Health, 101*(1), 94–100. https://doi.org/10.2105/AJPH.2009.176784

Galinsky, A. M., Simile, C., Zelaya, C. E., Norris, T., & Panapasa, S. V. (2019). Surveying strategies for hard-to-survey populations: Lessons from the Native Hawaiian and Pacific Islander national health interview survey. *American Journal of Public Health, 109*(10), 1384–1391. https://doi.org/10.2105/AJPH.2019.305217

Ghosh, C. (2010). A national health agenda for Asian Americans and Pacific Islanders. *JAMA, 304*(12), 1381. https://doi.org/10.1001/jama.2010.1358

Gomez, S. L., Von Behren, J., McKinley, M., Clarke, C. A., Shariff-Marco, S., Cheng, I., Reynolds, P., & Glaser, S. L. (2017). Breast cancer in Asian Americans in California, 1988–2013: Increasing incidence trends and recent data on breast cancer subtypes. *Breast Cancer Research and Treatment, 164*(1), 139–147. https://doi.org/10.1007/s10549-017-4229-1

Gomez, S. L., Noone, A.-M., Lichtensztajn, D. Y., Scoppa, S., Gibson, J. T., Liu, L., Morris, C., Kwong, S., Fish, K., Wilkens, L. R., Goodman, M. T., Deapen, D., & Miller, B. A. (2013). Cancer incidence trends among Asian American populations in the United States, 1990-2008. *Journal of the National Cancer Institute, 105*(15), 1096–1110. https://doi.org/10.1093/jnci/djt157

Gordon, N. P., Lin, T. Y., Rau, J., & Lo, J. C. (2019). Aggregation of Asian-American subgroups masks meaningful differences in health and health risks among Asian ethnicities: An electronic health record based cohort study. *BMC Public Health, 19*(1), 1551. https://doi.org/10.1186/s12889-019-7683-3

Heeringa, S. G., Wagner, J., Torres, M., Duan, N., Adams, T., & Berglund, P. (2004). Sample designs and sampling methods for the collaborative psychiatric epidemiology studies(Cpes). *International Journal of Methods in Psychiatric Research, 13*(4), 221–240. https://doi.org/10.1002/mpr.179

Holland, A. T., & Palaniappan, L. P. (2012). Problems with the collection and interpretation of Asian-American health data: Omission, aggregation, and extrapolation. *Annals of Epidemiology, 22*(6), 397–405. https://doi.org/10.1016/j.annepidem.2012.04.001

Holup, J. L., Press, N., Vollmer, W. M., Harris, E. L., Vogt, T. M., & Chen, C. (2007). Performance of the US Office of Management and Budget's revised race and ethnicity categories in Asian populations. *International Journal of Intercultural Relations, 31*(5), 561–573. https://doi.org/10.1016/j.ijintrel.2007.02.001

Ingram, M. (2020). Immigrants and access to care: Public health must lead the way in changing the nation's narrative. *American Journal of Public Health, 110*(9), 1260–1261. https://doi.org/10.2105/AJPH.2020.305790

Institute of Medicine. (2009). *Race, Ethnicity, and Language Data: Standardization for Health Care Quality Improvement.* The National Academies Press.

Islam, N. S., Khan, S., Kwon, S., Jang, D., Ro, M., & Trinh-Shevrin, C. (2010). Methodological issues in the collection, analysis, and reporting of granular data in Asian American populations: historical challenges and potential solutions. *Journal of Health Care for the Poor and Underserved, 21*(4), 1354–1381. https://doi.org/10.1353/hpu.2010.0939

Kanaya, A. M., Kandula, N., Herrington, D., Budoff, M. J., Hulley, S., Vittinghoff, E., & Liu, K. (2013). Mediators of atherosclerosis in South Asians living in America (Masala) study: Objectives, methods, and cohort description: Masala study methods and characteristics. *Clinical Cardiology, 36*(12), 713–720. https://doi.org/10.1002/clc.22219

Kennedy, C., & Ruiz, N. G. (2020) *Polling Methods are Changing, But Reporting the Views of Asian Americans Remains a Challenge.* https://pewrsr.ch/2YPlTaX.

King, L., & Deng, W. (2018). *Health Disparities among Asian New Yorkers. Epi Data Brief (100)*: New York City Department of Health and Mental Hygiene.

Koch-Weser, S., Liang, S. L., & Grigg-Saito, D. C. (2006). Self-reported health among Cambodians in Lowell, Massachusetts. *Journal of Health Care for the Poor and Underserved, 17*(2), 133–145. https://doi.org/10.1353/hpu.2006.0076

Kolonel, L. N., Henderson, B. E., Hankin, J. H., Nomura, A. M. Y., Wilkens, L. R., Pike, M. C., Stram, D. O., Monroe, K. R., Earle, M. E., & Nagamine, F. S. (2000). A multiethnic cohort in Hawaii and Los Angeles: Baseline characteristics. *American Journal of Epidemiology, 151*(4), 346–357. https://doi.org/10.1093/oxfordjournals.aje.a010213

Kuo, J., & Porter, K. (1998). Health status of Asian Americans: United States, 1992–94. *Advance Data,* (298), 1–16.

Lin-Fu J. S. (1993). Asian and Pacific Islander Americans: An Overview of Demographic Characteristics and Health Care Issues. *Asian American and Pacific Islander Journal of Health, 1*(1), 20–36.

Lopez, G., Ruiz, N., & Patten, E. (2017, September 8). *Key facts about Asian Americans, a diverse and growing population.* Pew Research Center. https://www.pewresearch.org/fact-tank/2017/09/08/key-facts-about-asian-americans.

Martinez, O. (2014). Immigration policy and access to health services. *Journal of Immigrant and Minority Health, 16*(4), 563–564. https://doi.org/10.1007/s10903-013-9864-y

Menke, A., Casagrande, S., Geiss, L., & Cowie, C. C. (2015). Prevalence of and Trends in Diabetes Among Adults in the United States, 1988-2012. *JAMA, 314*(10), 1021–1029. https://doi.org/10.1001/jama.2015.10029

Mui, P., Hill, S. E., & Thorpe, R. J. (2018). Overweight and obesity differences across ethnically diverse subgroups of Asian American men. *American Journal of Men's Health, 12*(6), 1958–1965. https://doi.org/10.1177/1557988318793259

Nguyen, T. T. (2014). Cancer in Asian American and Pacific Islander populations: Linking research and policy to identify and reduce disparities. *Cancer Epidemiology Biomarkers & Prevention, 23*(11), 2206–2207. https://doi.org/10.1158/1055-9965.EPI-14-0640

Park, S., Stimpson, J. P., Pintor, J. K., Roby, D. H., McKenna, R. M., Chen, J., & Ortega, A. N. (2019). The effects of the affordable care act on health care access and utilization among Asian American subgroups. *Medical Care, 57*(11), 861–868. https://doi.org/10.1097/MLR.0000000000001202

Parsons, V. L., Moriarity, C., Jonas, K., Moore, T. F., Davis, K. E., & Tompkins, L. (2014). Design and estimation for the national health interview survey, 2006–2015. *Vital and Health Statistics. Series 2, Data Evaluation and Methods Research,* (165), 1–53.

Pham, C., Fong, T.-L., Zhang, J., & Liu, L. (2018). Striking racial/ethnic disparities in liver cancer incidence rates and temporal trends in California, 1988–2012. *JNCI: Journal of the National Cancer Institute, 110*(11), 1259–1269. https://doi.org/10.1093/jnci/djy051

Ponce, N. (2009). *Health Issues in the Asian American Community.* Jossey-Bass.

Ponce, N. (2011). What a difference a data set and advocacy make for AAPI health. *AAPI Nexus, 9,* 159–162.

Ponce, N., Scheitler, A., & Shimkhada, R. (2016). *Understanding the Culture of Health for Asian American, Native Hawaiian, and Pacific Islanders (AANHPIs): What Do Population-Based Health Surveys Across the Nation Tell Us About the State of Data Disaggregation for AANHPIs?* A Report to the Robert Wood Johnson Foundation. https://www.policylink.org/sites/default/files/AANHPI-draft-Report-9-262016.pdf

Ponce, N. A., Bautista, R., Sondik, E. J., Rice, D., Bau, I., Ro, M. J., & Tseng, W. (2015). Championing partnerships for data equity. *Journal of Health Care for the Poor and Underserved, 26*(2A), 6–15. https://doi.org/10.1353/hpu.2015.0058

Quach, T., Liu, R., Nelson, D. O., Hurley, S., Von Behren, J., Hertz, A., & Reynolds, P. (2014). Disaggregating data on Asian American and Pacific Islander women to provide new insights on potential exposures to hazardous air pollutants in California. *Cancer Epidemiology Biomarkers & Prevention, 23*(11), 2218–2228. https://doi.org/10.1158/1055-9965.EPI-14-0468

Ro, M. (2002). Moving forward: Addressing the health of Asian American and Pacific Islander women. *American Journal of Public Health, 92*(4), 516–519. https://doi.org/10.2105/AJPH.92.4.516

Srinivasan, S., & Guillermo, T. (2000). Toward improved health: Disaggregating Asian American and Native Hawaiian/Pacific Islander data. *American Journal of Public Health, 90*(11), 1731–1734. https://doi.org/10.2105/AJPH.90.11.1731

Takeuchi, D. T., Gong, F., & Gee, G. (2012). The NLAAS Story: Some Reflections, Some Insights A commentary prepared for the special issue of the Asian American Journal of Psychology. *Asian American Journal of Psychology, 3*(2), 10.1037/a0029019. https://doi.org/10.1037/a0029019

UCLA Center for Health Policy Research. (2018a). *California Health Interview Survey Methodology Report 2017–18.* https://healthpolicy.ucla.edu/chis/design/Pages/methodology.aspx.

UCLA Center for Health Policy Research. (2018b). *A New Design for CHIS 2019–2020.* https://healthpolicy.ucla.edu/chis/design/Pages/2019-2020-methods.aspx.

Ye, J., Mack, D., Fry-Johnson, Y., & Parker, K. (2012). Health care access and utilization among US-born and foreign-born Asian Americans. *Journal of Immigrant and Minority Health, 14*(5), 731–737. https://doi.org/10.1007/s10903-011-9543-9

Zhang, Y., Misra, R., & Sambamoorthi, U. (2020). Prevalence of multimorbidity among Asian Indian, Chinese, and Non-Hispanic White adults in the United States. *International Journal of Environmental Research and Public Health, 17*(9), 3336. https://doi.org/10.3390/ijerph17093336

CHAPTER

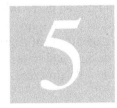

5

DEVELOPING RESEARCH INTERVENTIONS IN ASIAN AMERICAN SETTINGS

SHAHMIR H. ALI, NADIA S. ISLAM

LEARNING OBJECTIVES

By the end of this chapter, readers will be able to:

▪ Identify types of intervention study designs used to conduct research in Asian American communities and considerations for selecting particular study designs to meet the cultural, social, and health needs of different Asian American populations.

▪ Using multiple theoretical lenses, describe the key stages in the development, implementation, and evaluation of research interventions in Asian American communities.

▪ Explore how various stakeholders and partnerships may be engaged effectively to tailor research interventions for Asian American communities.

▪ Describe important sociocultural domains in diverse Asian American communities and identify methodologies for effectively addressing these factors to maximize intervention success.

Applied Population Health Approaches for Asian American Communities, First Edition. Edited by Simona C. Kwon, Chau Trinh-Shevrin, Nadia S. Islam, and Stella S. Yi.
© 2023 John Wiley & Sons, Inc. Published 2023 by John Wiley & Sons, Inc.
Companion Website: www.wiley.com/go/kwon/asianamerican

INTRODUCTION

In the last chapter, we explored population-based study designs and effective methods of collecting data to capture the diverse health needs of Asian Americans. In this chapter, we will explore different ways of assessing the impact of policies, program, and clinical interventions on the health of Asian American populations. Specifically, the aim of the section is to provide a practical guide on the steps and considerations needed to develop appropriate and effective research interventions to meet the needs of Asian American communities. We will begin by exploring different types of intervention study designs and how they have been applied in Asian American settings. We will then present an in-depth discussion of the processes involved in adapting these interventions to the needs of diverse Asian American populations.

INTERVENTION STUDY DESIGNS AND THEIR APPLICATION IN ASIAN AMERICAN COMMUNITIES

Overview of Key Intervention Study Designs and Their Objectives

The goal of all research intervention study designs is to evaluate how social, behavioral, or health-related outcomes in a population are impacted by implementing a treatment, preventive measure, or other specific action. Each type of study design achieves this goal through various techniques that are selected and implemented based on the specific aims of the research, the unique needs of the study population, and logistical constraints (Aggarwal & Ranganathan, 2019). Key considerations that drive differences between intervention study designs are included in Table 5.1.

TABLE 5.1 **Considerations in Intervention Design and Their Application in Asian American Health Research Interventions**

Component	Description	Example
Level of intervention	Are you allocating interventions to individual participants or to groups (or communities) of participants?	Tong et al. conducted an intervention aimed at increasing colorectal cancer screening among Hmong Americans in which lay health workers recruited participants through their own social networks and the different clusters of participants recruited by each lay health worker were then provided the educational intervention or the control intervention (Tong et al., 2017).
Control groups	Does your study involve a separate group of participants who will receive no intervention or a different intervention than the one you are investigating?	Kandula et al. conducted an intervention aimed at reducing atherosclerotic cardiovascular disease risk among South Asians in which an intervention group attended interactive group classes while a control group received only translated print education materials (Kandula et al., 2015).
Randomization	Does your study involve any randomization processes to guide recruitment and inclusion of participants, including both selection criteria for the study as a whole as well as distribution of participants within discrete components of the study	Fang et al. (2017) conducted a church-based intervention aimed at increasing cervical cancer screening among Korean American women in which each participating church was first matched with a church of similar size and geographic location, and then each church within a matched pair was assigned randomly to either the intervention or control group using a computerized coin flip (C. Y. Fang et al., 2017).

Masking/ Blinding/ Placebo	Will you be withholding or hiding any information from some or all study participants or research staff as part of your intervention?	Fang et al. (2013) conducted an intervention aimed at decreasing substance use among Asian American adolescent girls in which investigators and recruiting staff were blinded to participant assignment procedures (i.e., whether a participant was assigned to the intervention group or to the control group) in order to minimize potential investigator bias (L. Fang & Schinke, 2013).
Intra-intervention relationships	Does your study involve multiple interventions or do participants engage with the intervention(s) in specific sequences?	Taylor et al. (2002) conducted an intervention aimed at increasing cervical cancer screening among ethnic Chinese women in the United States and Canada that compared two different interventions and a control group. One intervention group received a health intervention delivered by outreach workers while the other group received the intervention materials by mail. The control group received usual care (Taylor et al., 2002).
Temporal sequencing	Does the sequencing of your intervention (or specific components of the intervention) across the study period play an important role?	Lopez et al. (2017) conducted an intervention aimed at improving hypertension management among South Asian Americans in which different participant groups received the electronic health record (EHR) component of the intervention at different, successive intervals during the study (i.e., stepped-wedge design) (P. M. Lopez et al., 2017).

Each of these different methodological dimensions seeks either to enhance the efficacy of the intervention or reduce biases in how post-intervention changes are evaluated. Additionally, different methodologies may be better suited to allow for more complex or multifaceted interventions to be assessed in different research contexts. Even the most commonly used study designs vary considerably. Quasi-experimental studies, for instance, generally do not involve any randomization of interventions; however, they may or may not include a control group and may involve different temporal sequencing or intra-intervention relationships (Harris et al., 2006). Similarly, the randomized controlled trial (RCT), traditionally considered the "gold standard" of health research, is centered on the principle of randomly allocating individuals or groups into two or more intervention arms, with one arm usually serving as a control group. An RCT may or may not involve participant masking or other methodological considerations based on the specific research aims and logistical demands of a study (Thiese, 2014). Although study designs must always be adapted to the unique needs of the diverse populations they intend to serve, these basic methodological dimensions must be considered as fundamental to all intervention research.

Individual versus cluster randomization must also be considered in RCT study designs (i.e., deciding to randomize either individuals or clusters of individuals into certain intervention arms). While individual-level randomization is common in traditional RCTs, the National Institutes for Health (NIH) suggests that cluster-level randomization should be considered if (1) the ultimate unit of interest is a system or broader collective (e.g., interventions focused on hospital-wide or neighborhood-wide change); and (2) there is a potential for contamination, a phenomenon that occurs when members of a control group receive the active intervention (e.g., if two neighbors are participating in an individual-level educational intervention, and one is in the control group and one is in the intervention group, the participant in the intervention group may share educational materials with the control group participant, resulting in contamination). Moreover, there are a number of practical considerations that must be weighed when selecting randomization procedures. True randomization procedures that employ groups or communities as units would require a substantial number of individuals to be recruited into and retained in such studies – a noteworthy challenge in any setting but one that is especially daunting in research implemented in Asian American communities where in-language, culturally relevant outreach strategies must be employed to reach diverse populations (Katz et al., 2001; Sunmin Lee et al., 2010; Pennell et al., 2011). In fact, scholars such as Katz et al. have argued that randomization is unethical in these settings because community-based studies often investigate interventions that offer only benefits to a community, with no significant recognizable risks (Katz et al., 2001). For example, a group-based educational intervention aim promoting healthy eating among hypertensive Filipino Americans potentially provides benefit to the intervention group, without any discernable potential harm; thus, randomizing individuals to a separate group that would not receive this intervention may be difficult to justify. One innovative method to address the randomization challenge in population health research interventions is the regression discontinuity design (RDD), sometimes termed the "cutoff design." In this quasi-experimental methodology, individuals or groups are assigned into intervention arms based on a quantitative indicator (e.g., blood pressure or cholesterol level) measured at baseline such that either all participants with measurements above an identified score cutoff receive the treatment and those below it do not ("sharp" RDD) or that the probability of being selected for treatment is higher for those participants with measurements above the cutoff versus those with measurements below the cutoff ("fuzzy" RDD) (Moscoe et al., 2015; Pennell et al., 2011). Such procedures allow researchers to assess the impact of an intervention reliably while maneuvering around many of the practical and ethical constraints of randomization.

Another novel, innovative, and increasingly popular intervention methodology is the stepped wedge cluster randomized trial. This study design builds on the cluster randomized trial, which involves randomization into intervention arms at the group level but with outcomes measured among individuals in each group (Hemming et al., 2015). Briefly, stepped wedge cluster randomized trials begin with an initial period in which none of the study sample clusters are provided with the intervention (i.e., all participants may be considered to be in the control group). Then, in regular and successive intervals (i.e., "steps"), one cluster after another is randomized to be exposed to the study intervention until all clusters have been exposed. Data collection occurs continuously such that clusters may serve as their own controls and outcomes may be compared to assess intervention impact in each cluster (Hemming et al., 2015). Similar to RDD, this methodology overcomes the practical and ethical dilemmas of working with community clusters allocated exclusively to either the control or intervention group. Additionally, this design provides the benefit of not having to implement an intervention to the full study sample at once, allowing researchers to avoid potential logistical challenges, such as limited staffing or other resource constraints.

Examples of Intervention Research Among Asian American Populations

Increasingly, researchers are applying innovations in ways that acknowledge and accommodate both logistical constraints and ethical considerations related to implementing intervention studies among Asian American populations. Table 5.2 presents examples of innovative research designs tailored to the needs of different Asian ethnic groups in diverse settings.

Among studies using randomization, both two- and three-arm study designs have been explored to assess the effectiveness of nonclinical interventions, such as educational sessions intended to increase health-related knowledge or change behavior. However, while a two-arm RCT involves two different intervention groups with one group typically assigned to "control" status (e.g., Lim et al.'s weight loss promotion study among South Asians at risk for diabetes had a CHW-led intervention arm and a usual care control arm), a three-arm RCT will involve three different intervention groups (e.g., Taylor et al.'s cervical cancer screening intervention among Chinese American women had an outreach worker intervention arm, a direct mail-based intervention arm, and a usual care control arm) (Lim et al., 2019; Taylor et al., 2002). Recent studies have also employed the crossover methodology to ensure that all participants benefit from the intervention being assessed (Lim et al., 2019; Padela et al., 2020; Taylor et al., 2002). For example, in their randomized crossover design, Padela et al. tested the effectiveness of an educational workshop for American Muslims about kidney donation. (Padela et al., 2020). The researchers established two trial arms, which they termed the "early" and "late" arms. In the first stage of the trial, the early arm received the intervention workshop (i.e., an in-depth, multi-method educational session about kidney donation) while the late arm received a control workshop detailing different aspects of end-of-life care. Subsequently, in the

TABLE 5.2 **Examples of Intervention Study Designs Applied in Asian American Settings**

Study Design	Author	Population	Setting	Aim	Intervention
Randomized controlled trial (two-arm, cluster-randomized)	(Lim et al., 2019)	South Asians at risk for diabetes	New York City (NYC), NY	Promote weight loss	Community health worker (CHW) coaching with EHR-based interventions
Randomized controlled trial (three-arm, individual-randomized)	(Taylor et al., 2002)	Chinese women underutilizing cervical cancer screening	Seattle, WA, and Vancouver, BC (Canada)	Promote cervical cancer screening	Tailored counseling, logistical assistance, and home visits by outreach workers along with written and audio-visual promotional resources or only receiving promotional resources by mail
Cross-over randomized controlled trial (two-arm, randomized)	(Padela, et al., 2020)	Muslim (majority South Asian) Americans	Washington, DC, and Chicago, IL	Promote knowledge about living kidney donation	Group workshops focused on expert-led and moderated panel presentations and peer-facilitated discussions
Quasi-experimental intervention (two-arm, nonrandomized)	(Bernstein et al., 2016)	Korean American women with depression	NYC, NY	Promote coping strategies for depression, lower depressive symptoms, and improve purpose in life	Group-based logo-autobiography program led by trained facilitator
Stepped-wedge quasi-experimental intervention (two-arm, nonrandomized)	(P. M. Lopez et al., 2017)	South Asian adults with hypertension	NYC, NY	Promote hypertension control	CHW health coaching or EHR-based interventions
Pre-post quasi-experimental intervention (one-arm, nonrandomized)	(Ma et al., 2019)	Members of Chinese, Korean, Vietnamese, and Filipino community-based organizations	Philadelphia, PA	Promote healthy food purchasing, cooking, and consumption behaviors and increase nutrition knowledge	Distribute promotional materials, train community-based organization leaders and members on healthy food preparation and nutrition guidelines, host food-related activities in the community

"crossover" stage of the trial, the early arm received the control workshop and the late arm received the intervention workshop. Survey assessments were conducted at three timepoints: before and after the intervention workshop and during the transition period between the two workshops. In this way, researchers were able to employ a randomized design to test the effectiveness of the intervention workshop while still delivering critical education to all participants. Given that the study results demonstrated the effectiveness of the intervention workshop, providing the intervention to all participants emerged as a particularly beneficial aspect of this design.

As an example of innovations using quasi-experimental design, Lopez et al. employed a stepped-wedge design to simultaneously analyze the effectiveness and implementation of a multi-component approach to improve hypertension control among South Asian American adult patients in 16 NYC primary care practices (P. M. Lopez et al., 2017). The model included integrating CHW-led health coaching with provider-led EHR-based interventions. Researchers established five clusters of practices and implemented the provider-led EHR-based components successively in each cluster over a two-year period. Nested within this larger stepped-wedge study design was an individual-level RCT in which patients were randomized to receive the CHW-led intervention or usual care. In this way, researchers developed a study design that allowed for a staggered delivery of the EHR and integrated EHR-CHW interventions to each cluster of practices, allowing for assessment of intervention effectiveness of both components while simultaneously ensuring that all patients at the practice level benefited from quality improvement efforts to support hypertension control.

DEVELOPING INTERVENTIONS FOR ASIAN AMERICANS

Successfully developing interventions for specific Asian American populations that reside in diverse geographic and socioeconomic settings and have unique linguistic and cultural characteristics requires researchers to identify appropriate theoretical foundations for their work and engage with the communities of interest to develop, implement, and evaluate the research. In this section, we will explore the unique factors that researchers must consider when working with Asian American communities and outline best practices to guide intervention studies within Asian American populations.

Theoretical Frameworks and Informative Models to Aid Intervention Development

Public health researchers have developed a number of conceptual and theoretical frameworks to help identify key constructs relevant for assessing different components of an intervention's effectiveness, appropriateness, and adaptability. These frameworks also assist researchers in identifying the barriers and facilitators that may emerge during the implementation of a study. In this section, we will briefly explore three such frameworks and examine how they may be applied in Asian American-focused health research settings.

The Reach, Effectiveness, Adoption, Implementation, and Maintenance (RE-AIM) framework, published in 1999 by Glasgow et al., was informed by the need for improved reporting of issues related to implementation and external validity of health promotion and health care interventions in the research literature, particularly for studies implemented in complex, "real-world" research settings as opposed to "optimal" laboratory or clinical conditions (Gaglio et al., 2013; Glasgow et al., 1999).The RE-AIM framework facilitates the evaluation of the impact of health promotion interventions on the individual, organization, and community levels through five dimensions that follow a logical sequence:

1. *Reach.* The number, proportion, and representativeness of individuals participating in an intervention.
2. *Effectiveness.* The impact of the intervention on outcomes of interest.
3. *Adoption.* The number, proportion, and representativeness of the research settings and intervention agents willing to implement the program or treatment.
4. *Implementation.* Consistency of the intervention's implementation and fidelity to protocol.
5. *Maintenance.* Extent to which the intervention becomes routine and integrated into the standard practices or polices of an institution or community. At the individual level, this can be long-term sustainability of the intervention as evidenced by outcomes lasting beyond six months following the last dose of the intervention.

The PRECEDE–PROCEED framework provides researchers with a multidirectional eight-phase process to inform the design, implementation, and evaluation of an intervention (Porter, 2016). PRECEDE refers to the first four phases of the framework: Predisposing, Reinforcing, and Enabling Constructs in Educational Diagnosis and Evaluation, three of which are described here:

- *Predisposing* constructs encompass the knowledge, beliefs, and personal characteristics related to the desired change.

- *Reinforcing* constructs are incentives or rewards designed to sustain the desired change.

- *Enabling* factors comprise the resources or skills that serve as facilitators or barriers to achieving the desired change.

All of these constructs may impact behaviors, attitudes, and environmental factors throughout the implementation of an intervention.

PROCEED refers to the last four phases of the framework: Policy, Regulatory, and Organizational Constructs in Educational and Environmental Development. These phases focus on an intervention's implementation (actually conducting the intervention components), process evaluation (assessing whether the intervention is being conducted as planned), impact evaluation (assessing the intervention's effectiveness in influencing intermediary behavioral or environmental outcomes), and outcome evaluation (assessing the extent to which the intervention helps achieve broader or central public health goal). In other words, PRECEDE provides a planning structure that relies on specific measurable objectives and baseline data to guide intervention development, while PROCEED focuses on monitoring and continuous quality improvement (Porter, 2016). Researchers may operationalize different components of the framework based on their needs at different stages of the planning, implementation, and evaluation process.

The Consolidated Framework for Implementation Research (CFIR) is meta-theoretical – that is, CFIR includes constructs from multiple existing theoretical frameworks (Damschroder et al., 2009). CFIR aims to consolidate the overlapping and missing components from earlier frameworks in a manner that may allow researchers to assess what works where and why across multiple contexts. In doing so, the framework focuses on five constructs:

1. *Intervention characteristics.* Complexity, adaptability, and perceived quality of the intervention are included.

2. *Outer setting.* This describes how the intervention is connected with broader community and other external policies and incentives.

3. *Inner setting.* The focus is on dynamics between intervention agents and readiness for implementation.

4. *Individual characteristics.* Traits of individuals refer to the knowledge, beliefs, and self-efficacy of participants.

5. *Process.* This includes procedures related to planning, fidelity of implementation, and evaluation.

To illustrate the application of these different frameworks, Table 5.3 presents an example of how each one has been applied to research conducted within Asian American communities.

The application of a particular theoretical framework may be guided by which constructs are most salient to specific populations. For instance, in applying the RE-AIM and CFIR frameworks, Saw et al. and Leong et al., respectively, observed that cultural and linguistic adaptations had to be made by intervention agents throughout each program. Kim & Sarna, using the PRECEDE–PROCEED framework, noted that acculturation-related concerns tied into predisposing factors relevant in the intervention design (Kim & Sarna, 2004; Leong et al., 2020; Saw et al., 2013). Ultimately, choosing a particular framework must be informed by how helpful it may be in capturing all the potential considerations and complexities involved in the study. The PRECEDE–PROCEED framework, for instance, may be particularly beneficial for complex, multicomponent, or long-term interventions requiring the identification of specific and multifaceted barriers and facilitators, while RE-AIM and CFIR may be more useful in guiding the implementation process and identifying considerations that may inform replication, scale, and sustainability of interventions (CFIR Research Team, 2020).

Stakeholders and Partnerships

Another key component in developing effective interventions for Asian American communities is collaboration between researchers and a diverse range of stakeholders to establish meaningful partnerships. Community-based participatory partnerships are an integral component of community-based participatory research (CBPR) – a methodology that is described in detail in Chapter 8. Partnerships may be defined as individuals and organizations who collaborate with researchers within the context of a shared goal or around an issue of importance to the community, forming mutually beneficial relationships wherein partners have shared responsibilities, privileges, and power (Connors et al., 2003; Giachello et al., 2007). These partnerships may directly benefit an intervention by (1) enhancing program design and efficacy through the solicitation and application of community

TABLE 5.3 **Examples of How Different Theoretical Frameworks Have Been Applied in the Development, Implementation, and Evaluation of Asian American-Focused Health Research**

Framework	Study characteristics	How framework was applied
RE-AIM	(Saw et al., 2013) **Population:** Asian Americans with severe mental illness **Aim:** Promoting smoking cessation **Design:** Quasi-experimental	RE-AIM guided the development and implementation of the intervention evaluation, which primarily centered on interviews with study staff but also included analysis of cross-sectional data. **Reach** - 20 of the 100 clients endorsing tobacco use attended at least one session. Those with higher psychosocial functioning, focus on well-being more likely to participate **Effectiveness** - Reduction/cessation of tobacco use, health-related quality of life change **Adoption** - At the staff level, all clinical study staff received minimum six hours training (abiding by funding agency recommendations) **Implementation** - Modifications of protocol were made by clinicians to better need the cultural, linguistic, and psychological needs of clients **Maintenance** - At the setting level, smoking cessation counseling is still being offered by clinic after the intervention, although it has been integrated into larger wellness program
PRECEDE–PROCEED	(Kim & Sarna, 2004) **Population:** Korean American women aged 40–75 **Aim:** Promoting mammography use **Design:** RCT	PRECEDE-PROCEED informed the development of the intervention content **Predisposing factors** - Breast cancer screening-related knowledge and attitudes, health history, acculturation, sociodemographic characteristics **Reinforcing factors** - Hearing from survivors, integrated religious and cultural reinforcements, and integrating these reinforcement mechanisms as part of intervention **Enabling factors** - Socioeconomic and health-related factors such as income level, health insurance status, and having a regular source of health care

CFIR	(Leong et al., 2020) **Population:** Asian and Pacific Islander Americans aged 55 and older **Aim:** Promoting well-balanced and low-sodium diet **Design:** Quasi-experimental (pre-/post-test)	CFIR guided the development and implementation of the evaluation, which centered on interviews with representatives of the community-based organizations participating in program: **Intervention Characteristics** - Adaptions were focused on cultural/linguistic needs, logistical considerations. Mixed perspectives on how easy the training material was to understand, with some noting it to be very complex and difficult to interpret. **Outer Setting** - Partnerships and trainings with local, regional, and national organizations were key in implementing the intervention as well as aligning its goals with community values and needs. **Inner Setting** - Organizational characteristics (maturity, social standing in the community, size) were important in facilitating implementation. Organizational culture and engagement with leadership were important in enhancing implementation success and program effectiveness. **Characteristics of Individuals** - Strong motivation on the part of program facilitators to learn, gain competency, and adjust materials based on needs of participants. **Process** - Actively finding and building new partnerships throughout intervention (e.g., working with local grocery stores) enhanced implementation.

perspectives throughout the development and implementation process; (2) facilitating resource and idea sharing to better meet the needs of the community; (3) building capacity within the community to support the long-term sustainability or scale up of the intervention; and (4) integrating existing services into intervention effort and reducing the amount of competing or fragmented programs (Giachello et al., 2007).

There are many different types of partnerships that may be created or leveraged as part of research interventions. Examples are presented in Table 5.4. Ultimately, the types of partnerships best suited to a particular intervention depend on the aim of the research, its foreseeable impact on a community, and the long-term goals for sustainability and scale-up of the intervention. For example, an intervention focused on preventing violence among South Asian youth through a school-based, peer-led educational program might benefit from collaborations with individual school sites or school/educational associations (e.g., Islamic school alliances) serving a high proportion of South Asian students. Developing a strong advisory committee to inform different stages of the intervention process is also an impactful partnership model. Specifically, building a community advisory board (CAB) to work hand in hand with researchers in a formal and consistent manner has been an effective methodology used in intervention research across diverse Asian American communities (Chaudhary et al., 2010; Kwon et al., 2012) (see Case 4 in the Appendix).

A number of considerations and potential obstacles to developing strong partnerships have been articulated in past research and should inform the development of new interventions (Giachello et al., 2007). First, to ensure that partners remain engaged in discussion and planning on a continuous basis, researchers must acknowledge

TABLE 5.4 **Examples of Community Based Participatory Partnerships in Asian American-Focused Research Interventions**

Type of Partnership	Definition/Composition	Example
Community advisory boards	Groups of opinion leaders from within the community of interest that provide suggestions and technical assistance to researchers and other outside agents of change.	Form a group of leaders of local Chinese American community-based organizations to have monthly team meetings with researchers in order to review study materials and implementation strategy.
Commissions and task forces	Formal groups of citizens appointed by official bodies. May be formed to accomplish a specific series of activities, often at the request of an overseeing body.	Collaborate with a state commission on Asian American affairs, comprised of individuals appointed by the state governor to be the voice of the Asian American community in that state, in order to enhance study implementation and sustainability.
Consortia and alliances	Semi-official membership organizations with broad, policy-oriented goals that may span large geographic areas. Typically consist of organizations and coalitions as opposed to individuals.	Collaborate with an alliance of Islamic schools in order to implement a widescale awareness-raising intervention focused on South Asian youth.
Networks	Loose-knit groups formed primarily for resource and information sharing.	Form a network of Asian American organizations or research partners involved in similar activities or with similar goals in order to support one another and share resources.

Source: Adapted from Cohen et al. (2002).

that collaborators are often more interested in the activities or outcomes of an intervention than in the granular planning or evaluation sessions essential to developing the research. Ensuring that results are visible and shared iteratively throughout the research process may prevent feelings of discouragement or concerns among partners that the process is not worth their time. Second, when building collaborations, researchers must recognize and respect potential partners' resource limitations (i.e., time, staff, money). Creating material or nonmaterial incentives for participation in these partnerships is one method of addressing this challenge. For example, researchers may provide stipends to individuals participating in regular CAB meetings or offer training and technical assistance to the staff members of partnering organizations. Finally, in order to build fruitful and productive relationships with partners, researchers must consider group dynamics and power relationships within any advisory or collaborating body. Establishing specific roles and responsibilities for each partner and remaining cognizant of organizational structures, histories, and cultural differences as well as intra-partner dynamics are vital to preventing miscommunication and conflict.

Cultural Factors That Impact Intervention Success

In the previous sections, we explored the critical role of theoretical frameworks in providing guidance for the design, implementation, and evaluation of an intervention and the importance of engaging stakeholders and building partnerships to ensure that an intervention is effective, relevant, and sustainable at the community level. In addition to these foundational components, researchers working within Asian American communities have identified cultural factors that are uniquely relevant to conducting research among diverse Asian American populations. As one of the most diverse populations in the United States, Asian Americans trace their ancestry from more than 20 countries across East, Southeast, and South Asia, with significant linguistic, religious, and ethnic differences (Lopez, Ruiz, & Patten, 2017). However, behind this complex community profile are a number of shared sociocultural domains impacting the Asian American population's experience in the United States overall. Although these domains may surface in different ways across diverse Asian American groups, they are salient to the population as a whole and, thus, are important considerations in the context of research interventions intended to serve Asian Americans.

Cultural factors underlie these domains. Culture is defined by the American Sociological Association to include "the language, customs, beliefs, rules, arts, knowledge, and collective identities and memories developed by members of all social groups that make their social environments meaningful" (American Sociological Association, 2020). Although Asian cultures are notable for their vast diversity and there is no single "Asian" culture *per se*, researchers have identified shared priorities and values across Asian American ethnic groups (Pew Research Center, 2012b). Accordingly, community-based health research is often geared toward the cultural adaptation of an evidence-based approach that has proven successful among the general U.S. population or among another non-Asian racial or ethnic group. Bernal et al. defined cultural adaptation as the systematic modification of an intervention to render it compatible with a population's cultural patterns, meanings, and values (Bernal & Domenech Rodríguez, 2009). While the cultural adaptation process is critical to developing appropriate interventions for small populations, an overemphasis on the impact of culture on help-seeking and other individual-level factors in health research may lead to researchers to ignore critical provider- and system-level factors that must be addressed in order to improve an intervention's reach, accessibility, and effectiveness. Therefore, as we explore cultural considerations within health research, it is vital to consider the many different facets of culture that influence the behavior of individuals or communities within a broader context of health service availability and accessibility.

Family

Family-related factors impact the health behaviors and outcomes of Asian Americans, often because family dynamics may facilitate or pose barriers to participation in health interventions (George et al., 2013). About 29% of Asian Americans reside in multigenerational households, a higher proportion compared to any other racial or ethnic group in the United States (Cohn & Passel, 2018). Within an Asian American population of interest, relationships between potential research participants and their mothers, fathers, siblings, children, grandparents, and other extended family members should be considered not only in the design and implementation of an intervention but also in establishing expectations for the long-term sustainability of the intervention in fostering positive health outcomes. For instance, in the context of mental health research, some researchers working with certain Asian ethnic groups have emphasized the role of stigmatization, judgment, and shame within the family setting as contributors to negative health outcomes (Kramer et al., 2002). Considering the potential impact of family dynamics on mental health is essential to developing interventions intended to serve Asian American individuals and, importantly, to exploring ways in which family members may be engaged as significant facilitators to enhance mental health outcomes. For example, Bae & Kung have proposed a model for family interventions tailored for Asian Americans with a schizophrenic patient in the family that specifically acknowledges the strong role family members play in the management and experience of schizophrenia (Bae & Kung, 2000). The three-component model includes home visits, family workshops, and support groups. First, mental health professionals visit patients' homes and build relationships and trust with family members. Second, mental health professionals provide regular psychoeducation workshops for the entire family unit in a culturally sensitive manner (i.e., acknowledging the unique stigmas and cultural abstractions of mental health in diverse Asian American communities). Third, mental health professionals conduct support groups with family members that exclude the patients themselves. In this way, they may create nonconfrontational spaces for family members to discuss their own experiences, coping mechanisms, and other interpersonal dynamics related to the health of a schizophrenic patient while navigating around stigmatized topics and respecting the interpersonal relationships of different family members in the household (Bae & Kung, 2000). The authors caution that the implementation of the model must be adapted to cultural specificities of different Asian American ethnic groups.

Family members can also be integrated into Asian American lifestyle behavior interventions to reinforce intervention aims and strengthen interpersonal support systems vital to ensure the sustainability of the behavioral goals. For example, as part of an innovative lifestyle intervention to promote cardiovascular health among South Asians, Kandula et al. hosted four heart-health *melas* for participants and their families. Melas are festive gatherings that may be cultural, religious, or social in tone and are common to many South Asian cultures. By including participants' families in the melas, researchers acknowledged the central role of family relationships in determining dietary patterns and physical activity behaviors among the participants in the study. The melas served to reinforce information delivered to participants in classes and coaching sessions and aimed to increase group cohesion and support (Kandula et al., 2013).

Gender

There has been a growing call for critical acknowledgment of the roles gender and sexuality play in the lived experiences of Asian Americans. Not only must researchers accord greater weight to the specific ways in which gender may influence certain health-relevant behaviors, but also researchers must investigate the stereotypes that have been constructed regarding Asian American gender roles and the harm these stereotypes may exert on individuals and communities within the context of health sciences, including public health research interventions (Wong & Jeffrey, 1999). At the most basic level, many health issues are experienced only – or disproportionately more intensely – by either men or women (see Chapter 3). At more complex levels, it is important to consider both the gender roles and stereotypes constructed within the Asian American community as well as those constructed outside the community, based on perceptions or assumptions held by non-Asian Americans. For example, within the Asian American community, across many Asian American cultures, gender influences household- and family-based responsibilities and expectations. These expectations may determine the behaviors that are considered more or less acceptable across gender lines within the household or community. Furthermore, while gender-based disparities in behavioral and social factors may be driven in part by cultural or religious traditions specific to each Asian ethnic group, gender roles and expectations across Asian American populations are impacted strongly by socioeconomic status, immigration status, and other factors. Specific knowledge-, attitude-, or behavior-related drivers behind health outcomes may also differ by gender – comprising a reason why lifestyle behavior interventions in Asian American settings typically have focused on either exclusively men or women (Ali et al., 2020; Zhou & Oh, 2012). For instance, while many components of the heart health intervention among South Asians designed by Kandula et al. involved group-based educational sessions that included both men and women, the researchers also designed a separate exercise intervention specifically for South Asian American mothers at risk for diabetes. The development of this additional component was driven, in part, by the desire of many South Asian women with diverse religious and cultural backgrounds to participate in women-only sessions in trusted community settings, particularly with respect to physical activities (Kandula et al., 2016; Kandula et al., 2013). These behavioral or social disparities may translate into specific practical concerns in the context of intervention design that may need to be addressed. For instance, a cervical cancer control intervention among Cambodian American women provided participants with assistance in transportation and childcare in order to facilitate Pap testing completion (Jackson et al., 2000).

Moreover, these internal gender dynamics within the Asian American community occur alongside many external perceptions of assumptions that may be held by non–Asian Americans on the role of gender in the community. For example, gender-based stereotypes regarding Asian American communities must also be acknowledged. While Asian Americans across the gender spectrum may experience ethnic or racial discrimination and its ramifications on personal health status, a survey among Asian American women specifically highlighted experiences of feeling perceived by others or the general public as submissive, expected to be agreeable, and easily controllable (Mukkamala & Suyemoto, 2018). On the other hand, Asian American men of South Asian, Western Asian, or Muslim descent have been observed to experience discrimination related to associations with terrorism or as perpetrators of violence (Ewing, 2008). Many of these gender-based perceptions and stereotypes impact the health experiences of Asian Americans by influencing the ways individuals interact with health providers and the health system. To conduct health research effectively within this context, researchers must work actively against assumptions about the role of gender in Asian American communities. Acknowledging gendered experiences of discrimination and conducting formative research prior to the development of an intervention to understand how participant-informed gender roles may impact the health issue of focus is a key example of operationalizing a community-centered approach to this challenge.

Community

Asian American individuals may belong simultaneously to multiple communities based on their ethnicity, place of residence, gender, religion, and personal preferences and characteristics. As with gender roles, community membership directly impacts health experiences and must be acknowledged by researchers and potentially incorporated into the design of research interventions. In some cases, "community" may be geographically defined, such as communities centered around "Chinatowns" or "Koreatowns" in U.S. cities (see Case 3 in the Appendix). However, community may be defined more generally as a diverse group of people linked together by certain social ties, shared perspectives, or common sociocultural backgrounds (MacQueen et al., 2001). The formation of community networks across Asian American settings provides the basis for resource sharing, connectedness, business development, advocacy for community needs, cultural and social activities, and other material and social support (Ling, 2009). Importantly, these community networks can occur both informally (e.g., friend-based and neighborhood-based social networks) or formally, through the establishment of community-based organizations. Despite having diverse structures and purpose, community-based organizations serve the common purpose of establishing networks of community support, organizing social and cultural activities, and strengthening and empowering communities through outreach efforts and resource connectivity (Chaudhary et al., 2010). As discussed in the context of stakeholders and partnerships, engaging with community networks or organizations may help researchers to design and implement more effective and meaningful research. For example, Korean Community Services of New York , the largest and older social service provider for Korean Americans in NYC, has participated in a robust array of community-based intervention studies, playing both a leading and collaborative role with academic agencies (Gore et al., 2019; Islam et al., 2013; Li et al., 2017; Pollack et al., 2014; Yi et al., 2019).

Communities are not limited to the local environment. Particularly in the case of smaller Asian ethnic populations that may be geographically dispersed, the formation of community may take place at the state or national levels. For example, Hmong Americans in Minnesota have developed various statewide community organizations to support resource sharing and social support for the diverse population of Hmong residents living across the state (Yang, 2012). Indeed, making an effort to understand how different types of communities at local, state, and national levels impact a particular Asian American population of interest may allow researchers to better understand that population's health-related needs and resources as well as how these networks may be integrated into research design to enhance an intervention's impact or sustainability. For instance, as part of a healthy diet intervention for Chinese, Vietnamese, Korean, and Filipino Americans in Philadelphia, Ma et al. conducted a capacity-building component that trained leaders of community-based organizations in healthy food preparation skills and nutrition guidelines to empower these leaders and their respective community networks with healthy lifestyle behaviors (Ma et al., 2019).

Religion

A diverse array of religions is practiced across Asian American communities, including Christianity, Buddhism, Islam, and Hinduism. Importantly, the adherents of many significant non-Abrahamic religions practiced across the United States, such as Buddhism and Hinduism, are majority-Asian American – underscoring the contribution of the Asian American population to religious diversity in the United States (Pew Research Center, 2012a). Religious affiliation also varies among Asian ethnic groups. One national study reported that over half (52%) of Chinese Americans were unaffiliated with a religion, while only 8% of Filipino Americans lacked religious affiliation (Pew Research Center, 2012a). To design successful health-related interventions, researchers must be aware of this diversity itself as well as the specific beliefs and rituals practiced by the population of interest. To ensure these factors are accounted for within research design, researchers have worked with religious organizations to develop interventions and/or conducted interventions in religious settings, including Muslim mosques, Hindu temples, Sikh gurdwaras, and Christian churches (Fang et al., 2017; Northridge et al., 2017; Patel et al., 2017). Such collaborative efforts have allowed researchers to understand and account for religious beliefs about health issues and practices within health interventions. Additionally, researchers may structure interventions around religious activities. For example, with a strong partnership in place between a research team and a faith-based organization or institution, the researchers may be able to conduct health promotion activities or education sessions before or after prayer services to maximize participation by a religious community of interest.

Moreover, religion may shape specific lifestyle factors or behaviors that have been associated with health disparities experienced by Asian Americans. Two key examples are dietary behaviors and sexual identity. Dietary behaviors, in particular, are impacted by religious guidelines and beliefs that differ vastly among communities. For example, some Muslim communities will not consume any pork or alcohol products. Some Hindu communities will not consume any meat, while others will not consume alcohol, and still others will consume certain types of meat but refuse beef products. To develop effective health-promoting dietary interventions, researchers must recognize dietary restrictions while also incorporating the preferences of the Asian American community of interest. For example, in a Hindu temple-based lifestyle intervention conducted among Gujarati Indian Americans, Patel et al. focused on helping participants identify components of a balanced vegetarian diet (Patel et al., 2017).

Regarding sexual health and gender identity, numerous researchers have explored ways to incorporate the health promoting aspects of religion into education and health service provision. Yet religious mores may constrain outreach to sexual and gender minorities, posing an obstacle to improving the health status of these populations. Although intervention studies specifically focused on the health needs of Asian American sexual minorities is limited, research among gay and lesbian Filipino Americans identified religion as a direct influence on identify formation and a psychological stressor (Nadal & Corpus, 2013). Formative research conducted through collaborative partnerships with key stakeholders is critical to understanding these issues and essential to identifying strategies to help researchers navigate religious influences on behavior, health, and identity.

Finally, it is important to remember that religious practices manifest in daily, weekly, or other regular activities within Asian American communities. For example, many Muslim Asian Americans (particularly men) may attend Friday *Jummah* prayers at their local mosques, while Catholic Asian Americans may attend Sunday mass at their local churches. Indeed, these activities and routines intersect with other sociocultural factors within the lived experiences of Asian American individuals such as family or gender (e.g., religion-informed family or gender roles), community (e.g., religion-based community formation), holidays (e.g., religious holidays), and even language (e.g., the greeting *As-salamu alaykum* is commonplace across Muslim communities across Asia, regardless of country of origin).

Holidays

Festivals and holidays play a central role in many Asian American communities. Researchers must familiarize themselves with the holidays that are significant to the population of interest in order to align intervention activities with the calendar that is meaningful to that community. Holidays traditionally celebrated in the United States such as Christmas, Thanksgiving, or Halloween may not be celebrated to the same extent in Asian American communities – or they may be celebrated in different ways, accompanied by special foods and activities unique to each Asian culture. Additionally, each of the many different ethnic groups that comprise the Asian American population may have their own cultural holidays that they prioritize. Some of these holidays are religious in origin, spanning countries and regions, while others are tied to specific geographic areas or ethnic communities. The kite flying festival of Basant, for example, is celebrated mainly by Punjabi communities in India and Pakistan, while the Bengali New Year (পহেলা বৈশাখ) is celebrated by those of Bengali heritage in Bangladesh and some of India's eastern states. Similarly, the Lunar New Year, also referred to as the Spring Festival, is celebrated across East and Southeast Asian countries, whereas the Dragon Boat Festival (端午節) is celebrated only by communities of Chinese descent. Researchers working within these communities must – at a minimum – account for these holidays in their planning and implementation activities. However, these holidays also offer opportunities for researchers to engage with the community of interest and enhance intervention implementation. As an example, Bhagat et al. organized a community event around the Punjabi holiday of *Basant*. By bringing women and children together in a fun, social environment, service providers were able to create a relaxed platform upon which to talk with community members about women's health and distribute flyers for their program (Bhagat et al., 2002). The event, which was attended by over 200 women and children, was identified as a central component in the study authors' efforts to mobilize community efforts to address prenatal health needs of immigrant Punjabi women. Specifically, the authors noted the value of "putting a face to the system" by introducing immigrant women and children to community health nurses and CHWs in an informal setting.

Language

Approximately 77% of Asian Americans speak a language other than English at home, more than any other racial or ethnic group in the United States (Ramakrishnan & Ahmad, 2014). Cultural adaptation of existing health interventions typically encompasses a linguistic component that includes translating study materials into participants' preferred language or hiring linguistically competent staff to implement interventions in the language of the population of interest. However, researchers have faced numerous challenges that stem from the distinct historical and cultural roots of these extremely different languages. Researchers may not be able to imbue concepts or terms with the same fundamental meanings when translating from English to Asian languages, leading to poor translations that do not convey the key messages of the intervention. Failing to consider linguistic barriers in a comprehensive manner or translating study materials without appropriate linguistic competency may result in the intervention being received by participants in a manner different to what was envisioned. These challenges are particularly salient when working on sensitive health issues, such as mental health, sexual health, or substance abuse. For instance, Leung et al. have argued that many existing translations of mental health terminology from English into Chinese fail to appropriately capture both accuracy and social acceptance (Leung et al., 2016). As an example, the authors argue that the term sometimes used when translating "mania" into Chinese, "zào kuáng (躁狂)," may be highly stigmatizing and carry a more negative connotation than its English counterpart because it combines two characters, the first of which signifies violence/insanity while the second denotes a particularly harsh form of madness. Instead, the authors suggest "jī zào (激躁)" as a less stigmatizing, more appropriate translation. More broadly, when designing interventions for Asian American populations with limited English proficiency, it is not sufficient to simply conduct word-by-word translation of the study materials into the language of the population of interest. Researchers must also consider how linguistic adaptations may impact the meaning of the materials and the intervention as a whole. Working with partner organizations to identify a process for reviewing translations prior to intervention implementation and making changes when needed is key to ensuring meaningful cultural adaptation of a health intervention (Ma et al., 2019). Process evaluations may also provide insights in any potential issues with translation procedures; for example, interviews with intervention agents, such as CHWs, may highlight any issues with interpretability of translated material.

Immigration

Most Asian Americans in the United States (59%) were born abroad, a proportion that rises to 73% among Asian American adults (G. Lopez et al., 2017). Significant differences in immigration experiences exist among Asian Americans. For example, only 27% of Japanese Americans are foreign-born, with many Japanese Americans having descended from plantation workers who migrated to the United States in the 19th century. By contrast, 92% of Bhutanese Americans are foreign-born and a majority arrived recently as refugees (G. Lopez et al., 2017). The immigration status of an individual (e.g., U.S. citizen, permanent resident, work or student visa holders, or undocumented immigrants) directly impacts access to health-related resources and services, which, in turn, influences health status and outcomes. For example, undocumented Asian Americans comprise approximately 16% of all undocumented immigrants in the United States and 8% of the Asian American population (Asian Americans Advancing Justice, 2019; United States Census Bureau, 2019). These individuals are more likely to experience health disparities, such as disproportionate occupational morbidity and mortality (Schenker, 2010) (see Chapter 3 for additional examples).

Likewise, immigration status impacts individual and household socioeconomic status. Asian Americans experience some of the starkest within-group socioeconomic disparities of any ethnic or racial group in the United States, with disparities increasing in recent years (Kochhar & Cilluffo, 2018). Various structural and social factors associated with immigration contribute to these socioeconomic disparities, including legal residency status, acculturation level, and English proficiency. Lueck (2018) observed that Asian Americans who immigrated to the United States between the ages of 18 and 34 had a 102% higher likelihood of socioeconomic success than those who immigrated at ages older than 34 years. Lueck linked this finding with the higher economic upward mobility among younger Asian immigrants, reasoning that they may manage the processes of linguistic and social acculturation more adeptly than older immigrants (Lueck, 2018).

In parallel, undocumented Asian Americans face many of the same issues experienced by undocumented immigrants in general in the United States, including constraints in accessing health services, fear of deportation, and distrust of government (Asian Americans Advancing Justice, 2019; Derose et al., 2007). Other noncitizen Asian Americans (e.g., permanent residents, work or student visa holders) may experience similar health disparities. For example, findings from the National Latino and Asian American Study observed that noncitizens as a whole – a population defined as including lawful permanent residents, refugees, students, temporary workers, and undocumented immigrants – were about 40% less likely than U.S.-born citizens to use mental health services (Lee & Matejkowski, 2012). Incorporating methodologies into research design that facilitate participation by noncitizens is an important aspect of developing more inclusive studies to inform policy and practice. For example, one study eschewed direct mail recruitment strategies in favor of CHW-led, in-person recruitment in order to encourage participation by undocumented Asian American domestic workers (Katigbak et al., 2016).

While most Asian Americans currently living in the United States are first-generation (foreign-born) immigrants, the population of second-generation Asian Americans (U.S.-born children of foreign-born parents) is increasing. Health researchers must consider unique socioeconomic, acculturation, and health behavior-related factors in the lives of second-generation communities and how they may be incorporated appropriately into intervention design (Ali, DiClemente, & Parekh, 2020). For example, second-generation Asian Americans typically demonstrate a higher level of English proficiency and greater facility and comfort with technology than their immigrant parents. Thus, health researchers may develop mHealth research interventions to address their health needs, whereas such interventions may not be as successful when implemented within first-generation communities that are less familiar with mobile- or web-based technologies (Ali, DiClemente, & Parekh, 2020).

Geography

The locations in which Asian Americans live across the United States similarly involve unique dynamics that must be considered in research interventions. At the national level, the proportion of Asian American residents is particularly high in the urban centers of states such as New York, Hawaii, California, and Washington (United States Census Bureau, 2012). Importantly, Asian American communities have often clustered around certain neighborhoods within cities. In NYC, for example, the neighborhood of Flushing, in the borough of Queens, is home to a large Chinese American community, while the neighborhood of Jackson Heights, Queens, has a notably numerous South Asian American population (McGovern & Frazier, 2015). These residential disparities among specific Asian American groups may be incorporated into intervention design by identifying settings in each neighborhood to serve as intervention sites (see Case 4 in the Appendix).

Asian Americans living in different U.S. regions, states, or cities may display starkly different sociodemographic profiles. In particular, Asian American populations experience extremely diverse poverty rates. For example, in NYC, the Asian American poverty rate in some Brooklyn community districts is as high as 59%, whereas in some Manhattan districts, the rate is only 20% (Asian American Federation, 2008). Additionally, the places in which Asian Americans live have been associated with distinct health outcomes and health disparities. For instance, in large part due to disparities in residential location, Asian Americans in New York State are exposed to twice as much air pollution, measured as particulate matter (PM2.5), as non-Hispanic Whites (Union of Concerned Scientists, 2019). Foreign-born Asian Americans and those living in urban centers often reside in ethnic enclaves with other Asian Americans (see Case 3 in the Appendix) (Logan & Zhang, 2013; Walton, 2015). This residential clustering is often accompanied by a concentration of culturally adapted services or resources, such as ethnic groceries and in-language health and social service providers. An awareness of the residential landscape may inform the selection of appropriate intervention settings for a specific Asian American population. For example, research interventions focused on Chinese American communities often implement recruitment efforts (e.g., distribution of flyers and posters) in urban Chinatown districts (Huang & Garcia, 2020; Ying, 2009).

As the size and diversity of the Asian American population increases, it is also important to consider the ways in which new communities of Asian Americans experience the health system. Research conducted among Asian Americans in rural settings has highlighted experiences of discrimination, hostility, and struggles with racial identity and belonging that are distinct to those environments (Walton, 2018). Self-reported negative experiences related to racial or ethnic identity may also be more pronounced among Asian Americans in rural settings than among urban-dwelling Asian Americans. Research interventions in rural settings must consider the impact of residential context on health, including unique intra- and inter-community social dynamics and greater role of geographical barriers in issues such as health care access. Additionally, researchers must adapt recruitment methodologies and implementation approaches (e.g., telehealth) to ensure inclusivity and meet the needs of rural populations.

These eight sociocultural domains provide building blocks for researchers to consider in the development, implementation, and evaluation of effective and appropriately tailored interventions to meet the needs of Asian American communities across the United States (for more details on the integration of these domains in an intervention, see Case 4 in the Appendix). Recognizing intersectionality among these factors and within Asian American health research in general is an important aspect of a broader effort to disaggregate studies related to specific Asian American populations (see Chapter 4) (Srinivasan & Guillermo, 2000). *Intersectionality* refers to the overlap of different social categorizations, such as race, class, and gender, which interact to create unique experiences or systems of disadvantage (Collins & Bilge, 2020). It is important to acknowledge the role of intersectionality in understanding each of the aforementioned cultural factors in Asian American research intervention design because an individual's experience of one factor may be moderated or directly driven by another. Gender roles and expectations, for example, may be directly influenced by religion and family structure, while immigration status may impact an individual's use of community-based networks to fulfill basic needs. Similarly, Asian American immigrants may choose to settle in areas close to family members or members of their ethnic group, driving the geographic clustering of distinct Asian American populations. Intersectionality impacts intervention design because researchers must identify and accommodate diverse interactions between multiple cultural factors the Asian American population of interest in the study. For example, Patel (2007) provides a set of guidelines for culturally competent mental health interventions for South Asian American women in which she argues that the unique confluence of experiences related to gendered racism in the United States and gendered South Asian traditions must be considered in how researchers design counseling initiatives. Researchers have a responsibility not only to acknowledge this fundamental power imbalance but also to integrate gender empowerment into interventions to meet the mental health needs of South Asian American women in more effective, sustainable ways (Patel, 2007). Intersectionality is discussed more extensively in Chapter 12.

Finally, researchers must also consider the pervasive impact of the model minority myth on individual Asian American communities and the Asian American population as a whole. The *model minority myth,* a term coined in the early 20th century, refers to a cultural stereotype that characterizes Asian Americans as an educated, law-abiding, high-income, hardworking, and monolithic community. The model minority myth has shaped the lives of Asian Americans and contributed to health disparities in this population by reinforcing systemic racism and discriminatory structures (see Chapter 2) (Yi et al., 2016). Because the model minority myth has masked health disparities in Asian American communities, this construct is essential to consider in designing health research interventions for Asian Americans. Conducting formative or observational research that disaggregates Asian American health data by ethnic group and highlights the extent of specific health disparities among distinct populations will not only inform the design of more successful research interventions but also combat stereotypes by providing health-related data that may be used in advocacy efforts to raise awareness of community needs, garner funding, and develop and implement supportive services. Similarly, it is important to consider variations in socioeconomic and educational status among and within Asian American communities to effectively tailor intervention strategies, particularly given the socioeconomic diversity of this population and the bimodal distribution of income and educational attainment within certain communities (see Chapter 1).

SUMMARY AND RECOMMENDATIONS

In this chapter, we sought to provide a practical guide on the steps and considerations essential to developing, implementing, and evaluating research interventions to meet the needs of the diverse spectrum of Asian American communities. Specifically, when conducting intervention research in Asian American communities, researchers must ask themselves:

- What type of study design will be most appropriate and feasible to meet the goal of the intervention?
- What theoretical frameworks may be employed to help guide the development, implementation, and evaluation of the intervention?
- Which stakeholders should be engaged to ensure the intervention is tailored to the unique needs of the specific Asian American community of interest?

■ How are the influences of family, gender, community, religion, holidays, language, immigration, and geography acknowledged or incorporated within the intervention?

Answering these questions at the outset of the study design process will ensure that research is conceptualized with Asian Americans as active partners and centers community voices and priorities. The principles, frameworks, and illustrative examples offered throughout the chapter may provide further guidance in moving research from conceptualization to community-based implementation, evaluation, and long-term sustainability. Ultimately, efforts to advance health equity in Asian American communities will rely on the implementation of both scientifically rigorous and community-centered, culturally contextualized interventions.

DISCUSSION QUESTIONS

1. What are some benefits, limitations, and ethical dilemmas associated with conducting RCTs in Asian American communities?

2. What are some different ways the fidelity of an intervention's implementation may be evaluated? Consider how the RE-AIM, PRECEDE-PROCEED, and CFIR frameworks strive to address these challenges. What are some unique challenges associated with intervention fidelity in Asian American research interventions?

3. How might a CAB prove beneficial to achieving research goals in an Asian American community of interest? How can researchers initiate the formation of a CAB to advise a particular research initiative?

4. What are some ways that the design of a research intervention can acknowledge the interaction of factors related to family, gender, community, religion, holidays, language, immigration, and geography?

REFERENCES

Aggarwal, R., & Ranganathan, P. (2019). Study designs: Part 4 – Interventional studies. *Perspectives in Clinical Research, 10*(3), 137. https://doi.org/10.4103/picr.PICR_91_19

Ali, S. H., DiClemente, R. J., & Parekh, N. (2021). Changing the landscape of South Asian migrant health research by advancing second-generation immigrant health needs. *Translational Behavioral Medicine, 11*(6), 1295–1297. https://doi.org/10.1093/tbm/ibaa084

Ali, S. H., Misra, S., Parekh, N., Murphy, B., & DiClemente, R. J. (2020). Preventing type 2 diabetes among South Asian Americans through community-based lifestyle interventions: A systematic review. *Preventive Medicine Reports, 20*, 101182. https://doi.org/10.1016/j.pmedr.2020.101182

American Sociological Association. (2020). Culture. Retrieved from https://www.asanet.org/topics/culture#:~:text=topic%2Dimage_culture.&text=Sociology%20understands%20culture%20as%20the,make%20their%20social%20environments%20meaningful.

Asian American Federation. (2008). Working but Poor: Asian American Poverty in New York City. Retrieved from http://www.aafny.org/doc/WorkingButPoor.pdf

Asian Americans Advancing Justice. (2019). Inside the Numbers: How Immigration Shapes Asian American and Pacific Islander Communities. Retrieved from https://advancingjustice-aajc.org/sites/default/files/2019-06/1153_AAJC_Immigration_Final_Pages_LR-compressed.pdf

Bae, S.W., & Kung, W. W.M. (2000). Family intervention for Asian Americans with a schizophrenic patient in the family. *American Journal of Orthopsychiatry, 70*(4), 532–541. https://doi.org/10.1037/h0087789

Bernal, G., & Domenech Rodríguez, M. M. (2009). Advances in Latino family research: Cultural adaptations of evidence-based interventions. *Family Process, 48*(2), 169–178. https://doi.org/10.1111/j.1545-5300.2009.01275.x

Bernstein, K., Park, S.-Y., Hahm, S., Lee, Y. N., Seo, J. Y., & Nokes, K. M. (2016). Efficacy of a culturally tailored therapeutic intervention program for community dwelling depressed korean american women: A non-randomized quasi-experimental design study. *Archives of Psychiatric Nursing, 30*(1), 19–26. https://doi.org/10.1016/j.apnu.2015.10.011

Bhagat, R., Johnson, J., Grewal, S., Pandher, P., Quong, E., & Triolet, K. (2002). Mobilizing the community to address the prenatal health needs of immigrant Punjabi women. *Public Health Nursing, 19*(3), 209–214. https://doi.org/10.1046/j.0737-1209.2002.19309.x

CFIR Research Team. (2020). *Tools.* Retrieved from https://cfirguide.org/tools/

Chaudhary, N., Vyas, A., & Parrish, E. B. (2010). Community based organizations addressing South Asian American health. *Journal of Community Health, 35*(4), 384–391. https://doi.org/10.1007/s10900-010-9256-3

Cohen, L., Baer, N., & Satterwhite, P. (2002). Developing effective coalitions: an eight step guide. In M. E. Wurzbach (Ed.), *Community Health Education & Promotion: A Guide to Program Design and Evaluation* (2nd ed., pp. 161–178). Gaithersburg, MD: Aspen Publishers Inc.

Cohn, D. V., & Passel, J. S. (2018). A record 64 million Americans live in multigenerational households. *Pew Research Center.* Retrieved from https://www.pewresearch.org/fact-tank/2018/04/05/a-record-64-million-americans-live-in-multigenerational-households/

Collins, P. H., & Bilge, S. (2020). *Intersectionality:* John Wiley & Sons.

Connors, K. M., Cashman, S. B., Seifer, S. D., & Unverzagt, M. (2003). *Advancing the Healthy People 2010 objectives through community-based education.*

Damschroder, L. J., Aron, D. C., Keith, R. E., Kirsh, S. R., Alexander, J. A., & Lowery, J. C. (2009). Fostering implementation of health services research findings into practice: A consolidated framework for advancing implementation science. *Implementation Science, 4*(1), 50. https://doi.org/10.1186/1748-5908-4-50

Derose, K. P., Escarce, J. J., & Lurie, N. (2007). Immigrants and health care: Sources of vulnerability. *Health Affairs, 26*(5), 1258–1268. https://doi.org/10.1377/hlthaff.26.5.1258

Ewing, K. P. (2008). *Being and Belonging: Muslims in the United States Since 9/11: Russell Sage Foundation.*

Fang, C. Y., Ma, G. X., Handorf, E. A., Feng, Z., Tan, Y., Rhee, J., Miller, S. M., Kim, C., & Koh, H. S. (2017). Addressing multilevel barriers to cervical cancer screening in Korean American women: A randomized trial of a community-based intervention. *Cancer, 123*(6), 1018–1026. https://doi.org/10.1002/cncr.30391

Fang, L., & Schinke, S. P. (2013). Two-year outcomes of a randomized, family-based substance use prevention trial for Asian American adolescent girls. *Psychology of Addictive Behaviors, 27*(3), 788–798. https://doi.org/10.1037/a0030925

Gaglio, B., Shoup, J. A., & Glasgow, R. E. (2013). The re-aim framework: A systematic review of use over time. *American Journal of Public Health, 103*(6), e38–e46. https://doi.org/10.2105/AJPH.2013.301299

George, S., Duran, N., & Norris, K. (2014). A systematic review of barriers and facilitators to minority research participation among African Americans, Latinos, Asian Americans, and Pacific Islanders. *American Journal of Public Health, 104*(2), e16–e31. https://doi.org/10.2105/AJPH.2013.301706

Giachello, A., Ashton, D., Kyler, P., Rodriguez, E., Shanker, R., & Umemoto, A. (2007). *Making Community Partnerships Work: A Toolkit.* White Plains, NY: March of Dimes Foundation.

Glasgow, R. E., Vogt, T. M., & Boles, S. M. (1999). Evaluating the public health impact of health promotion interventions: The RE-AIM framework. *American Journal of Public Health, 89*(9), 1322–1327. https://doi.org/10.2105/AJPH.89.9.1322

Gore, R., Patel, S., Choy, C., Taher, M., Garcia-Dia, M. J., Singh, H., Kim, S., Mohaimin, S., Dhar, R., Naeem, A., Kwon, S. C., & Islam, N. (2019). Influence of organizational and social contexts on the implementation of culturally adapted hypertension control programs in Asian American-serving grocery stores, restaurants, and faith-based community sites: A qualitative study. *Translational Behavioral Medicine,* ibz106. https://doi.org/10.1093/tbm/ibz106

Harris, A. D., McGregor, J. C., Perencevich, E. N., Furuno, J. P., Zhu, J., Peterson, D. E., & Finkelstein, J. (2006). The use and interpretation of quasi-experimental studies in medical informatics. *Journal of the American Medical Informatics Association, 13*(1), 16–23. https://doi.org/10.1197/jamia.M1749

Hemming, K., Haines, T. P., Chilton, P. J., Girling, A. J., & Lilford, R. J. (2015). The stepped wedge cluster randomised trial: Rationale, design, analysis, and reporting. *BMJ, 350,* h391–h391. https://doi.org/10.1136/bmj.h391

Huang, Y. C., & Garcia, A. A. (2020). Culturally-tailored interventions for chronic disease self-management among Chinese Americans: A systematic review. *Ethnicity & Health, 25*(3), 465–484. https://doi.org/10.1080/13557858.2018.1432752

Islam, N. S., Zanowiak, J. M., Wyatt, L. C., Chun, K., Lee, L., Kwon, S. C., & Trinh-Shevrin, C. (2013). A randomized-controlled, pilot intervention on diabetes prevention and healthy lifestyles in the New York City Korean community. *Journal of Community Health, 38*(6), 1030–1041. https://doi.org/10.1007/s10900-013-9711-z

Jackson, J. C., Taylor, V. M., Chitnarong, K., Mahloch, J., Fischer, M., Sam, R., & Seng, P. (2000). Development of a Cervical Cancer Control Intervention Program for Cambodian American Women. *Journal of Community Health, 25*(5), 359–375. https://doi.org/10.1023/A:1005123700284

Kandula, N. R., Dave, S., De Chavez, P. J., Bharucha, H., Patel, Y., Seguil, P., Kumar, S., Baker, D. W., Spring, B., & Siddique, J. (2015). Translating a heart disease lifestyle intervention into the community: The South Asian Heart Lifestyle Intervention (Saheli) study; a randomized control trial. *BMC Public Health, 15*(1), 1064. https://doi.org/10.1186/s12889-015-2401-2

Kandula, N. R., Dave, S., De Chavez, P. J., Marquez, D. X., Bharucha, H., Mammen, S., Dunaif, A., Ackermann, R. T., Kumar, S., & Siddique, J. (2016). An exercise intervention for south asian mothers with risk factors for diabetes. *Translational Journal of the American College of Sports Medicine, 1*(6), 52–59.

Kandula, N. R., Patel, Y., Dave, S., Seguil, P., Kumar, S., Baker, D. W., Spring, B., & Siddique, J. (2013). The South Asian Heart Lifestyle Intervention (Saheli) study to improve cardiovascular risk factors in a community setting: Design and methods. *Contemporary Clinical Trials, 36*(2), 479–487. https://doi.org/10.1016/j.cct.2013.09.007

Katigbak, C., Foley, M., Robert, L., & Hutchinson, M. K. (2016). Experiences and lessons learned in using community-based participatory research to recruit Asian American immigrant research participants: CBPR to recruit Asian immigrants. *Journal of Nursing Scholarship, 48*(2), 210–218. https://doi.org/10.1111/jnu.12194

Katz, D. L., Nawaz, H., Jennings, G., Chan, W., Ballard, J., Comerford, B., Spargo, K., & Walsh, J. (2001). Community health promotion and the randomized controlled trial: Approaches to finding common ground: *Journal of Public Health Management and Practice, 7*(2), 33–40. https://doi.org/10.1097/00124784-200107020-00006

Kim, Y. H., & Sarna, L. (2004). An intervention to increase mammography use by Korean American women. *Oncology Nursing Forum, 31*(1), 105–110. https://doi.org/10.1188/04.ONF.105-110

Kochhar, R., & Cilluffo, A. (2018). Income inequality in the U.S. is rising most rapidly among Asians. Retrieved from https://www.pewsocialtrends.org/2018/07/12/income-inequality-in-the-u-s-is-rising-most-rapidly-among-asians/

Kramer, E. J., Kwong, K., Lee, E., & Chung, H. (2002). Cultural factors influencing the mental health of Asian Americans. *The Western Journal of Medicine, 176*(4), 227–231.

Kwon, S., Rideout, C., Tseng, W., Islam, N., Cook, W. K., Ro, M., & Trinh-Shevrin, C. (2012). Developing the community empowered research training program: Building research capacity for community-initiated and community-driven research. *Progress in Community Health Partnerships: Research, Education, and Action, 6*(1), 43–52. https://doi.org/10.1353/cpr.2012.0010

Lee, S. (2010). Barriers to health care access in 13 Asian American communities. *American Journal of Health Behavior, 34*(1). https://doi.org/10.5993/AJHB.34.1.3

Lee, S., & Matejkowski, J. (2012). Mental health service utilization among noncitizens in the united states: Findings from the National Latino and Asian American study. *Administration and Policy in Mental Health and Mental Health Services Research, 39*(5), 406–418. https://doi.org/10.1007/s10488-011-0366-8

Leong, J., Jang, S. H., Bishop, S. K., Brown, E. V. R., Lee, E. J., & Ko, L. K. (2021). "We understand our community": Implementation of the Healthy Eating Healthy Aging program among community-based organizations. *Translational Behavioral Medicine, 11*(2), 462–469. https://doi.org/10.1093/tbm/ibaa049

Leung, C.-M., Ungvari, G. S., & Xiang, Y.-T. (2016). Conceptual issues behind the Chinese translations of the term 'Bipolar Disorder': Bipolar disorder in China. *Asia-Pacific Psychiatry, 8*(4), 256–259. https://doi.org/10.1111/appy.12253

Li, S., Sim, S.-C., Lee, L., Pollack, HenryJ., Wyatt, L. C., Trinh-Shevrin, C., Pong, P., & Kwon, S. C. (2017). Hepatitis b screening & vaccination behaviors in a community-based sample of Chinese & Korean Americans in New York City. *American Journal of Health Behavior, 41*(2), 204–214. https://doi.org/10.5993/AJHB.41.2.12

Lim, S., Wyatt, L. C., Mammen, S., Zanowiak, J. M., Mohaimin, S., Goldfeld, K. S., Shelley, D., Gold, H. T., & Islam, N. S. (2019). The DREAM Initiative: Study protocol for a randomized controlled trial testing an integrated electronic health record and community health worker intervention to promote weight loss among South Asian patients at risk for diabetes. *Trials, 20*(1), 635. https://doi.org/10.1186/s13063-019-3711-y

Ling, H. (2009). *Asian America Forming New Communities,* Expanding Boundaries: Rutgers University Press.

Logan, J. R., & Zhang, W. (2013). Separate but Equal: Asian Nationalities in the U.S. *US2010 Project.* Retrieved from https://s4.ad.brown.edu/Projects/Diversity/Data/Report/report06112013.pdf

Lopez, G., Ruiz, N. G., & Patten, E. (2017). Key facts about Asian Americans, a diverse and growing population. *Pew Research Center.* Retrieved from https://www.pewresearch.org/fact-tank/2017/09/08/key-facts-about-asian-americans/

Lopez, P. M., Zanowiak, J., Goldfeld, K., Wyka, K., Masoud, A., Beane, S., Kumar, R., Laughlin, P., Trinh-Shevrin, C., Thorpe, L., & Islam, N. (2017). Protocol for project IMPACT (Improving millions hearts for provider and community transformation): A quasi-experimental evaluation of an integrated electronic health record and community health worker intervention study to improve hypertension management among South Asian patients. *BMC Health Services Research, 17*(1), 810. https://doi.org/10.1186/s12913-017-2767-1

Lueck, K. (2018). Socioeconomic success of Asian immigrants in the United States. *Journal of Ethnic and Migration Studies, 44*(3), 425–438. https://doi.org/10.1080/1369183X.2017.1320940

Ma, G. X., Zhu, L., Shive, S. E., Zhang, G., Senter, Y. R., Topete, P., Seals, B., Zhai, S., Wang, M., & Tan, Y. (2019). The evaluation of ideal-reach program to improve nutrition among Asian American community members in the Philadelphia metropolitan area. *International Journal of Environmental Research and Public Health, 16*(17), 3054. https://doi.org/10.3390/ijerph16173054

MacQueen, K. M., McLellan, E., Metzger, D. S., Kegeles, S., Strauss, R. P., Scotti, R., Blanchard, L., & Trotter, R. T. (2001). What is community? An evidence-based definition for participatory public health. *American Journal of Public Health, 91*(12), 1929–1938. https://doi.org/10.2105/AJPH.91.12.1929

McGovern, B., & Frazier, J. W. (2015). Evolving ethnic settlements in queens: Historical and current forces reshaping human geography. *Focus on Geography, 58*(1), 11–26. https://doi.org/10.1111/foge.12045

Moscoe, E., Bor, J., & Bärnighausen, T. (2015). Regression discontinuity designs are underutilized in medicine, epidemiology, and public health: A review of current and best practice. *Journal of Clinical Epidemiology, 68*(2), 132–143. https://doi.org/10.1016/j.jclinepi.2014.06.021

Mukkamala, S., & Suyemoto, K. L. (2018). Racialized sexism/sexualized racism: A multimethod study of intersectional experiences of discrimination for Asian American women. *Asian American Journal of Psychology, 9*(1), 32–46. https://doi.org/10.1037/aap0000104

Nadal, K. L., & Corpus, M. J. H. (2013). "Tomboys" and "baklas": Experiences of lesbian and gay Filipino Americans. *Asian American Journal of Psychology, 4*(3), 166–175. https://doi.org/10.1037/a0030168

Northridge, M. E., Kavathe, R., Zanowiak, J., Wyatt, L., Singh, H., & Islam, N. (2017). Implementation and dissemination of the Sikh American families oral health promotion program. *Translational Behavioral Medicine, 7*(3), 435–443. https://doi.org/10.1007/s13142-017-0466-4

Padela, A. I., Duivenbode, R., Quinn, M., & Saunders, M. R. (2021). Informing American Muslims about living donation through tailored health education: A randomized controlled crossover trial evaluating increase in biomedical and religious knowledge. *American Journal of Transplantation, 21*(3), 1227–1237. https://doi.org/10.1111/ajt.16242

Patel, N. R. (2007). The construction of south-asian-american womanhood: Implications for counseling and psychotherapy. *Women & Therapy, 30*(3–4), 51–61. https://doi.org/10.1300/J015v30n03_05

Patel, R. M., Misra, R., Raj, S., & Balasubramanyam, A. (2017). Effectiveness of a group-based culturally tailored lifestyle intervention program on changes in risk factors for type 2 diabetes among asian indians in the united states. *Journal of Diabetes Research, 2017*, 1–13. https://doi.org/10.1155/2017/2751980

Pennell, M. L., Hade, E. M., Murray, D. M., & Rhoda, D. A. (2011). Cutoff designs for community-based intervention studies. *Statistics in Medicine, 30*(15), 1865–1882. https://doi.org/10.1002/sim.4237

Pew Research Center. (2012a). Asian Americans: A Mosaic of Faiths. Retrieved from https://www.pewforum.org/2012/07/19/asian-americans-a-mosaic-of-faiths-overview/

Pew Research Center. (2012b). Chapter 5: Family and Personal Values. In *The Rise of Asian Americans*: Pew Research Center.

Pollack, H. J., Kwon, S. C., Wang, S. H., Wyatt, L. C., Trinh-Shevrin, C., & on behalf of the AAHBP Coalition. (2014). Chronic hepatitis b and liver cancer risks among asian immigrants in New York city: Results from a large, community-based screening, evaluation, and treatment program. *Cancer Epidemiology Biomarkers & Prevention, 23*(11), 2229–2239. https://doi.org/10.1158/1055-9965.EPI-14-0491

Porter, C. M. (2016). Revisiting Precede–Proceed: A leading model for ecological and ethical health promotion. Health Education Journal, 75(6), 753–764. https://doi.org/10.1177/0017896915619645

Ramakrishnan, K., & Ahmad, F. Z. (2014). Language diversity and English proficiency. *Center for American Progress, 27.*

Saw, A., Kim, J., Lim, J., Powell, C., & Tong, E. K. (2013). Smoking cessation counseling for asian immigrants with serious mental illness: Using re-aim to understand challenges and lessons learned in primary care–behavioral health integration. Health Promotion Practice, 14(5_suppl), 70S-79S. https://doi.org/10.1177/1524839913483141

Schenker, M. B. (2010). A global perspective of migration and occupational health. American *Journal of Industrial Medicine, 53*(4), 329–337. https://doi.org/10.1002/ajim.20834

Srinivasan, S., & Guillermo, T. (2000). Toward improved health: disaggregating Asian American and Native Hawaiian/Pacific Islander data. *American Journal of Public Health, 90*(11), 1731–1734. https://doi.org/10.2105/AJPH.90.11.1731

Taylor, V. M. (2002). A randomized controlled trial of interventions to promote cervical cancer screening among chinese women in north america. *CancerSpectrum Knowledge Environment, 94*(9), 670–677. https://doi.org/10.1093/jnci/94.9.670

Thiese, M. S. (2014). Observational and interventional study design types; an overview. *Biochemia Medica, 24*(2), 199–210. https://doi.org/10.11613/BM.2014.022

Tong, E. K., Nguyen, T. T., Lo, P., Stewart, S. L., Gildengorin, G. L., Tsoh, J. Y., Jo, A. M., Kagawa-Singer, M. L., Sy, A. U., Cuaresma, C., Lam, H. T., Wong, C., Tran, M. T., & Chen, M. S. (2017). Lay health educators increase colorectal cancer screening among Hmong Americans: A cluster randomized controlled trial: Hmong Colorectal Cancer Screening Trial. *Cancer, 123*(1), 98–106. https://doi.org/10.1002/cncr.30265

Union of Concerned Scientists. (2019). Inequitable Exposure to Air Pollution from Vehicles in New York State. Retrieved from https://www.ucsusa.org/sites/default/files/attach/2019/06/Inequitable-Exposure-to-Vehicle-Pollution-NY.pdf

United States Census Bureau. (2012). The Asian Population: 2010. Retrieved from https://www.census.gov/prod/cen2010/briefs/c2010br-11.pdf

United States Census Bureau. (2019). Asian-American and Pacific Islander Heritage Month: May 2019. Retrieved from https://www.census.gov/newsroom/facts-for-features/2019/asian-american-pacific-islander.html#:~:text=22.2%20million,the%20United%20States%20in%202017.

Walton, E. (2015). Making sense of asian american ethnic neighborhoods: A typology and application to health. *Sociological Perspectives, 58*(3), 490–515. https://doi.org/10.1177/0731121414568568

Walton, E. C. (2018). Asian Americans in Small-Town America. *Contexts, 17*(4), 18-23.

Wong, S.-l. C., & Jeffrey, J. S. A. (1999). Gender and Sexuality in Asian American Literature. *Signs, 25*(1), 171-226. Retrieved from http://www.jstor.org/stable/3175619

Yang, S. (2012). The evolution of Hmong self-help organizations in Minnesota. *Hmong Studies Journal, 13*(1), 1.

Yi, S. S., Kwon, S. C., Sacks, R., & Trinh-Shevrin, C. (2016). Commentary: Persistence and health-related consequences of the model minority stereotype for asian americans. *Ethnicity & Disease, 26*(1), 133. https://doi.org/10.18865/ed.26.1.133

Yi, S. S., Wyatt, L. C., Patel, S., Choy, C., Dhar, R., Zanowiak, J. M., Chuhan, H., Taher, M. D., Garcia, M., Kavathe, R., Kim, S., Kwon, S. C., & Islam, N. S. (2019). A faith-based intervention to reduce blood pressure in underserved metropolitan New York immigrant communities. *Preventing Chronic Disease, 16*, 180618. https://doi.org/10.5888/pcd16.180618

Ying, Y.-W. (2009). Strengthening Intergenerational/Intercultural Ties in Immigrant Families (SITIF): A Parenting Intervention to Bridge the Chinese American Intergenerational Acculturation Gap. In N.-H. Trinh, Y. C. Rho, F. G. Lu, & K. M. Sanders (Eds.), *Handbook of Mental Health and Acculturation in Asian American Families* (pp. 45-64). Totowa, NJ: Humana Press.

Zhou, Q. P., & Oh, K. M. (2012). Comparison of lifestyle behaviors and related factors between Asian American and White adults with prediabetes: Lifestyles in Asians with prediabetes. *Nursing & Health Sciences, 14*(1), 58–66. https://doi.org/10.1111/j.1442-2018.2011.00664.x

PART

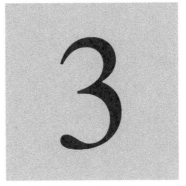

3

APPROACHES

CHAPTER

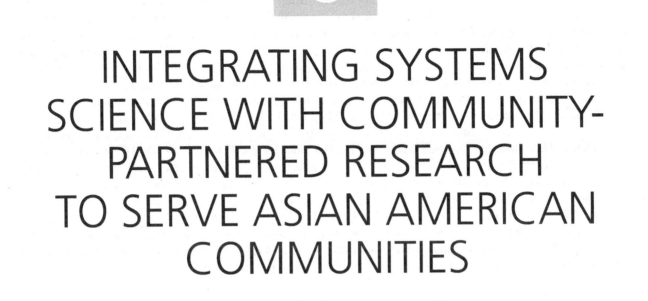

INTEGRATING SYSTEMS SCIENCE WITH COMMUNITY-PARTNERED RESEARCH TO SERVE ASIAN AMERICAN COMMUNITIES

STELLA S. YI, MATTHEW LEE, YAN LI, RIENNA G. RUSSO, SARA S. METCALF

LEARNING OBJECTIVES

By the end of this chapter, readers will be able to:

- Recognize the importance of applying systems science approaches to improve health equity.
- Describe the basic concepts of three systems science approaches in public health, including system dynamics, agent-based modeling, and group modeling building.
- Inspect the potential of integrating community-based participatory research, systems science, and implementation science in health equity research through a concrete example – the Healthy Aging Collaboratives led by the NYU Center for the Study of Asian American Health (CSAAH) at NYU Grossman School of Medicine.

Applied Population Health Approaches for Asian American Communities, First Edition. Edited by Simona C. Kwon, Chau Trinh-Shevrin, Nadia S. Islam, and Stella S. Yi.
© 2023 John Wiley & Sons, Inc. Published 2023 by John Wiley & Sons, Inc.
Companion Website: www.wiley.com/go/kwon/asianamerican

INTRODUCTION

Racial/ethnic minorities currently make up nearly one third of the U.S. population, and this proportion is increasing at a rapid pace (Humes et al., 2010; U.S. Census Bureau, 2017). The population growth of minorities accounted for 98% of overall population growth in the 100 largest U.S. metropolitan areas from 1990 to 2010 (Frey, 2011). Yet racial/ethnic minority groups remain vastly underrepresented in medical research, leading to poor generalizability of evidence-based interventions (EBIs) for these populations – including Asian Americans (Lee et al., 2013; Oh et al., 2015).

For population health researchers interested in implementing EBIs for racial/ethnic minority populations, few options exist other than to develop new approaches from scratch. However, developing new approaches through the design and implementation of clinical or community trials and longitudinal cohort studies is time-consuming and costly, requiring significant investment of financial, human, and logistical resources – all of which are increasingly difficult to secure for studies of any population. Similarly, the cultural adaptation and testing of an intervention that has been evaluated and shown to be effective in a majority non-Hispanic white (white) population for specific racial/ethnic minority populations is a significant undertaking.

Given these constraints, how can we accelerate the translation of research for diverse populations?

To answer this question, we propose an integrated approach that combines methods from three disciplines in public health research: systems science, community-based participatory research (CBPR), and implementation science. This integrated approach is currently being applied by researchers at the NYU Center for the Study of Asian American Health (CSAAH) at NYU Grossman School of Medicine, where we work with partners locally, regionally, and nationally to accelerate the translation of disparities research for diverse communities. In this chapter, we will describe the components and application of our integrated approach. Because CBPR methods and implementation science are discussed in Chapters 8 and 7, we will focus on systems science, limiting our discussion of CBPR and implementation science to the aspects of those disciplines that apply specifically to the integrated approach. We will also provide an illustration of how CSAAH is applying the integrated approach to accelerate community-based translational research in Asian American communities.

SYSTEMS SCIENCE METHODS COMMONLY USED IN PUBLIC HEALTH

Systems science generally refers to a variety of computational research approaches that may be used to study complex connections and interactions between multi-level determinants of health and health outcomes. Population health researchers have applied systems science approaches such as system dynamics (SD), agent-based modeling (ABM), group model building (GMB), and social network analysis to develop models that inform public health intervention design and policymaking (Luke & Stamatakis, 2012).

In congruence with the scientific method, most approaches to systems science begin with the task of problem definition. Indeed, Jay W. Forrester, the founder of system dynamics, famously admonished aspiring modelers to "model the problem, not the system." Why? A model should be focused on responding to a particular problem so that key aspects of the problem may be prioritized and addressed during the model development process. The boundaries of the system modeled may then be drawn in terms of components included as well as the model's temporal and spatial extent. "Modeling the system," rather than the modeling the problem, results in a lack of clarity around why the system is being modeled and what aspects of the model are most important to ensure its successful application.

System Dynamics

System dynamics is a structured approach to simulation modeling that involves articulation of feedback mechanisms and delays caused by accumulations in the system. The field of SD emerged as an outgrowth of control theory as applied to social systems, such as industrial organizations (Forrester, 1961). The underlying tenet of SD is that the structure of the system is the cause of its behavior over time. The core structures of SD models are stocks and flows (Sterman, 2000). Stocks are state variables that accumulate changes over time. Flows are the rates of change over time. A given stock may have any number of flows into and out of it. Mathematically, a stock is expressed as the integral of its net inflow, so that the stock may only be changed through its constituent flows.

The units of a given flow are the same as those of the stock to which it is connected, divided by the unit of time used in the model. To illustrate this concept: for a population stock, the units are people; in a model of annual demographic change, flows of births, deaths, or migration would have units of people/year.

In the standard SD modeling process, a characteristic pattern of behavior is first identified and graphed for the state variable that is most central – endogenous – to the problem being modeled. These characteristic trends are known as behavior over time graphs (BOTGs) or reference modes. Classic reference modes include S-shaped diffusion, exponential growth or decay, or overshoot and collapse. If the pattern of behavior over time for the key problem variable is flat (constant), then the problem is not actually dynamic and would be inappropriate for the application of SD. Constant variables may, however, be included in a model as exogenous parameters that influence the system but are not changed by it. These parameters may be uniquely configured to specify "what-if" scenarios for model simulation and to identify leverage points through virtual experimentation, which, when changed from one simulation run to another, have the greatest influence on simulated model outcomes.

After patterns of behavior have been graphed and key variables have been identified, connections between variables may be mapped using causal loop diagrams (CLDs). CLDs comprise a visual approach that helps to identify reinforcing (positive) and balancing (negative) feedback loops among the elements of the system. The development of CLDs is often conducted iteratively with the articulation of stock-flow diagrams (SFDs). Although both CLDs and SFDs are qualitative representations, each stock identified is a specific quantitative representation, since it is predefined as an integral and may only be modulated through changes in its flows. Therefore, regardless of how the conceptual phase of model development unfolds, specification of stock and flow structures is a fundamental step toward formalization of a SD model.

Agent-Based Modeling

While the tradition of SD emerged with Forrester's pioneering work in the 1950s using the earliest computers, the advent of agent-based modeling (ABM) was enabled by the expansion of computational power available for running simulation experiments. ABM is characterized by bottom-up representations of individuals that interact with each other and their simulated environment (Bonabeau, 2002; Epstein, 2006). ABM is a powerful tool for modeling real-world phenomena because agents may represent a wide range of entities (e.g., individuals, retailers, organizations) and have many sophisticated properties such as adaptability, mobility, heterogeneity, and the ability to interact with each other. For example, when ABM is used to evaluate the impact of different food policies, agents can represent human individuals who may make dietary decisions based on their socioeconomic characteristics, the influence of their peers, and the food environment in their community (Li, Zhang, et al., 2016).

Whereas the stocks of traditional SD models generally represent aggregates and averages, the agents in ABM represent individual idiosyncrasies and, thereby, heterogeneity within a population. Thus, ABM can complement SD models by answering questions in which differences between individual characteristics are of particular importance. For example, an agent-based model that captures the progression of cardiovascular disease has been used to assess how a lifestyle intervention would have different impacts on populations in different geographical areas (Li et al., 2015). For a given stock-flow SD model, equivalent (but more computationally intensive) ABM could be undertaken. However, only ABM that implements feedback mechanisms and accounts for delays in the system may be considered the same as SD modeling.

Group Model Building

Group model building (GMB) allows for a better understanding of the variables, relationships, and feedback loops that comprise complex systems to inform causal mapping and SD simulation models (Langellier et al., 2019). Community stakeholders, decision makers, trained modelers, and researchers are involved in developing causal maps, which enable insight into how various strategies, policies, and activities are related and may impact a community (Hovmand et al., 2014). Using these maps as a basis for GMB may result in a more realistic representation of the pathways connecting policy changes to behavior changes among the population of interest. Additionally, inviting the involvement of decision makers throughout this process may promote buy-in, facilitating uptake of the prevention policy recommendations that emerge (Hovmand et al., 2014). The development process is described below.

Planning a GMB Workshop

In preparation for the GMB workshops, experienced systems science modelers and members of the research team should convene planning meetings to discuss SD models, review GMB facilitation manuals, and identify additional stakeholders and subject matter experts (SMEs) who should be included in the workshops. Workshop organizers may reach out to community partnerships and research collaborators to help identify these additional members. Potential participants may include private sector stakeholders, elected policy makers, members of civil society, community-based organizations, and nonprofit organizations employees and researchers (Langellier et al., 2019). For example, if the subject matter relates to healthy aging, workshop organizers may request that community partnerships identify older adults who may be interested and available to participate in the GMB workshops. However, as the GMB process relies on small group work and open discussions, workshops should limit the number of participants to a manageable size.

Considerations regarding the location, duration, and language of the workshops should be based on the identified participants. Some workshops may take place over two days, whereas others may be held on a single day. For example, if a workshop is convened in a location that requires long car or public transport for participants invited to attend, a single-day session may facilitate participation, whereas a two-day session might be preferable for larger gathering requiring airline travel. If linguistic interpretation services are needed, translators should be identified in coordination with community partnerships. The format and schedule of the sessions and preference for simultaneous or consecutive interpretation should be discussed with community partners and other stakeholders prior to the workshop (Hovmand et al., 2014).

At the time of writing this chapter, concerns related to the novel coronavirus (COVID-19) pandemic have created an imperative for conducting remote and virtual GMB workshops. This imperative has seeded rapid innovation to expand online opportunities for collaboration using GMB. Effective opportunities for virtual GMB are likely to persist following the pandemic and may be used as stand-alone delivery methods or as hybrid enhancements to traditional GMB workshops.

Team Roles and Responsibilities

The following roles are typically involved in traditional GMB workshops implemented as part of a community-based SD project. Depending on team size and expertise, some roles may be combined. The *community facilitator* is responsible for leading the GMB session, serving to draw out knowledge and insights from the group. This person should be familiar with the problem being modeled, the local context and community norms related to the problem, and how to facilitate dialogue across participants. The *model facilitator* focuses on the model that is being built and the *wall builder* is primarily responsible for grouping the BOTGs and CLDs based on the facilitated discussion. Both roles should be filled by individuals who are familiar with SD and able to relay information and assumptions back to the group and restructure the processes as appropriate. The *recorder* writes down, sketches, or photographs the important parts of the proceedings to allow for a later reconstruction of the thought processes involved in the session. The *gatekeeper* helps frame the problem, identifies the appropriate participants, and works to support the modeling team (Hovmand et al., 2014; Langellier et al., 2019; Richardson & Andersen, 1995).

Workshop Structure

The structure of a GMB workshop commonly involves an introduction, a variable elicitation exercise, a behavior over time graphs exercise, a CLD exercise, a structure and behavior review, an action ideas session, concluding remarks, and an internal evaluation (Hovmand et al., 2014; Langellier et al., 2019). At the start, the *gatekeeper* convenes the group and introduces the identified problem, goals of the session, and modeling team. At this point, consent to participate is confirmed and documented. Following the introduction, a variable elicitation session begins, perhaps using dot stickers to prioritize EBIs. During this session, the group identifies key variables for inclusion in the CLD. These variables are factors that affect or are affected by policy, systems, and environmental changes in the community of interest. Given the potential to identify numerous variables, the goal of this session is to sift through the possible choices and select the variables most important to the participant group. The *community facilitator* instructs participants to place dots beside the issues they deem most important.

The next exercise is conducted to develop reference modes as BOTGs. These graphs help groups visualize important variables and how they move or change over time. This session serves as a springboard for deeper discussion about the problem to be modeled. The *community facilitator* provides examples of different time horizons and instructs participants to create graphs of how behavior changes over time for as many variables as possible. Participants are instructed to sort their graphs over time from most important/favorite to least important/favorite and then explain their decision. The *wall builder* clusters the BOTGs on the wall based on participants' discussion. The *wall builder* or *model facilitator* identifies a few key variables named by participants and begins to link the variables on sheets of paper to create the causal link diagram for the seed structure model.

The causal loop diagramming exercise involves the creation of a CLD based on key variables identified during the prior sessions. The purpose of this session is to make connections between variables and identify feedback loops to represent how variables are related in the target community. The *community facilitator* reviews the variables identified and the *model facilitator* introduces the basic conventions of the CLDs highlighting polarity, variable definition, feedback, and delays. The *model facilitator* reviews the preliminary model s/he created and asks for participants to work in small groups to create their own CLD by adding other variables and drawing connections from their CLD to the *model facilitator* CLD. The *community facilitator* then asks the small groups to present their CLDs and discuss potential conclusions based on their models. During the discussion, the *model facilitator* draws the CLD on a white erase board or paper for all participants to see.

Following the creation of the CLDs, there is a structure and behavior review. The *model facilitator* reviews the CLD and seeks validation from the participants that the variables and relationships have been accurately represented. Participants are encouraged to provide feedback and make adjustments.

After a model has been developed, the action ideas session is used to identify and prioritize actions. The *community facilitator* asks participants to describe ways in which they can intervene in the systems depicted by the CLDs, to assess the potential impact and feasibility of proposed interventions, and to consider the unintended or secondary consequences of such interventions.

During the closing of the session, the *gatekeeper* outlines the next steps and thanks participants. The *community facilitator* reviews the activities completed during the session, describes major products created, and explains how these products will be used to develop a clean, electronic version of the CLD. This electronic version will be shared with the participants to confirm the structure. Individuals are then asked to share their action ideas and how they relate to the model. The *wall builder* places these action ideas on the wall, ranking them based on the feasibility and potential impact.

After the workshop, the research team conducts an evaluation of the workshop products. A team member transfers the CLD to a computer program. Major aspects of the CLD, such as the feedback loops, direction of arrows and polarities, are verified using transcriptions of conversations during the GMB exercises and notes alongside the original drawings. The model is then shared with participants to further validate the model generated.

INTEGRATING METHODOLOGIES TO ADVANCE HEALTH EQUITY

In recent years, leaders in systems science and implementation science have called for greater attention toward addressing community-level health disparities and health equity. Together with local and national partners, CSAAH is applying an integrated approach to accelerate the translation of disparities research for diverse communities. This approach combines research methods from systems science and implementation science, leverages mixed-methods data, and is driven by CBPR principles. Figure 6.1 depicts the integrated approach.

Underlying Research Disciplines: CBPR, Systems Science, Implementation Science

As described above, systems science is a computational research approach that can be used to study complex connections and interactions between multi-level determinants of health and health outcomes. Our approach focuses specifically on the use of GMB, due to its participatory nature, and ABM, because this method better captures individual level behaviors and health outcomes than other techniques and is able to examine the complex nature of health inequalities (McAuley et al., 2016; Speybroeck et al., 2013). In addition, use of well-designed agent-based models may improve the prediction of outcomes related to an intervention under different

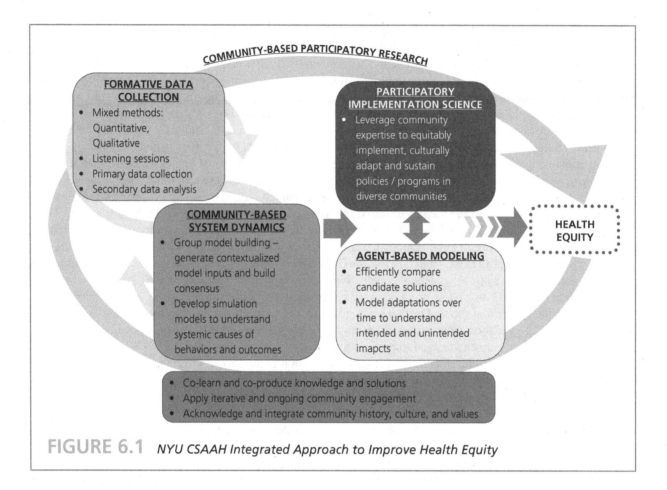

FIGURE 6.1 *NYU CSAAH Integrated Approach to Improve Health Equity*

scenarios and identify alternate policies and programs that may result in the desired outcomes (Auchincloss & Diez, 2008; Marshall & Galea, 2015). ABM has been increasingly used to study the development and consequences of chronic health conditions and for the comparison of health interventions (Li, Berenson, et al., 2016; Li, Kong, et al., 2015; Li, Lawley, et al., 2016; Nianogo & Arah, 2015; Zhang et al., 2015).

CBPR is defined by the W.K. Kellogg Foundation Community Health Scholars Program as "a collaborative approach to research that equitably involves all partners in the research process and recognizes the unique strengths that each brings. CBPR begins with a research topic of importance to the community and has the aim of combining knowledge with action and achieving social change to improve health outcomes and eliminate health disparities" (W.K. Kellogg Health Scholars, 2016). Unlike traditional health research, CBPR calls for the active and equal partnership of community stakeholders throughout the research process, including selecting health concerns and research questions, determining study design, recruiting participants, designing instruments, implementing research/interventions, and disseminating findings. If done well, CBPR promotes benefits such as increased trust between researchers and communities, enhanced quantity and quality of collected data, and stronger infrastructure building and sustainability (Green, 1995; Schulz et al., 1998). CBPR suggests that researchers' knowledge (e.g., research design, measurement tools, and data analysis) works in concert with community stakeholders' knowledge (e.g., cultural norms and values, community dynamics, organizational politics) to ensure the successful development and implementation of research and interventions. CBPR is further discussed in Chapter 8.

Dissemination and implementation (D&I) science is defined as "a growing field of study that examines the process by which scientific evidence is adopted, implemented, and sustained in typical community or clinical settings" (Estabrooks et al., 2018). *Dissemination research* is the scientific study of active and targeted distribution of information and materials from EBIs to audiences through specific channels and using planned strategies. *Implementation research* is the scientific study of using strategies to integrate evidence-based health interventions in specific settings, with the goals of improving outcomes and advancing population health. These concepts are described in greater detail in Chapter 7, along with additional key terms and definitions essential to understanding and conducting D&I research. The integrated framework presented in Figure 6.1 seeks to operationalize a *participatory implementation science* approach, grounded in CBPR principles, that seeks to integrate community-based organizations and stakeholders as research partners (not just study participants) by leveraging their unique expertise and honoring local culture, history, and knowledge (Ramanadhan et al., 2018). In this way, the approach aims to shift the research paradigm to co-produce knowledge and systems-level change to integrate research evidence into community settings and address health inequities.

Intersection of Systems Science, CBPR, and Implementation Science

GMB, ABM, CBPR, and implementation science are complementary. To maximize their utility, these methodologies may be employed together in an integrated approach that explores research questions in a nuanced, comprehensive manner. The goal of the integrated approach is to develop meaningful responses to complex questions about health disparities and determine efficient ways to advance health equity.

Systems Science and CBPR. The promise of combining systems science and CBPR approaches, and the potential synergies to be gained from the integration of these two methodologies, has been described (Frerichs et al., 2016). However, excluding a unique example of the application of these methods by a single research group toward the development of obesity prevention interventions, the full potential of combining these two methods to benefit racial/ethnic minority populations has not yet been realized (Gittelsohn et al., 2015). Both methodologies take a holistic view of problems and consider communities in context, focus on capacity and knowledge building and co-learning, and are geared toward the production of action-oriented solutions (Frerichs et al., 2016). Compared to community intervention trials that are costly and often challenging to implement in real-world settings, simulation analyses such as ABM provide important insights regarding changes in health behaviors and health outcomes across populations of interest amidst constantly evolving social, political, and economic contexts (Zhang et al., 2017). Further, while experimental or observational approaches may identify the relationship between a single risk factor and health outcomes after controlling for other factors, we propose to model behaviors, risk factors, and health outcomes as a complex system in which heterogeneous individuals interact with each other and their environment and adapt their behaviors dynamically.

Systems Science and Mixed Methods Data Collection. Systems science has been combined with mixed methods data collection in two notable examples. First, Gittelsohn et al. described a longstanding project in Baltimore in which a series of agent-based models were combined with extensive administrative and community-based data, including community input, to test the effects of obesity interventions and inform program selection (Gittelsohn et al., 2015). Second, Zhang et al. reported the effects of an agent-based model to evaluate the impact of different social network interventions on children's physical activity in two afterschool programs (Zhang et al., 2015). In that study, qualitative data from structured interviews were used in combination with quantitative data to build an agent-based model to simulate consumer behaviors in a food hub (Krejci et al., 2016). These two examples demonstrate that it is technically viable to combine CBPR with ABM by (1) applying primary data collected using a CBPR approach to model development; (2) using ABM to engage community partners and equip them with the necessary systems science tools and methods to allow for analysis of quantifiable program outcomes; and (3) promoting effective communication and collaboration among different stakeholders to design implementable, culturally sensitive programs.

As leaders in both fields have highlighted, systems thinking and methods hold great promise both for answering key implementation science questions as well as clarifying the relationships and interactions between key domains and contextual factors. Yet, to date, these methodologies have been underutilized thus far in D&I research. One key opportunity to address this gap is the application of GMB as a method for selecting and tailoring implementation strategies (Powell et al., 2017). This particular application appears in our integrated framework (Figure 6.1) in the green box in the lower left-hand side of the figure. Conducting GMB activities that are grounded in and driven by CBPR principles not only creates opportunities to generate *contextualized model inputs* driven by community and stakeholder perspectives and grounded in localized knowledge but also may lead to selecting implementation strategies that have optimal fit and greater buy-in from partner organizations and community members. In our conceptualization, generating contextualized model inputs refers to selecting relevant factors of interest (and estimating the size and range of their effects) in a manner that reflects and resonates with the lived experiences of communities and decision makers. Additionally, while implementation research to date has made great advances in identifying and focusing on contextual factors in one type of setting (e.g., clinical, community, schools, local health departments) or partnership at a time, implementation studies can and should start to engage with dynamic factors spanning multiple settings and sectors – a core facet of systems thinking and systems science. Opportunities to bridge sectors and account for contextual factors across multiple sectors are highlighted in the following case study.

APPLYING THE INTEGRATED APPROACH: HEALTHY AGING

CSAAH'S recent healthy aging collaboratives, developed in partnership with Asian American and Native Hawaiian and Pacific Islander (NH/PI) communities nationally and in New York City (NYC), provide an illustrative example of the application of the integrated approach described above. Our integrated approach consists of five segments: (1) CBPR; (2) formative research; (3) participatory implementation science; (4) community-based SD; and (5) AMB.

Driving the integrated approach are the *CBPR principles* that have been integral to CSAAH's efforts since we were first established in 2003 as a National Institutes of Health (NIH) National Institute on Minority Health & Health Disparities (NIMHD) Project Excellence in Partnership Outreach Reach and Training (EXPORT) Center. These include co-learning and co-producing knowledge and solutions, applying iterative and ongoing community engagement, and acknowledging and integrating community history, culture, and values. As described in previous publications, as we apply a community action-oriented model of advancing health equity, our primary mission is to address, alleviate, and eliminate health disparities among Asian American communities through a transdisciplinary and CBPR approach (Trinh-Shevrin et al., 2015). Applying this model includes maintaining our regional and national community and our academic partner base – a network that includes leading national organizations that serve the Asian American and NH/PI communities in the United States. In line with this emphasis, the development of our healthy aging section was first pursued in response to a request in 2012 from our partners to include aging-related questions within our ongoing Community Health Resources Needs Assessment (CHRNA). Figure 6.2 below depicts a timeline that begins with this request and details how our healthy aging work has progressed since then, with ongoing collaborations across sectors (e.g., academic, primary care, local government), as well as multiple grants secured to support this work across multiple dimensions of healthy aging.

Recent community-facing activities relevant to our healthy aging collaboratives include 1) the launch of a digital stories project, wherein we use short video vignettes to raise awareness of health disparities within Asian American and NH/PI populations through interactive storytelling; and 2) the development and delivery of linguistically appropriate information sessions for specific Asian American and NH/PI ethnic groups on topics related to the vignettes (e.g., oral health, nutrition).

Our mixed methods **formative research** activities have served both to build consensus among partners regarding project goals and priority activities as well as generate contextualized inputs for current and future GMB (see Case 5 in the Appendix).

We are also incorporating **participatory implementation science** into the structure this project via the cultural adaptation of an evidence-informed screening toolkit for early detection of cognitive decline. Adaptation of materials and messaging is a core process in implementation science that applies thoughtful and planned alterations to the design and/or delivery of an EBI or tool with the explicit goal of improving fit or effectiveness in a specific context (e.g., ethnic enclaves in NYC). More specifically, cultural adaptation refers to prioritizing cultural factors within the adaptation process and accounts for cultural patterns, meanings, and values within each context of interest. The screening toolkit for early cognitive decline, known as the Kickstart Assess Evaluate Refer (KAER) Toolkit, was developed by the Gerontological Society of America for use with aging adults in the general U.S. population. To date, there is no culturally adapted version of KAER for Asian American or any other racial/ethnic minority groups. CSAAH partnered with the Gerontological Society of America to carry out this adaptation for Asian Americans and the final toolkit will be delivered by CSAAH staff and partners to Chinese, Korean, and Bangladeshi American groups in community settings in NYC.

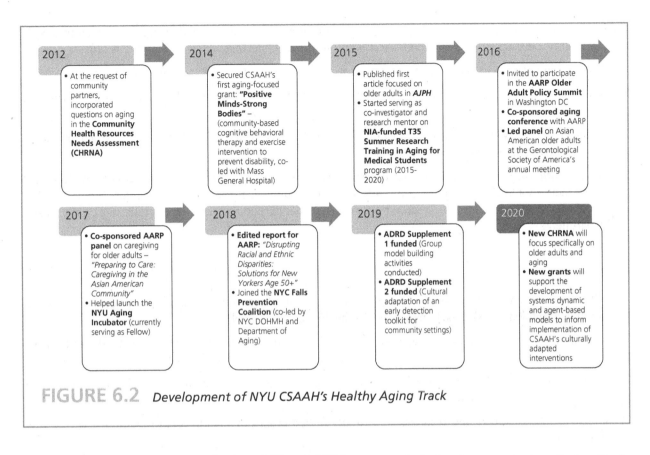

FIGURE 6.2 *Development of NYU CSAAH's Healthy Aging Track*

Activities to develop **community-based SD** and **ABM** are currently in development. As described earlier in this chapter, the purpose of the community-based SD work is to co-build capacity and co-develop simulation models that examine complex health behaviors and outcomes within community contexts. Our formative mixed methods data collection generated relevant initial inputs for these models and, at the time of writing this chapter, we are in the process of building capacity to conduct ABM. At this stage, we have modeled the theoretical impact of planned long-term construction in Manhattan's Chinatown on fruit and vegetable access and consumption for the neighborhood's older residents. Ultimately, our goal is to use ABM to inform our participatory implementation science work on the ground.

Preliminary findings from CSAAH's healthy aging collaboratives demonstrate that it is possible to achieve meaningful integration of calls to action in systems science and implementation science while simultaneously valuing the culture, history, and values of communities. Combining systems science with CBPR and implementations science, our integrated approach is a potentially powerful tool for prioritizing interventions for racial/ethnic minority communities. Because programs identified through our collaborative process are likely to have high acceptability in the populations of interest and prove feasible for community-based partners to implement, the translation of interventions to diverse populations may be accelerated. Moreover, describing the steps supporting the practical applications of our integrated approach to address health disparities in one culture-specific setting – in this case, healthy aging among Asian Americans in NYC – may inform broader dissemination and application of the approach to address health disparities in other real-world settings.

SUMMARY AND RECOMMENDATIONS

Public health problems – for all communities – are complex. Increasingly, these problems require multi-sector, multidisciplinary solutions that blend methodology, expertise, and lived experiences to address health inequity. For Asian American communities and other understudied populations (e.g., other racial/ethnic minority groups, sexual and gender minority groups, older adults), integrating systems science with community-partnered research and implementation science represents a potential way to improve efficiency, strengthen multi-sector partnerships, and, ultimately, develop feasible and more sustainable and acceptable approaches to improve health.

Recommendations for developing studies that operationalize an integrated approach include:

1. *Start small.* Reach out to local community-based organizations and listen to their priorities, concerns, and lived experiences.

2. *Learn in pieces.* Systems science is a vast field. Begin by selecting and understanding one particular method (e.g., ABM) to help make it more digestible.

3. *Build relationships with others across different academic fields of study.* For example, community-based researchers should develop partnerships with implementation science researchers. Epidemiologists should work with engineers and with practitioners in non-academic public health institutions (e.g., local health departments).

DISCUSSION QUESTIONS

1. Why is the systems science approach helpful for health equity research? What are some new solutions that could be provided by using systems science for health equity research?

2. How do the three systems science approaches described in the chapter (i.e., SD, ABM, GMB) differ from each other?

3. In addition to the healthy aging field, are there any other areas of health equity research that could benefit from applying an integrated approach?

4. Other than Asian Americans, what are some understudied groups that could benefit from this type of integrated approach?

REFERENCES

Auchincloss, A. H., & Diez Roux, A. V. (2008). A new tool for epidemiology: the usefulness of dynamic-agent models in understanding place effects on health. *American Journal of Epidemiology, 168*(1), 1–8. https://doi.org/10.1093/aje/kwn118

Bonabeau E. (2002). Agent-based modeling: methods and techniques for simulating human systems. *Proceedings of the National Academy of Sciences of the United States of America, 99 Suppl 3*(Suppl 3), 7280–7287. https://doi.org/10.1073/pnas.082080899

Epstein, J.M. (2006). *Generative social science: studies in agent-based computational modeling.* Princeton University Press.

Estabrooks, P. A., Brownson, R.C., Pronk, N.P. (2018). Dissemination and implementation science for public health professionals: An overview and call to action. *Preventing Chronic Disease, 15.* https://doi.org/10.5888/pcd15.180525

Forrester, J. (1961). *Industrial Dynamics.* Wiley.

Frerichs, L., Lich, K. H., Dave, G., & Corbie-Smith, G. (2016). Integrating Systems Science and Community-Based Participatory Research to Achieve Health Equity. *American Journal of Public Health, 106*(2), 215–222. https://doi.org/10.2105/AJPH.2015.302944

Frey, W. H. (2011). *The New Metro Minority Map: Regional Shifts in Hispanics, Asians, and Blacks from Census 2010.* Brookings. https://www.brookings.edu/research/the-new-metro-minority-map-regional-shifts-in-hispanics-asians-and-blacks-from-census-2010/

Gittelsohn, J., Mui, Y., Adam, A., Lin, S., Kharmats, A., Igusa, T., & Lee, B. Y. (2015). Incorporating Systems Science Principles into the Development of Obesity Prevention Interventions: Principles, Benefits, and Challenges. *Current Obesity Reports, 4*(2), 174–181. https://doi.org/10.1007/s13679-015-0147-x

Green, L.W. (1995). *Study of Participatory Research in Health Promotion: Review and Recommendations for the Development of Participatory Research in Health Promotion in Canada.* Royal Society of Canada.

Hovmand P., Brennan L., Kemner A. (2014). *Healthy kids, Healthy Communities group model building facilitation handbook.* http://www.transtria.com/pdfs/HKHC%20Group%20Model%20Building%20Handbook.pdf

Humes K.R., Jones N.A., Ramirez R.R. (2011). *Overview of Race and Hispanic Origin:* 2010. 2010 Census Briefs. https://www.census.gov/prod/cen2010/briefs/c2010br-02.pdf.

Krejci, C. C., Stone, R. T., Dorneich, M. C., & Gilbert, S. B. (2016). Analysis of Food Hub Commerce and Participation Using Agent-Based Modeling: Integrating Financial and Social Drivers. *Human Factors, 58*(1), 58–79. https://doi.org/10.1177/0018720815621173

Langellier, B. A., Kuhlberg, J. A., Ballard, E. A., Slesinski, S. C., Stankov, I., Gouveia, N., Meisel, J. D., Kroker-Lobos, M. F., Sarmiento, O. L., Caiaffa, W. T., Diez Roux, A. V., & SALURBAL Group (2019). Using community-based system dynamics modeling to understand the complex systems that influence health in cities: The SALURBAL study. *Health & Place, 60,* 102215. https://doi.org/10.1016/j.healthplace.2019.102215

Lee, H., Fitzpatrick, J. J., & Baik, S. Y. (2013). Why isn't evidence based practice improving health care for minorities in the United States?. *Applied Nursing Research, 26*(4), 263–268. https://doi.org/10.1016/j.apnr.2013.05.004

Li, Y., Berenson, J., Gutierrez, A., Pagan, J.A. (2016). everaging the Food Environment in Obesity Prevention: the Promise of Systems Science and Agent-Based Modeling. *Current Nutrition Reports, 5*(4):245–254. https://doi.org/10.1007/s13668-016-0179-1

Li, Y., Kong, N., Lawley, M., Weiss, L., & Pagán, J. A. (2015). Advancing the use of evidence-based decision-making in local health departments with systems science methodologies. *American Journal of Public Health, 105 Suppl 2*(Suppl 2), S217–S222. https://doi.org/10.2105/AJPH.2014.302077

Li, Y., Lawley, M. A., Siscovick, D. S., Zhang, D., & Pagán, J. A. (2016). Agent-Based Modeling of Chronic Diseases: A Narrative Review and Future Research Directions. *Preventing chronic Disease, 13*, E69. https://doi.org/10.5888/pcd13.150561

Li, Y., Zhang, D., & Pagán, J. A. (2016). Social Norms and the Consumption of Fruits and Vegetables across New York City Neighborhoods. *Journal of Urban Health: Bulletin of the New York Academy of Medicine, 93*(2), 244–255. https://doi.org/10.1007/s11524-016-0028-y

Luke, D. A., & Stamatakis, K. A. (2012). Systems science methods in public health: dynamics, networks, and agents. *Annual Review of Public Health, 33*, 357–376. https://doi.org/10.1146/annurev-publhealth-031210-101222

Marshall, B. D., & Galea, S. (2015). Formalizing the role of agent-based modeling in causal inference and epidemiology. *American Journal of Epidemiology, 181*(2), 92–99. https://doi.org/10.1093/aje/kwu274

McAuley, A., Denny, C., Taulbut, M., Mitchell, R., Fischbacher, C., Graham, B., Grant, I., O'Hagan, P., McAllister, D., & McCartney, G. (2016). Informing Investment to Reduce Inequalities: A Modelling Approach. *PloS One, 11*(8), e0159256. https://doi.org/10.1371/journal.pone.0159256

Nianogo, R. A., & Arah, O. A. (2015). Agent-based modeling of noncommunicable diseases: a systematic review. *American Journal of Public Health, 105*(3), e20–e31. https://doi.org/10.2105/AJPH.2014.302426

Oh, S. S., Galanter, J., Thakur, N., Pino-Yanes, M., Barcelo, N. E., White, M. J., de Bruin, D. M., Greenblatt, R. M., Bibbins-Domingo, K., Wu, A. H., Borrell, L. N., Gunter, C., Powe, N. R., & Burchard, E. G. (2015). Diversity in Clinical and Biomedical Research: A Promise Yet to Be Fulfilled. *PLoS Medicine, 12*(12), e1001918. https://doi.org/10.1371/journal.pmed.1001918

Powell, B. J., Beidas, R. S., Lewis, C. C., Aarons, G. A., McMillen, J. C., Proctor, E. K., & Mandell, D. S. (2017). Methods to Improve the Selection and Tailoring of Implementation Strategies. *The Journal of Behavioral Health Services & Research, 44*(2), 177–194. https://doi.org/10.1007/s11414-015-9475-6

Ramanadhan, S., Davis, M. M., Armstrong, R., Baquero, B., Ko, L. K., Leng, J. C., Salloum, R. G., Vaughn, N. A., & Brownson, R. C. (2018). Participatory implementation science to increase the impact of evidence-based cancer prevention and control. *Cancer Causes & Control, 29*(3), 363–369. https://doi.org/10.1007/s10552-018-1008-1

Richardson, G. P., & Andersen, D. F. (1995). Teamwork in group model building. *System Dynamics Review, 11*(2), 113–137. https://doi.org/10.1002/sdr.4260110203

Speybroeck, N., Van Malderen, C., Harper, S., Müller, B., & Devleesschauwer, B. (2013). Simulation models for socioeconomic inequalities in health: a systematic review. *International Journal of Environmental Research and Public Health, 10*(11), 5750–5780. https://doi.org/10.3390/ijerph10115750

Sterman, J. (2000). *Business dynamics: Systems thinking and modeling for a complex world.* Irwin/McGraw-Hill.

Trinh-Shevrin, C., Kwon, S. C., Park, R., Nadkarni, S. K., & Islam, N. S. (2015). Moving the dial to advance population health equity in New York City Asian American populations. *American Journal of Public Health, 105 Suppl 3*(Suppl 3), e16–e25. https://doi.org/10.2105/AJPH.2015.302626

U.S. Census Bureau. (2017). *Newsroom: The Nation's Population is Becoming More Diverse.* https://www.census.gov/newsroom/press-releases/2017/cb17-100.html.

W.K. Kellogg Health Scholars (2016). *Community Track.* http://www.kellogghealthscholars.org/about/community.php

Zhang, J., Shoham, D. A., Tesdahl, E., & Gesell, S. B. (2015). Network interventions on physical activity in an afterschool program: an agent-based social network study. American *Journal of Public Health, 105 Suppl 2*(Suppl 2), S236–S243. https://doi.org/10.2105/AJPH.2014.302277

Zhang, X., Pérez-Stable, E. J., Bourne, P. E., Peprah, E., Duru, O. K., Breen, N., Berrigan, D., Wood, F., Jackson, J. S., Wong, D., & Denny, J. (2017). Big Data Science: Opportunities and Challenges to Address Minority Health and Health Disparities in the 21st Century. *Ethnicity & Disease, 27*(2), 95–106. https://doi.org/10.18865/ed.27.2.95

CHAPTER

PARTICIPATORY DISSEMINATION AND IMPLEMENTATION RESEARCH IN COMMUNITY SETTINGS

MATTHEW LEE, SIMONA C. KWON

LEARNING OBJECTIVES

By the end of this chapter, readers will be able to:

- Define key concepts from dissemination and implementation science and how they relate to community health and health disparities research.
- Identify models and frameworks used to conduct dissemination and implementation research in community settings.
- Describe opportunities and future directions for implementation science to advance and sustain health equity for underserved populations.

Applied Population Health Approaches for Asian American Communities, First Edition. Edited by Simona C. Kwon, Chau Trinh-Shevrin, Nadia S. Islam, and Stella S. Yi.
© 2023 John Wiley & Sons, Inc. Published 2023 by John Wiley & Sons, Inc.
Companion Website: www.wiley.com/go/kwon/asianamerican

INTRODUCTION

There are well-documented gaps between what is known to work in research (e.g., evidence-based interventions [EBIs], including programs, practices, policies, guidelines) and practice (e.g., translation into clinical and community settings), particularly for underserved racial/ethnic minorities and immigrant populations (Clarke et al., 2013; Institute of Medicine, 2001; Purnell et al., 2016). Dissemination and implementation (D&I) science in health has emerged as a rapidly growing field to address these research-to-practice gaps, focused on enhancing the overall quality and quantity of evidence and accelerating its translation into real-world uptake to impact equitable and sustainable outcomes (Estabrooks et al., 2018; Lobb & Colditz, 2013). In recent years, tremendous developments in the field have encouraged greater attention to contextual factors that impact the successful and equitable reach, adoption, implementation, and sustainability of EBIs as well as strategies that may improve these processes and outcomes (Chinman et al., 2017; Woodward et al., 2019). However, much of D&I research has focused on clinical and practice settings, with less emphasis on understanding how many of these contextual factors and implementation strategies are also shaped by community dynamics, including culture, history, values, and capacity (DuMont et al., 2019; Minkler et al., 2018; Ramanadhan et al., 2018). This chapter provides an introduction to conducting community-based and community-partnered D&I research, with an emphasis on the importance of cultural adaptation to enhance the relevance, acceptability, appropriateness, reach, fit, and sustainability of EBIs for underserved populations. We begin with an overview of key terminology and frameworks from implementation science that have been used to conduct D&I research in community settings and present our own process framework of participatory cultural adaptation for implementation research (see Figure 7.1). To conclude, we provide recommendations for leveraging community-partnered and participatory implementation science to shift the paradigm of intervention research toward prioritizing marginalized populations within the EBI development process and building community capacity to sustain EBIs to reduce gaps and inequities in health.

KEY TERMINOLOGY

Dissemination and implementation (D&I) science has been defined succinctly by leaders in the field as "a growing field of study that examines the process by which scientific evidence is adopted, implemented, and sustained in typical community or clinical settings" (Estabrooks et al., 2018). Specifically, *dissemination research* is the scientific study of active and focused distribution of information and materials from EBIs to audiences through specific channels and using planned strategies. *Implementation research* is defined as the scientific study of using strategies to integrate EBIs successfully within specific settings in order to improve outcomes and advance population health. More recently, experts have also advanced *participatory implementation science* as an approach within the field that can more explicitly call attention to the need for coordinated and effective action by supporting "iterative, ongoing engagement between stakeholders and researchers to improve the pathway between research and practice, create system change, and address health disparities and health equity" (Ramanadhan et al., 2018).

Despite the importance of ensuring that research evidence is communicated effectively and clearly to key public health audiences, particularly community leaders and advocates, dissemination remains an understudied domain within implementation science. *Dissemination strategies* refer to the specific mechanisms and channels used to package and spread information about EBIs to reach key stakeholders and decision makers in a particular setting, including potential adopters and opinion leaders. In contrast to passive approaches to diffusing information (e.g., expecting community practitioners, leaders, and advocates to identify and digest research publications on their own), dissemination is planned, active, focused, and may be either very broad (e.g., mass media campaigns) or very narrow (e.g., intensive one-on-one technical assistance) in its scope.

Purtle and colleagues outlined *data-driven dissemination* as a novel approach that focuses on specifying three concrete areas within the broad scope of dissemination research and practice: (1) *formative audience research* to characterize the awareness, adoption, and attitudes of a particular audience toward an intervention as well as how they prefer to receive information about their community and their health; (2) *audience segmentation research* to identify and meaningfully engage subgroups within an audience to tailor dissemination strategies for each segment; and (3) *dissemination effectiveness research* to test and evaluate the outcomes of each

TABLE 7.1 **Examples of Data-Driven Dissemination Research Focused on Asian American Communities and Health**

Formative audience research	• Conduct a national survey of community-based organizations that primarily serve Asian Americans and immigrant populations to understand how they seek information about and identify resources to deliver EBIs to the communities they serve. • Interview local policy makers about their beliefs, knowledge, and attitudes toward health disparities that disproportionately impact Asian Americans in their jurisdiction and whom they would contact about issues regarding Asian American health.
Audience segmentation research	• First: Conduct key informant interviews at faith-based organizations (e.g., mosques) in the local community to identify relevant subgroups in the setting (e.g., imams, elders, adolescents). • Second: Conduct focus groups with each subgroup to identify who/what are the trusted sources of health information for them.
Dissemination effectiveness research	• Test whether airing segments on a local Korean-language radio station to promote a smoking cessation program being offered at a Korean-serving community-based organization increases the program's recruitment, participation, and completion rates. • Evaluate whether distributing a culturally appropriate and relevant plate planning tool at ethnic supermarkets increases dietary knowledge and supports behavior change for Chinese youth and their parents.

individual strategy and the dissemination plan as a whole (Purtle et al., 2020). Table 7.1 provides an overview of this approach with specific community-focused examples for each of the three areas.

Implementation researchers have focused a great deal of attention on building conceptual clarity and consensus in specifying implementation strategies and implementation outcomes. *Implementation strategies* are defined as "systematic processes or methods, techniques, activities, and resources that support the adoption, integration, and sustainment of [EBIs] into usual settings" (Rabin & Brownson, 2018). Powell and colleagues (2015) conducted a modified Delphi process with implementation experts to compile and refine implementation strategies and their definitions into a discrete list of 73 strategies referred to as the Expert Recommendations for Implementing Change (ERIC) compilation or compendium. Some of these strategies include discrete actions such as *obtaining formal commitments* from community partners on their roles and responsibilities related to implementing change or *conducting dynamic trainings*, while others focus on generating more structural change and systems-level action such as *building coalitions, accessing new funding,* and *capturing and sharing local knowledge.*

Implementation strategies are selected to support successful implementation, which may be assessed by explicitly identifying and assessing *implementation outcomes,* defined as "the effects of deliberate and purposive actions to implement new treatments, practices, and services" (Proctor et al., 2011). Importantly, implementation outcomes must be understood as distinct from intervention outcomes at the clinical, treatment, behavioral, or service levels. However, they are also a necessary precursor to intervention success: failing to achieve implementation outcomes will result in poor intervention outcomes. Table 7.2 highlights some of the key differences between conceptualizing implementation versus intervention outcomes in community settings.

Closely related to implementation is the potential need for *de-implementation* in a setting. Specifically, de-adoption and unlearning of prior programs and practices may be necessary in order to make space and free up resources for the adoption of new evidence-based changes. For underserved and marginalized communities, in particular, out-of-date or even harmful practices and programs may be in place because of lack of access to newer guidelines and recommendations and/or the resources needed to implement them.

Often, an EBI may have been developed or evaluated in a community or setting in which resources and/or capacity differed from the conditions in which the current D&I research is being conducted. In these instances, adaptation may be necessary to tailor the EBI to local needs and the real-world context of the community. A key

TABLE 7.2 Examples of Outcomes in Community-Based Implementation Research

Implementation Outcomes	Intervention Effectiveness, Efficiency, Equity, and Impacts on:
• **Feasibility** given community capacity and available resources • **Acceptability** of the selected EBI for community leaders and members • **Appropriateness** of the selected strategies and communication channels • **Adoption** of the EBI by community leaders, opinion leaders, and members • **Fidelity** to EBI protocol and core functions • **Dose** or amount delivered to key community subgroups • **Reach** or penetration of the program • **Sustainability** of the change effort within the community setting • **Costs** of implementing and sustaining the EBI	– Community knowledge, attitudes, and practices – Health behaviors + behavioral outcomes – Neighborhood access – Social cohesion and social networks – Community advocacy and collective action – Quality of care + clinical outcomes

domain in implementation science, *adaptation,* is defined by Stirman and colleagues (2019) as "the process of thoughtful and deliberate alteration to the design or delivery of an intervention, with the goal of improving its fit or effectiveness in a given context." *Cultural adaptation,* more specifically, refers to modifications that pay explicit attention to the importance of cultural patterns, meanings, and values within the community context and seeks to integrate both observable and cognitive aspects of a local culture into intervention content (Barrera et al., 2013). As defined by Bernal and colleagues (2009), cultural adaptation is "the systematic modification of an evidence-based treatment (EBT) or intervention protocol to consider language, culture, and context in such a way that it is compatible with the client [and community's] cultural patterns, meanings, and values."

While modifications to intervention delivery are common in dynamic settings and occur for a variety of reasons, these changes are not always documented or reported (Escoffery et al., 2018). Important considerations when adapting and culturally adapting EBIs include the *scale* of the adaptation (e.g., from small tweaks and refinements to major changes, such as adding/removing/re-ordering elements), the *timing* of the adaptation (e.g., pre-adoption, pre-implementation, during implementation, during sustainment), whether the adaptation was *planned/proactive* or *unplanned/reactive,* who participated in the decision and process to adapt (e.g., community leaders and members), as well as the baseline *capacity* (e.g., structures, processes, and resources available in the setting) – and whether additional *capacity building* might be necessary to foster successful adaptation, implementation, and sustainability. *Capacity building* describes activities or strategies that aim to build resources and enable a community setting to deliver an EBI, especially after the initial support and funding for the EBI has concluded, and is a critical consideration when working with underserved communities and partnering with community-based organizations (Ramanadhan et al., 2020; Ramanadhan et al., 2021).

As D&I researchers seek to make adaptations explicit by documenting and reporting them, it is essential for researchers and practitioners to set clear *goals and reasons* for the adaptation and adapted elements, identify exactly *which elements* were modified and at *what level,* and, finally, to what extent fidelity to the core elements or functions of the original EBI was preserved. *Fidelity* is defined as the degree to which an intervention is implemented as intended. In the case of complex and multilevel interventions, fidelity describes the degree to which the core functions and processes of the intervention – rather than its specific components – were respected. Experts have differentiated between *fidelity-consistent modifications* (changes that preserve core elements needed for the intervention to be effective) and *fidelity-inconsistent modifications* (changes that alter the intervention in a manner that fails to preserve core elements) (Stirman et al., 2015; Shelton et al., 2018).

Most D&I research to date has focused on identifying factors and testing strategies that are critical to successful adoption and initial implementation of EBIs, with less attention focused on examining longer-term *sustainment* and *sustainability* (Birken et al., 2020; Shelton et al., 2018; Shelton & Lee, 2019; Stirman et al., 2012).

Leaders in the field have argued that sustainability research should be seen as a distinct and dynamic stage in translation science and that lack of knowledge about the conditions that sustain EBIs and their benefits and impacts is currently one of the most significant translational research problems facing the field (Chambers et al., 2013; Proctor et al., 2015; Scheirer & Dearing, 2011). Others have highlighted that better understanding, measuring, and communicating the value of sustainability may enhance the population return on investment (ROI) of public health research (Shelton et al., 2018; Shelton & Lee, 2019). Despite these calls to action, studying sustainment and sustainability remains challenging because the definitions and related concepts continue to evolve over time. Advancing methods for sustainability research is difficult due to the lack of clarity and consensus on what factors should be measured and which determinants and outcomes matter, particularly in community and other real-world settings. The most recent effort to compile a comprehensive definition of sustainability to advance D&I research came from Moore and colleagues (2017):

> (1) after a defined period of time, (2) the program, clinical intervention, and/or implementation strategies continue to be delivered and/or (3) individual behavior change (i.e., clinician, patient) is maintained; (4) the program and individual behavior change may evolve or adapt while (5) continuing to produce benefits for individuals/systems.

Building on this definition, in a review of reviews focused on sustainment studies, Birken and colleagues (2020) drew a distinction between sustainment – defined as "continuous evidence-based practice use, as intended, over time in ongoing operations, often involving adaptation to dynamic contexts" – and sustainability, which they described as "preparedness for sustained use or the characteristics of a new practice which will enhance its sustainment." Related to these definitions is the concept of sustainability capacity, which Schell and colleagues (2013) defined as "the existence of structures and processes that allow a program to leverage resources to effectively implement and maintain evidence-based policies and activities" and operationalized as a set of planning tools first with the development of the Program Sustainability Assessment Tool (PSAT) and, later, the Clinical Sustainability Assessment Tool (CSAT) (Center for Public Health Systems Science, 2021).

Lastly, the concepts of scaling-up and scaling-out are both relevant to implementation and sustainability research in community settings, particularly since the continuation of an EBI will likely involve some spread to additional similar or even new settings in the area. As defined by Aarons and colleagues (2017), *scale-up* is "the deliberate effort to broaden the delivery of an EBI with the intention of reaching larger numbers of a target audience" whereas *scale-out* is "an extension of scale-up and uniquely refers to the deliberate use of strategies to implement, test, improve, and sustain an EBI as it is delivered to new populations and/or through new delivery systems that differ from those in effectiveness trials." One community-based example of scaling-up would be to take an EBI focused on preventing cardiovascular disease that was designed for delivery by community health workers (CHWs) at local faith-based organizations (e.g., three mosques in Brooklyn, New York) and try to roll out that intervention to all other mosques in New York City or New York State. Extending this example, a related scale-out effort could involve exploring the relevance of bringing that same cardiovascular disease prevention program to nearby Korean churches, given that the churches have structures in place similar to those found in the mosques (e.g., communal meals prepared and served at the faith-based organization several days a week). When implementing an EBI in a new setting or focusing its delivery on a new community, it is essential to consider whether there is sufficient justification to expect that the EBI would have similar benefits to those found in earlier trials.

THEORIES, MODELS, AND FRAMEWORKS

As a rapidly growing field, D&I science has developed an astonishing array of theories, frameworks, and models (TMFs). These TMFs have been useful in identifying and describing potential barriers and facilitators associated with adoption, implementation, and sustainment and in informing planning, measurement, and evaluation in D&I studies. Recent reviews have categorized TMFs as being focused either on processes, determinants, outcomes, evaluation, or pragmatic considerations – or as hybrid frameworks serving multiple purposes (Damschroder, 2020; Shelton et al., 2020). These reviews have also summarized common elements across the TMFs most commonly used in D&I research.

Several frameworks highlight important domains or phases within D&I science. For example, the EPIS framework by Aarons and colleagues (2011) highlights four iterative phases: Exploration, Preparation/Adoption, Implementation, and Sustainment. Similarly, Koh and colleagues (2020) introduced five key domains within D&I science, including Context Assessment/EBI selection, Dissemination, Adaptation, Implementation, and Sustainability.

Other frameworks have focused on compiling and organizing contextual factors across implementation theories. For example, the Consolidated Framework for Implementation Research (CFIR) describes 39 theoretical constructs across five contextual domains: outer context, inner context, implementation processes, interventionist characteristics; intervention characteristics (Damschroder et al., 2009). In our work at the NYU Center for the Study of Asian American Health (CSAAH) at NYU Grossman School of Medicine, we applied four CFIR domains to analyze factors influencing implementation outcomes in our Racial and Ethnic Approaches to Community Health for Asian Americans (REACH FAR) project to deliver culturally adapted, evidence-based hypertension prevention programs across ethnic grocery stores, restaurants and faith-based organizations. Specifically, we focused on understanding site leaders' and champions' perceptions about adopting, adapting, and sustaining the program at the inner and outer settings to inform future translation and sustainability (Gore et al., 2019). Case 1 in the Appendix describes the implementation of REACH FAR.

Another implementation science framework that has demonstrated great versatility in informing intervention and implementation design, planning, and evaluation is the RE-AIM framework. As described more extensively in Chapter 6, RE-AIM stands for Reach; Effectiveness; Adoption; Implementation; and Maintenance (Glasgow et al., 2019; Glasgow et al., 1999). A robust framework developed to facilitate transparency in reporting, RE-AIM has become one of the most widely used frameworks in implementation science. Importantly, additional extensions were developed recently to guide assessment of contextual factors (PRISM – Practical Robust Implementation and Sustainability Model) (McCreight et al., 2019) to support pragmatic application in community and clinical settings (Glasgow & Estabrooks, 2018), integrate qualitative assessments of contextual factors (McCreight et al., 2019), and enhance sustainability and promote health equity (Shelton et al., 2020).

While some of these TMFs have been tested and applied in community settings, numerous opportunities exist for D&I researchers to investigate TMFs in community-partnered and participatory implementation science. Specifically, by co-selecting which TMFs to use to guide action and co-identifying how to meaningfully operationalize domains and constructs in the TMFs, researchers and community partners may advance understanding of the applicability and transferability of these TMFs in real-world settings. For example, despite the vast array of TMFs available to guide D&I researchers, few studies have focused explicitly on integrating principles from community-based participatory research (CBPR) to guide cultural adaptation processes in order to enhance successful dissemination, implementation, and sustainability of EBIs for underserved communities to eliminate health disparities.

PARTICIPATORY CULTURAL ADAPTATION FRAMEWORK FOR IMPLEMENTATION RESEARCH (PCAFIR)

Informed by years of conducting community-partnered and participatory implementation research focused on advancing health equity and building community capacity, we present a novel framework called the Participatory Cultural Adaptation Framework for Implementation Research (PCAFIR) (Figure 7.1).

1. Community Engagement and Promotion

Structured as a process framework for planned/proactive cultural adaptation, the PCAFIR encourages implementation researchers to begin by undergirding and supporting the entire process of culturally adapting, implementing, and sustaining EBIs by not just understanding but also respecting and upholding community priorities, history, values, and capacity. This emphasis is essential to maintaining ongoing community engagement and buy-in and to ensuring that implementation costs do not pose undue burdens to available community resources, infrastructure, and support structures. One potential research action step to inform this dimension of the process model comes from the *data-driven dissemination* approach described earlier from Purtle and colleagues (2020).

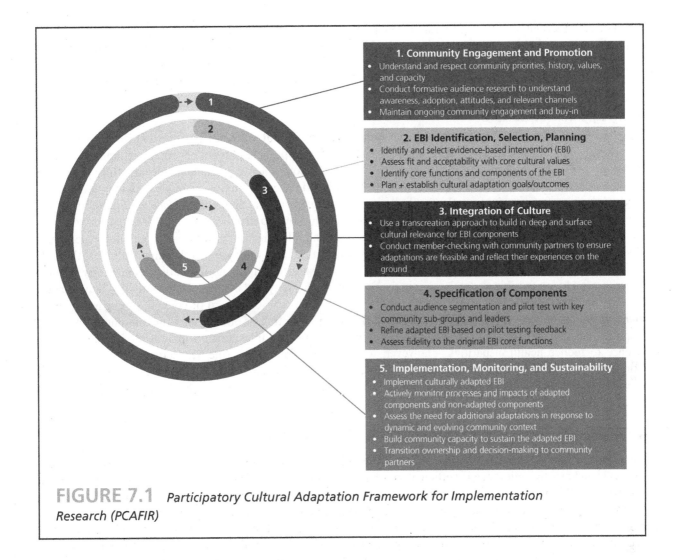

FIGURE 7.1 *Participatory Cultural Adaptation Framework for Implementation Research (PCAFIR)*

Using this approach, formative audience research may be conducted to identify the attitudes and beliefs that community leaders and members hold toward a particular health issue or disparity, available EBIs to address them, and preferred channels to receive trusted information about them.

2. EBI Identification, Selection, and Planning

In the next phase, grounded in that baseline understanding of current community capacity, awareness, and attitudes, researchers must identify potential EBIs to adapt to the culture, logistical realities, and budgetary constraints of the specific community setting and population. Several databases of EBIs are available to guide community-based researchers in identifying relevant programs that may demonstrate fit and acceptability to community partners and that also provide access to program materials. These databases include the National Cancer Institute's Evidence-Based Cancer Control Programs (EBCCP) website (formerly known as the RTIPS – Research-Tested Intervention Programs database), the Guide to Community Preventive Services (also known as The Community Guide), and the Pew Results First Clearinghouse Database, which contains information on the effectiveness of over 3,068 social policy programs.

A key aspect of determining the feasibility of delivering EBIs is identifying the costs associated with obtaining program materials and supporting implementation (Dopp et al., 2019). Although some EBI databases currently include some components of this critical costing data, many intervention researchers have neglected to detail these important aspects of program development and implementation, making program costs difficult to estimate, particularly in community settings. Once the EBI with the best initial fit has been selected together with community partners, it is important that researchers and their partners work together to co-identify goals for the adaptation process and set outcomes of interest to measure and evaluate when testing the adapted EBI.

3. Integration of Culture

The third phase of the PCAFIR process focuses on integrating cultural relevance into existing EBI components. We strongly encourage D&I researchers to use a *transcreation* approach, moving beyond the simple and literal *translation* of intervention materials. By transcreating the EBI components, researchers meaningfully imbue the adapted materials with the same implications for the new audience/community of interest as they did for the original audience/community by reflecting both surface and deep cultural domains. *Surface culture* refers to elements that may be observed about a community and its culture from a distance, whereas *deep culture* refers to elements that emerge only through meaningful interactions and relationship-building with community members. Once the transcreated materials are developed, researchers must carry out member-checking activities, through which the researchers circle back to the community and ensure that the materials reflect community partner experiences and are feasible to deliver within the community capacity and context. These activities may include conducting focus group discussions, giving a presentation to an advisory board or council, or engaging informally with the community (e.g., asking for feedback during a meeting or phone call with community leaders). Nápoles and colleagues (2018) have also recently called for bringing a transcreation approach to implementation science to reduce health disparities – however, whereas their framework (the Transcreation Framework for Community-engaged Behavioral Interventions to Reduce Health Disparities) is focused on guiding the design and delivery of a new transcreated intervention, our framework applies transcreation to focus on guiding the cultural adaptation of EBIs.

4. Specification of Components

Once the EBI components, messages, and materials have been transcreated, it is important to ensure that the symbolic and emotive relevance is sufficient to achieve the desired reach and penetration across key community subgroups within the population of interest. Drawing again from the data-driven dissemination approach, one recommendation is to use an audience segmentation approach to pilot test the culturally adapted EBI. Doing so ensures that key subgroups have not been overlooked. Once the pilot testing feedback from each segment has been used to further refine the culturally adapted EBI components, a critical next step is to conduct a fidelity assessment to compare the original EBI to the culturally adapted EBI in order to characterize whether and to what extent the core functions are preserved and recognizable (*fidelity consistent*) or whether those core elements and functions have changed (*fidelity inconsistent*) (Stirman et al., 2019).

5. Equitable Implementation, Monitoring, and Sustainability

At this point in the PCAFIR process, the culturally adapted EBI is ready to be delivered in the community setting for which it was intentionally and specifically adapted. Using the products developed during the previous phases, in which the adaptation process was explicitly documented, actively monitor the processes and impacts of the adapted components from initial implementation through sustainment. If any original components were not adapted, compare their performance to the adapted components and explore the need for additional or further adaptation. We recognize that community settings are dynamic and constantly evolving, so it is critical to regularly assess the need for additional planned adaptation as well as to document and report any unplanned/reactive adaptations that are made with the same rigor that was applied to the original cultural adaptation. Given our grounding in participatory approaches, our vision of sustaining culturally adapted EBIs includes the need to continuously build community capacity (e.g., to ensure sufficient resources to meet the demands and costs of continued implementation) as well as gradual transition of ownership of the program to the community. Engaging community partners not just as key stakeholders but also as key implementers throughout the full process helps to center community expertise and reduces the risk of reproducing power imbalances that often occur in community-partnered research. As we have learned from our extensive work with CHW-led interventions and longstanding partnerships with community-based organizations, implementation success is often predicated on (and can be sustained by) meaningful and ongoing engagement with actions on the ground at the community-level.

SUMMARY AND RECOMMENDATIONS

To conclude, the authors advocate for a paradigm shift in intervention and implementation research. There is a critical need to reassess the criteria used to evaluate whether or not an intervention is deemed "evidence-based." This reassessment centers on two points. First, we argue that researchers must review and critically assess existing EBIs, placing health equity principles at the center of that process. This requires us to ask three core questions of EBIs:

1. *Effective for whom?* Has the effectiveness of the EBI been demonstrated within marginalized populations or communities bearing the brunt of health disparities? Were marginalized and minoritized communities included in the efficacy and effectiveness trials?

2. *Based on what evidence?* Were the goals and outcomes used to evaluate the intervention measured only based on researcher values and priorities, or were community and cultural values and priorities meaningfully integrated as relevant evidence?

3. *What happens as dynamic contexts change over time?* Does the evidence base sufficiently recognize that an intervention's effectiveness is likely to shift in response to evolving contexts and population dynamics?

Second, at an even more fundamental level, researchers must recognize and remedy the inequity inherent in the current EBI development process. Typically, interventions are designed and tested for effectiveness and efficiency among better-resourced and well-reached populations before they are adapted and scaled-down for less-resourced and less-reached communities. This unidirectional design and testing of interventions with the expectation that "one-size-fits-all" approaches will achieve sufficient or equitable reach and impact for populations that are disproportionately and unfairly burdened by health disparities is unrealistic. Instead, EBIs should be designed explicitly for populations bearing the brunt of health disparities, accounting for the logistical issues, budgetary constraints, and cultural specificities that emerge in communities with complex and unique needs and strengths. Once an EBI is shown to be effective and efficient in a harder-to-reach population, then scale-up and scale-out of the EBI to better-resourced communities in the general population may be considered and is likely to be more successful and sustainable.

Introducing this type of progressive approach to EBI development could prove effective not only in improving health outcomes but also in increasing the cost-effectiveness of public health interventions. If an EBI were developed to accommodate the complex needs and limited budgets of lower-resourced communities, adapting that intervention for better-resourced populations with less intensive needs would be less demanding in terms of both scope and cost – benefiting research, policy, and practice priorities simultaneously. Conversely, resisting this change is likely to perpetuate and expand health inequities, preventing progress toward our goal of advancing population health equity and eliminating health disparities.

DISCUSSION QUESTIONS

1. What are some of the key challenges and factors affecting the translation of research findings into equitable real-world impacts, particularly for underserved communities?

2. How would you communicate the concept of "evidence-based interventions" to a community partner without using public health jargon? What about "implementation" or "dissemination"?

3. Drawing from the communities you have either lived or worked in (or currently live/work in), identify two or three reasons why cultural adaptation of EBIs would be necessary to optimize successful and equitable implementation and sustainment in that setting.

REFERENCES

Aarons, G. A., Hurlburt, M., & Horwitz, S. M. (2011). Advancing a conceptual model of evidence-based practice implementation in public service sectors. *Administration and Policy in Mental Health and Mental Health Services Research*, *38*(1), 4–23. https://doi.org/10.1007/s10488-010-0327-7

Aarons, G. A., Sklar, M., Mustanski, B., Benbow, N., & Brown, C. H. (2017). "Scaling-out" evidence-based interventions to new populations or new health care delivery systems. *Implementation Science*, *12*(1), 111. https://doi.org/10.1186/s13012-017-0640-6

Barrera Jr., M., Castro, F. G., Strycker, L. A., & Toobert, D. J. (2013). Cultural adaptations of behavioral health interventions: A progress report. *Journal of Consulting and Clinical Psychology*, *81*(2), 196. https://doi.org/10.1037/a0027085

Bernal, G., Jimenez-Chafey, M. I., & Domenech Rodríguez, M. M. (2009). Cultural adaptation of treatments: A resource for considering culture in evidence-based practice. *Professional Psychology: Research and Practice*, *40*, 361–368. https://doi.org/10.1037/a0016401

Birken, S. A., Haines, E. R., Hwang, S., Chambers, D. A., Bunger, A. C., & Nilsen, P. (2020). Advancing understanding and identifying strategies for sustaining evidence-based practices: a review of reviews. *Implementation Science*, *15*(1), 88. https://doi.org/10.1186/s13012-020-01040-9

Center for Public Health Systems Science. (2021). *Rate the sustainability capability of your program or clinical practice to help plan for the future.* Retrieved from Washington University of St. Louis, https://www.sustaintool.org.

Chambers, D. A., Glasgow, R. E., & Stange, K. C. (2013). The dynamic sustainability framework: addressing the paradox of sustainment amid ongoing change. *Implementation Science*, *8*(1), 117. https://doi.org/10.1186/1748-5908-8-117

Chinman, M., Woodward, E. N., Curran, G. M., & Hausmann, L. R. (2017). Harnessing implementation science to increase the impact of health disparity research. *Medical care*, *55*(Suppl 9 2), S16–S23. https://doi.org/10.1097/MLR.0000000000000769

Clarke, A. R., Goddu, A. P., Nocon, R. S., Stock, N. W., Chyr, L. C., Akuoko, J. A., & Chin, M. H. (2013). Thirty years of disparities intervention research: what are we doing to close racial and ethnic gaps in health care?. *Medical Care*, *51*(11), 1020–1026. https://doi.org/10.1097/MLR.0b013e3182a97ba3

Damschroder, L. J. (2020). Clarity out of chaos: use of theory in implementation research. *Psychiatry Research*, *283*, 112461. https://doi.org/10.1016/j.psychres.2019.06.036

Damschroder, L. J., Aron, D. C., Keith, R. E., Kirsh, S. R., Alexander, J. A., & Lowery, J. C. (2009). Fostering implementation of health services research findings into practice: a consolidated framework for advancing implementation science. *Implementation Science*, *4*, 50. https://doi.org/10.1186/1748-5908-4-50

Dopp, A. R., Mundey, P., Beasley, L. O., Silovsky, J. F., & Eisenberg, D. (2019). Mixed-method approaches to strengthen economic evaluations in implementation research. *Implementation Science*, *14*(2). https://doi.org/10.1186/s13012-018-0850-6

DuMont, K., Metz, A., & Woo, B. (2019, April 05). *Five recommendations for how implementation science can better advance equity.* Blog Post, Academy Health. https://academyhealth.org/blog/2019-04/five-recommendations-how-implementation-science-can-better-advance-equity

Escoffery, C., Lebow-Skelley, E., Haardoerfer, R., Boing, E., Udelson, H., Wood, R., Hartman, M., Fernandez, M. E., & Mullen, P. D. (2018). A systematic review of adaptations of evidence-based public health interventions globally. *Implementation Science*, *13*(1), 125. https://doi.org/10.1186/s13012-018-0815-9

Estabrooks, P. A., Brownson, R. C., & Pronk, N. P. (2018). Dissemination and implementation science for public health professionals: an overview and call to action. *Preventing Chronic Disease*, *15*, E162. https://doi.org/10.5888/pcd15.180525

Glasgow, R. E., & Estabrooks, P. E. (2018). Peer reviewed: Pragmatic applications of RE-AIM for health care initiatives in community and clinical settings. *Preventing Chronic Disease*, *15*, E02. https://doi.org/10.5888/pcd15.170271

Glasgow, R. E., Harden, S. M., Gaglio, B., Rabin, B., Smith, M. L., Porter, G. C., Ory, M. G., & Estabrooks, P. A. (2019). Re-aim planning and evaluation framework: Adapting to new science and practice with a 20-year review. *Frontiers in Public Health*, *7*, 64. https://doi.org/10.3389/fpubh.2019.00064

Glasgow, R. E., Vogt, T. M., & Boles, S. M. (1999). Evaluating the public health impact of health promotion interventions: the RE-AIM framework. *American Journal of Public Health*, *89*(9), 1322–1327. https://doi.org/10.2105/ajph.89.9.1322

Gore, R., Patel, S., Choy, C., Taher, M., Garcia-Dia, M. J., Singh, H., Kim, S., Mohaimin, S., Dhar, R., Naeem, A., Kwon, S. C., & Islam, N. (2019). Influence of organizational and social contexts on the implementation of culturally adapted hypertension control programs in Asian American-serving grocery stores, restaurants, and faith-based community sites: a qualitative study. *Translational Behavioral Medicine*, ibz106. Advance online publication. https://doi.org/10.1093/tbm/ibz106

Institute of Medicine (US) Committee on Quality of Health Care in America. (2001). *Crossing the quality chasm: A new health system for the 21st century.* National Academy Press (US).

Koh, S., Lee, M., Brotzman, L. E., & Shelton, R. C. (2020). An orientation for new researchers to key domains, processes, and resources in implementation science. *Translational Behavioral Medicine*, *10*(1), 179–185. https://doi.org/10.1093/tbm/iby095

Lobb, R., & Colditz, G. A. (2013). Implementation science and its application to population health. *Annual Review of Public Health*, *34*, 235–251. https://doi.org/10.1146/annurev-publhealth-031912-114444

McCreight, M. S., Rabin, B. A., Glasgow, R. E., Ayele, R. A., Leonard, C. A., Gilmartin, H. M., Frank, J. W., Hess, P. L., Burke, R. E., & Battaglia, C. T. (2019). Using the Practical, Robust Implementation and Sustainability Model (Prism) to qualitatively assess multilevel contextual factors to help plan, implement, evaluate, and disseminate health services programs. *Translational Behavioral Medicine*, *9*(6), 1002–1011. https://doi.org/10.1093/tbm/ibz085

Minkler, M., Salvatore, A.L., & Chang, C. (2018). Participatory approaches for study design and analysis in dissemination and implementation research. In R.C. Brownson, G.A. Colditz, E.K. Proctor (Eds.) *Dissemination and Implementation Research in Health: Translating Science to Practice (2nd ed., pp. 175–190).* Oxford University Press. https://doi.org/10.1093/acprof:oso/9780199751877.003.0010

Moore, J.E., Mascarenhas, A., Bain, J., & Straus, S.E. (2017). Developing a comprehensive definition of sustainability. *Implementation Science*, *12*, 110. https://doi.org/10.1186/s13012-017-0637-1

Nápoles, A. M., & Stewart, A. L. (2018). Transcreation: an implementation science framework for community-engaged behavioral interventions to reduce health disparities. *BMC Health Services Research*, *18*(1), 710. https://doi.org/10.1186/s12913-018-3521-z

Powell, B. J., Waltz, T. J., Chinman, M. J., Damschroder, L. J., Smith, J. L., Matthieu, M. M., Proctor, E. K., & Kirchner, J. E. (2015). A refined compilation of implementation strategies: Results from the Expert Recommendations for Implementing Change (Eric) project. *Implementation Science, 10*(1), 21. https://doi.org/10.1186/s13012-015-0209-1

Proctor, E., Luke, D., Calhoun, A., McMillen, C., Brownson, R., McCrary, S. & Padek, M. (2015). Sustainability of evidence-based health-care: research agenda, methodological advances, and infrastructure support. *Implementation Science, 10*:88. https://doi.org/10.1186/s13012-015-0274-5

Proctor, E., Silmere, H., Raghavan, R., Hovmand, P., Aarons, G., Bunger, A., Griffey, R., & Hensley, M. (2011). Outcomes for implementation research: Conceptual distinctions, measurement challenges, and research agenda. *Administration and Policy in Mental Health and Mental Health Services Research, 38*(2), 65–76. https://doi.org/10.1007/s10488-010-0319-7

Purnell, T. S., Calhoun, E. A., Golden, S. H., Halladay, J. R., Krok-Schoen, J. L., Appelhans, B. M., & Cooper, L. A. (2016). Achieving health equity: closing the gaps in health care disparities, interventions, and research. *Health Affairs, 35*(8), 1410–1415. https://doi.org/10.1377/hlthaff.2016.0158

Purtle, J., Marzalik, J. S., Halfond, R. W., Bufka, L. F., Teachman, B. A., & Aarons, G. A. (2020). Toward the data-driven dissemination of findings from psychological science. *American Psychologist, 75*(8), 1052–1066. https://doi.org/10.1037/amp0000721

Rabin, B. A., & Brownson, R. C. (2018). Terminology for dissemination and implementation research. In *Dissemination and Implementation Research in Health: Translating Science to Practice* (2nd edition), 19–45. https://doi.org/10.1093/oso/9780190683214.001.0001

Ramanadhan, S., Aronstein, D., Martinez-Dominguez, V., Xuan, Z., & Viswanath, K. (2020). Designing Capacity-Building Supports to Promote Evidence-Based Programs in Community-Based Organizations Working with Underserved Populations. *Progress in Community Health Partnerships: Research, Education, and Action, 14*(2), 149–160. https://doi.org/10.1353/cpr.2020.0027

Ramanadhan, S., Davis, M. M., Armstrong, R., Baquero, B., Ko, L. K., Leng, J. C., Salloum, R. G., Vaughn, N. A., & Brownson, R. C. (2018). Participatory implementation science to increase the impact of evidence-based cancer prevention and control. *Cancer Causes & Control, 29*(3), 363–369. https://doi.org/10.1007/s10552-018-1008-1

Ramanadhan, S., Galbraith-Gyan, K., Revette, A., Foti, A., Rackard James, C., Martinez-Dominguez, V., Miller, E., Tappin, J., Tracy, N., Bruff, C., Donaldson, S. T., Minsky, S., Sempasa, D., Siqueira, C., & Viswanath, K. (2021). Key considerations for designing capacity-building interventions to support evidence-based programming in underserved communities: A qualitative exploration. *Translational Behavioral Medicine, 11*(2), 452–461. https://doi.org/10.1093/tbm/ibz177

Scheirer, M.A. & Dearing, J.W. (2011). An agenda for research on the sustainability of public health programs. *American Journal of Public Health, 101*(11): 2059–2067. https://doi.org/10.2105/AJPH.2011.300193

Schell, S.F., Luke, D.A., Schooley, M.W., Elliott, M.B., Herbers, S.H., Mueller, N.B., & Burger, A.C. (2013). Public health program capacity for sustainability: a new framework. *Implementation Science, 8*:15. https://doi.org/10.1186/1748-5908-8-15

Shelton, R. C., Chambers, D. A., & Glasgow, R. E. (2020). An Extension of RE-AIM to Enhance Sustainability: Addressing Dynamic Context and Promoting Health Equity Over Time. *Frontiers in Public Health, 8*, 134. https://doi.org/10.3389/fpubh.2020.00134

Shelton, R. C., Cooper, B. R., & Stirman, S. W. (2018). The sustainability of evidence-based interventions and practices in public health and health care. *Annual Review of Public Health, 39*, 55–76. https://doi.org/10.1146/annurev-publhealth-040617-014731

Shelton, R. C. & Lee, M. (2019). Sustaining Evidence-Based Interventions and Policies: Recent Innovations and Future Directions in Implementation Science. *American Journal of Public Health, 109*(S2), S132–S134. https://doi.org/10.2105/AJPH.2018.304913

Shelton, R. C., Lee, M., Brotzman, L. E., Wolfenden, L., Nathan, N., & Wainberg, M. L. (2020). What Is Dissemination and Implementation Science?: An Introduction and Opportunities to Advance Behavioral Medicine and Public Health Globally. *International Journal of Behavioral Medicine, 27*(1), 3–20. https://doi.org/10.1007/s12529-020-09848-x

Stirman, S. W., Baumann, A. A., & Miller, C. J. (2019). The FRAME: an expanded framework for reporting adaptations and modifications to evidence-based interventions. *Implementation Science, 14*(1), 58. https://doi.org/10.1186/s13012-019-0898-y

Stirman, S. W., Gutner, C. A., Crits-Christoph, P., Edmunds, J., Evans, A. C., & Beidas, R. S. (2015). Relationships between clinician-level attributes and fidelity-consistent and fidelity-inconsistent modifications to an evidence-based psychotherapy. *Implementation Science, 10*, 115. https://doi.org/10.1186/s13012-015-0308-z

Stirman, S.W., Kimberly, J., Cook, N., Calloway, A., Castro, F., Charns, M. (2012). The sustainability of new programs and innovations: a review of the empirical literature and recommendations for future research. *Implementation Science, 7*, 17. https://doi.org/10.1186/1748-5908-7-17

Woodward, E. N., Matthieu, M. M., Uchendu, U. S., Rogal, S., & Kirchner, J. E. (2019). The health equity implementation framework: proposal and preliminary study of hepatitis C virus treatment. *Implementation Science, 14*(1), 26. https://doi.org/10.1186/s13012-019-0861-y

CHAPTER

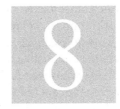

8

COMMUNITY ENGAGEMENT AND COMMUNITY-BASED PARTICIPATORY RESEARCH APPROACHES

PERLA CHEBLI, SIMONA C. KWON

LEARNING OBJECTIVES

By the end of this chapter, readers will be able to:

- Define key concepts underpinning community engagement (CE) and community-based participatory research (CBPR) and describe how they relate to health disparities research and the health equity framework.

- Identify models and frameworks used to conduct community-engaged research (CEnR) and CBPR and to translate evidence-based strategies and programs into community settings.

- Describe opportunities and future directions for CEnR to advance health equity for underserved populations.

Applied Population Health Approaches for Asian American Communities, First Edition. Edited by Simona C. Kwon, Chau Trinh-Shevrin, Nadia S. Islam, and Stella S. Yi.
© 2023 John Wiley & Sons, Inc. Published 2023 by John Wiley & Sons, Inc.
Companion Website: www.wiley.com/go/kwon/asianamerican

INTRODUCTION

Health disparities refer to inequalities observed in health care and health outcomes across different population groups, including among racial/ethnic minority groups (Artiga et al., 2020). Over the past 30 years, health disparities research has underscored the ways in which outcomes are impacted by the social determinants of health – the conditions within which individuals live, work, learn, and play (*Social Determinants of Health, CDC*, 2020). More recently, researchers have built on this work to establish the health equity framework. As described in Chapter 2, the health equity framework prioritizes the elimination of health disparities within racial/ethnic minority populations in order to advance the health of all (Srinivasan & Williams, 2014; Trinh-Shevrin et al., 2015).

Underlying the concept of health equity is a commitment to social justice (Braveman, 2014). Health researchers have an important role to play in fulfilling that commitment, particularly for racial/ethnic minority populations. To date, racial/ethnic minority and immigrant populations remain the most disadvantaged groups among the U.S. population in terms of health outcomes and with respect to the social determinants of health (Frieden & Centers for Disease Control and Prevention (CDC), 2013; Ward et al., 2004). In 2020, the novel coronavirus pandemic (COVID-19) provided glaring examples of these disadvantages as racial and ethnic minority populations bore a vastly disproportionate burden of COVID-19 infections, hospitalization, and mortality as compared to non-Hispanic Whites (Whites). For example, in New York City (NYC), from March 8 through April 10, 2020, Asian Americans had the second-highest COVID-19 diagnostic test positivity rates as compared to other racial/ethnic minority groups (Reichberg et al., 2020). Asian Americans also experienced a 35% increase in mortality attributed to COVID-19 in NYC between January and July, 2020 – a rate second only to Hispanic Americans (Rhee & Press, 2020). These disproportionate rates of infection and mortality were likely impacted by lower rates of health care access and utilization by Asian Americans – factors that have been documented in other disease areas, such as cancer (Jun & Nan, 2018; Trinh et al., 2016). Yet even as researchers have focused successfully on describing disparities and improving outcomes for some diseases and some populations, health equity remains a distant goal.

Employing CE strategies and CBPR methods in health research has the potential to accelerate progress toward the goal of health equity by allowing rapid translation of evidence-based interventions from the laboratory to real-world settings, particularly for racial/ethnic minority communities. However, successfully applying CE and CBPR requires a fundamental disruption to the traditional research paradigm in which knowledge has been presumed to flow unidirectionally, from an academic institution to the population of interest. By contrast, in CEnR and CBPR, knowledge is bidirectional, flowing back and forth between researchers and the populations of interest. Instead of designing studies *for* a specific population, researchers engage *with* the population to help the community identify its own priorities and design research that serves those aims. Researchers also report results back to the community and, wherever possible, support community leaders to integrate findings into community-based programs and policies.

In this chapter, we will focus on how CE may support knowledge generation as well as the translation of new evidence into real-world settings. That is, we will address the dual need to clarify the social determinants of health from the community's perspective *and* identify interventions that work in specific community contexts. We will provide an overview of key concepts in CE, describe the most commonly used frameworks and approaches in CEnR, and propose future directions for research. Throughout the chapter, we will use examples from our work at the NYU Center for the Study of Asian American Health (CSAAH) at NYU Grossman School of Medicine to illustrate concepts and provide directions for further study.

KEY CONCEPTS IN COMMUNITY ENGAGEMENT

Defining the Community

The first step in developing CEnR is to contemplate how and by whom the *community* is defined. Typically, a community is viewed as a group of individuals with *something in common*. This commonality could be related to spatial geographic boundaries (e.g., neighborhoods, schools), race or ethnicity, or a common interest or issue (e.g., patients with diabetes) (Simmons et al., 2011). With the emergence and ubiquity of communications technology, communities are no longer confined to spatial locations and often form online, as in the example of communities of support for patients coping with chronic conditions (Johnson & Ambrose, 2006). In all cases, researchers interested in CEnR should avoid ascribing meaning to a community and instead allow communities to self-determine what their shared identity is and what it means to them (Jewkes & Murcott, 1996). The *validity* of any CEnR is contingent on community participation (Jewkes & Murcott, 1996). For example, the Arab American population, a diverse group hailing from 22 countries in North Africa and the Middle East, is classified as White by the U.S. Office of Management and Budget. This classification is considered inaccurate by Arab Americans, who have led numerous lobbying and advocacy efforts to be recognized as an ethnic group separate from Whites (Abboud et al., 2019; Abuelezam et al., 2017). Therefore, outreach, engagement, and research with Arab American communities should be informed by their unique immigration history, cultural values, and experiences, rather than their assigned racial identity. This example illustrates the importance of thoughtful and participatory community definition as a precursor to CEnR.

Community Engagement

Community engagement is defined as "the process of *working collaboratively* with and through groups of people affiliated by geographic proximity, special interest, or similar situations to address issues affecting the well-being of those people. CE is a powerful vehicle for bringing about environmental and behavioral changes that will improve the health of the community and its members. It often involves partnerships and coalitions that help mobilize resources and influence systems, change relationships among partners, and serve as catalysts for changing policies, programs, and practices" (McCloskey et al., 2011). This definition incorporates three key components: (1) collaborating with community groups; (2) leveraging existing community assets and building capacity; and (3) advancing population health. Community groups may include community- and faith-based organizations, organizational leaders, community/neighborhood associations, school-based representatives, and community leaders, among others. Formative work with communities (e.g., multimethod assessments) is essential to understand how issues of interests are shaped and which community groups should be engaged in the research process. "Working collaboratively" is a rather broad definition, for CE is neither monolithic nor static but rather exists along a spectrum from low to high community participation. Generally, researchers refer to five levels of CE that comprise a framework for appraising the level of community participation: inform, consult, involve, collaborate, and empower (*Core Values, Ethics, Spectrum – The 3 Pillars of Public Participation*, n.d.; Kwon et al., 2018). Advancement through these five levels engenders bidirectional communication, enhanced community participation, and equitable partnership structures. This process is described below and illustrated in Figure 8.1.

1. *Inform.* At this initial level of CE, the community is involved only marginally in the research process. Communication is unidirectional, from researchers to the community.

2. *Consult.* The community provides feedback/answers to questions generated externally by researchers or administrators within the academic entity or funding agency. Bidirectional communication between researchers and the community begins.

3. *Involve.* The community cooperates with the academic entity; community feedback is considered in decision-making. This stage marks the beginning of community participation in the research process.

4. *Collaborate.* The community participates in all aspects of the research project as an equal partner; community input is key to decision-making. CBPR principles begin to apply.

5. *Empower.* At this highest level of CE, strong partnerships are established; decision-making happens at the community level. CBPR principles apply fully.

Reaching higher levels of CE requires an intentional and often slow process of trust building with communities. This process is especially tenuous with underserved immigrant and racial/ethnic minority groups for whom research may be tainted by historical exploitation and mistrust of academic and other institutions. For example, the egregiously unethical and abusive Tuskegee Study, which began in the 1930s and continued for four decades, still inspires fear and mistrust of the medical establishment among Black communities nationwide (Freimuth et al., 2001). In addition, the time and effort required for building relationships and infrastructure as well as the

INCREASING COMMUNITY INVOLVEMENT, TRUST, COMMUNICATION, JOINT OWNERSHIP, SHARED LEADERSHIP →

	INFORM	CONSULT	INVOLVE	COLLABORATE	EMPOWER
Relationship dynamics	Academic entity provides information to community	Academic entity obtains community feedback Beginning of bidirectional communication with the community	Community and academic entities cooperate Beginning of community participation in research process	Community-academic partnerships are formed Community participates in all aspects of project	Strong bidirectional relationships are established Decision making at the community
Academic entity's position	"We will keep you informed."	"We will consider your input and give feedback on how if informed our decisions."	"We will ensure your input is considered among the choices we implement."	"We will work together and incorporate your views as much as possible." [CBPR]	"We will implement what you decide." [CBPR]

FIGURE 8.1 *Spectrum of Community Engagement*

Source: Adapted from Kwon et al. (2018).

need for flexibility to accommodate community partners' goals may conflict with project timelines, budgets, and mandates (Staley, 2009). In light of these challenges, *why bother with CEnR, when easier research approaches exist?* For researchers committed to health equity and improving health outcomes for all populations, the answer is simple: CE is instrumental to understanding the socioecological context of health issues and, in turn, developing effective and contextually responsive interventions and implementation strategies.

There are no definitive guidelines for selecting the level of CE in a research project, as the decision will depend on the funding mechanism and the requirements of the project itself. Regardless of the level of CE, researchers have a responsibility to report community participation and CE strategies in the scholarly literature with honesty and transparency. Conversely, *tokenism,* or giving communities a symbolic role in the research process, should be avoided to prevent reinforcing mistrust in researchers and academic institutions and perpetuating biases and stereotypes.

Capacity Building

Capacity building is an integral element of CE and is defined as "the development of knowledge, skills, commitment, structures, systems and leadership to enable effective health promotion. It involves actions to improve health at three levels: the advancement of knowledge and skills among practitioners; the expansion of support and infrastructure for health promotion in organizations; and the development of cohesiveness and partnerships for health in communities" (Smith et al., 2006). To facilitate a capacity-building process, researchers convene meetings with community stakeholders as a necessary precondition to bidirectional learning. A potential pitfall of capacity building relates to its potential to view a community through a lens of *deficiency* – that is, researchers may view the community as fundamentally *deficient* in basic skills or capacity to conduct research or implement interventions. Researchers should focus, instead, on existing capacity within the community and develop strategies that leverage and strengthen existing community assets and resources. An example of a tool to support this process is collaborative asset-mapping exercises, in which communities inventory strengths and resources that could be mobilized to achieve the goals of a given project. Equitable engagement (e.g., through CBPR) reflects a belief that both community and academic partners have unique strengths that may be harnessed and enhanced through bidirectional learning methodologies embedded within capacity-building activities. A further benefit of this approach is its potential for developing research infrastructure within the community. Once established, this infrastructure may be leveraged in future research engagements, multiplying capacity gains. This additive and cyclical process of capacity building is illustrated in Figure 8.2.

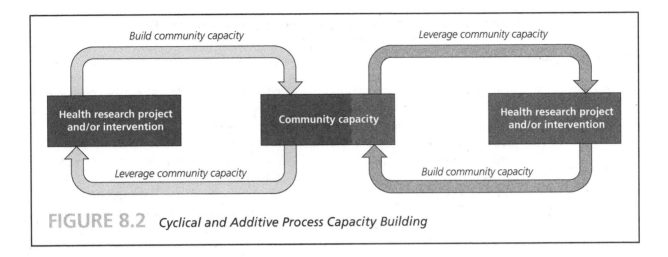

FIGURE 8.2   *Cyclical and Additive Process Capacity Building*

Successful capacity-building activities carried out within Asian American communities have been documented in the public health literature. One example is the Community Empowered Research Training (CERT) program, developed by CSAAH and its academic and community partners, which aimed to increase the research infrastructure capacity of community-based organizations serving Asian American communities across the United States (Kwon et al., 2012). The CERT curriculum priorities and content were informed by feedback from community partners, who identified the need for capacity-building activities focused on strengthening organizational skills in grant writing, leveraging data to enhance program and service development, and program evaluation (Kwon et al., 2012). Another example is Project AsPIRE, through which an existing cadre of community health workers (CHWs) were trained to deliver a hypertension intervention within the Filipino American community in NYC (Ursua et al., 2018).

A key benefit for researchers engaging in bidirectional learning through capacity-building activities is the strengthening of their skills and capacity to frame health issues in the relevant sociocultural contexts of their partner communities. Researchers may also benefit from enhanced community capacity to document health care experiences and other life experiences related to the social determinants of health. Including compelling community stories to illustrate either an urgent health problem or the benefits of an intervention are important elements of the policy briefs that form critical components of advocacy efforts to effect policy change. The current CBPR literature describing interventions with Asian Americans rarely reports policy action steps (Trinh-Shevrin et al., 2009). Thus, by encouraging and supporting community members to document and report these stories, researchers simultaneously may build capacity within the community while facilitating the development of valuable products in support of their own research and policy advocacy goals. Furthermore, forging new partnerships with community advocacy groups may facilitate the dissemination of research findings through nonacademic channels, including the policy arena, which could help researchers to magnify project impact (Brownson et al., 2018). Examples of strategies to build capacity for academic and community stakeholders are included in Table 8.1.

Coalition Building

Coalitions are defined as "inter-organizational, cooperative, and synergistic working alliances" that are organized in formal, structured ways for a common purpose, often in response to an emergent opportunity (e.g., funding) or threat (e.g., health concern in a specific community) (Butterfoss et al., 1993; Zakocs & Edwards, 2006). Building coalitions between community and academic partners is an effective strategy to pool expertise, perspectives, and resources to develop and sustain innovative approaches to affect community health (Trinh-Shevrin et al., 2011). Given the diversity of members who may join community coalitions (e.g., individuals, health service organizations, social service agencies, faith-based and community-based organizations), coalitions are well-positioned to facilitate a participatory process of elucidating and addressing the socioecological etiologies of health issues. Determinants of coalition effectiveness include establishing formal governance protocols, fostering leadership and participation, promoting group cohesion, and facilitating intergroup collaborations (Zakocs & Edwards, 2006).

TABLE 8.1 **Examples of Goals and Strategies for Capacity Building Activities**

Stakeholder group	Goals	Strategies
Researchers	Understand the social determinants of a health condition identified as a key concern by the community. Select intervention strategies to address relevant determinants. Include a policy action step as a dissemination strategy.	Conduct multimethod formative assessments that leverage community knowledge (e.g., asset-based assessment). Engage in participatory decision-making around intervention aims and implementation strategies. Establish partnerships with policy advocacy groups. Collect community stories to illustrate the impact of a health problem or provide evidence of success for a community intervention.
Community	Enhance infrastructure for research participation. Foster ownership of the research process or intervention.	Participate in training on research methods. Engage the community in decision-making around research conduct and processes. Participate in training on grant writing. Hold leadership position in project steering committee. Share intervention implementation responsibility (e.g., engage and train existing CHWs).

A notable example of an effective coalition is the CBPR-informed Asian American Hepatitis B Program (AAHBP), comprising community (e.g., Charles B. Wang Community Health Center) and academic partners (i.e., CSAAH), developed to address the high prevalence of the Hepatitis B virus among NYC's Asian American population. Community partners invited CSAAH to serve as the scientific/research arm of the coalition, designing the research and data collection efforts. This community-driven coalition guided the development and implementation of the initiative, from recognizing the community's urgent need to identifying relevant partners and developing the intervention (Trinh-Shevrin et al., 2011). CSAAH contributed content expertise to develop a health intervention embedded within existing community-based service organizations to foster acceptability and sustainability. AAHBP used trusted CHWs, patient navigators, and community based organizations to successfully reach medically underserved and limited English proficient communities (Pollack et al., 2011). CSAAH supported the development of a centralized registry by collecting, managing and analyzing de-identified data from multiple clinical sites through secured platforms that were linked via unique identifiers. In a 2020 systematic review of the effectiveness of viral hepatitis interventions (Ortiz et al., 2020), AAHBP was identified as a successful participatory multistrategy model that *"reached a high proportion of [limited English proficient] and immigrant communities by providing continual education, awareness, free screening, vaccination and treatment, in collaboration of a wide range of stakeholders and thus facilitating access to care."* In addition, program evaluation demonstrated the synergistic and additive efforts of academic and community partners: approximately 9,000 high-risk individuals were successfully navigated into hepatitis B screening, vaccination, and treatment (Pollack et al., 2011; Pollack et al., 2014). In recognition of this large-scale impact, the AAHBP was designated as a CDC Center of Excellence in the Elimination of Disparities (CEED) from 2007 to 2012, charged with identifying best practices in CE based on the experiences, successes, and lessons learned from the AAHBP.

CE MODELS AND FRAMEWORKS

Philosophical Underpinnings of CEnR

CEnR represents a departure from conventional scientific paradigms. Positivist science conceptualizes reality as singular and predictable through objective experimental research *on* participants. In contrast, CEnR shifts to a

TABLE 8.2 Components of Positivist and Social Constructivist Paradigms

Issue	Positivism	Social constructivism
Ontology	Reality is singular and objective	Reality is relative and socially constructed
Epistemology	Objectivist	Subjectivist
Methodology	Experimental, mostly quantitative	Interpretive, dialectical, methodological pluralism
Research purpose	Explain, predict	Understand, reconstruct
Role of the community	Research subjects	Research partners

Source: Adapted from Denzin & Lincoln. (2017).

social constructivist epistemology that views reality as plural and socially constructed. Research participants are collaborators in this paradigm, reflecting an appreciation of their perspectives and lived experiences as valid data (Table 8.2).

This shift in scientific paradigm is especially salient in health disparities research that is informed by social determinants of health. CEnR allows community members to describe their own health priorities and explain multilevel influences – an approach that directly contrasts with the conventional scientific method. That traditional paradigm may oversimplify the world for the sake of parsimony and, in so doing, inadvertently reinforce historical oppressions by bestowing on the researcher the unique authority to assert "the world is that way" (i.e., the "coerciveness of Truth"). In CEnR, the researcher and the community co-create multiple descriptors for coexistent experiences or "truths" (Denzin & Lincoln, 2017).

The Researcher in CEnR

Adopting a social constructivist paradigm also changes the role of the researcher. Positivist science imagines an invisible researcher, whose identity and beliefs are irrelevant or should be "neutralized" to preserve scientific rigor. In contrast, social constructivism and CEnR acknowledge that researchers hold multiple identities that invariably are brought into the research process. These identities place researchers on an insider–outsider continuum, having both similarities and differences with the communities with whom they work (Dwyer & Buckle, 2009). For example, Asian American researchers may share common characteristics with Asian immigrant communities, such as racial/ethnic identity and language. These shared characteristics may confer greater trust and acceptance from the community on the researchers and facilitate steps in the design and implementation of interventions, from relationship building to data collection. Yet racially/ethnically concordant researchers may also struggle to separate their personal assumptions and experiences from those of the community, which may bias data collection and analysis. For example, despite racial/ethnic concordance, researchers may have higher educational attainment and socioeconomic status than members of the communities of interest, which lead to differential experiences and privileges compared to the larger community. In addition, researchers' affiliations with academic institutions may create a power imbalance, making them relative "outsiders" to their own racial/ethnic communities (Kerstetter, 2012; Wallerstein et al., 2017). Therefore, researchers are not necessarily either insiders or outsiders in the research setting; rather, their position exists in the "space between" (Dwyer & Buckle, 2009). Importantly, this position is not static throughout the entire research project, but rather mutates in response to new interactions and findings.

Reflecting on the researchers' positionality relative to communities is an important aspect of CEnR. This process, called *reflexivity* or *reflecting critically on the self as researcher* (Denzin & Lincoln, 2017), prompts researchers to question how their unique identities may affect the development of partnerships with community members as well as the research process and its outcomes (Kerstetter, 2012; Muhammad et al., 2015). This reflexive exercise should be continuous to ensure that researchers are constantly working on identifying their assumptions and addressing them in a deliberate manner as they design and implement their research.

Translational Research

The pervasiveness of health disparities stems in part from the limited translation of evidence-based research into clinical and community practice (Glasgow & Emmons, 2007; Green, 2014). The effectiveness of interventions in tightly controlled clinical trials is not necessarily transferrable to real-world community and clinical settings. Indeed, the research-to-practice chasm has been estimated as requiring an average of 17 years from bench to community (Balas et al., 2000). CEnR is ideally suited to shorten this time frame by prioritizing collaboration with communities and patients to understand *what works for them*. The National Institutes of Health (NIH) National Center for Advancing Translational Sciences (NCATS) defines translation as "the process of turning observations in the laboratory, clinic and community into interventions that improve the health of individuals and the public – from diagnostics and therapeutics to medical procedures and behavioral changes" (*Translational Science Spectrum*, 2015). NCATS's translational science spectrum highlights the translational "bridges" needed to move evidence from bench to bedside and communities. The subsequent sections introduce the translational CEnR approaches that may be leveraged in community and clinical settings.

Community-Based Participatory Research

CBPR includes communities in all stages of the research process to foster joint ownership over data and interventions. Although often used as an umbrella term for participatory research, CBPR is, in fact, a distinct approach requiring a high level of CE. CBPR is defined as "systematic investigation with the participation of those affected by an issue for purposes of education and action or affecting social change" (McGowan & Green, 1995). Simply put, CBPR represents a collaborative process of inquiry and praxis that equitably involves community partners in the process. As a result, findings are grounded in local contexts and have potential for translatability (Ammerman et al., 2014; Israel et al., 1998; Wallerstein et al., 2017). Israel and colleagues proposed a set of nine core principles for CBPR, informed by evidence from the CBPR literature (Israel et al., 1998, 2001):

1. Recognize that the community is a unit of identity.

2. Leverage the community's existing strengths and capacity.

3. Foster collaborative and equitable partnership in all phases of research.

4. Facilitate co-learning and capacity building for all partners.

5. Balance knowledge generation and program/policy development to benefit the community.

6. Explore locally relevant multilevel determinants of health.

7. Engage in systems and intervention development through a cyclical and iterative process.

8. Disseminate research findings to all partners and engage partners in broader dissemination.

9. Commit to and plan for long-term sustainability.

Examples of strategies to operationalize each principle are provided in Table 8.3.

CBPR is especially impactful with Asian Americans and other historically marginalized communities that may be wary of top-down research approaches or face language and cultural barriers to participation in research. Indeed, the democratization of the research process through CBPR elevates community members from "participants" or "subjects" to "collaborators," which may start to mend historical mistrust in research institutions. Furthermore, CBPR allows for a granular exploration of subgroup differences in health outcomes and social determinants of health – a factor that is especially beneficial when working with a population as ethnically, linguistically, and socioeconomically diverse as Asian Americans. In the previous edition of this textbook, we published a systematic review of the literature that found CBPR facilitated greater participation by Asian Americans in research, specifically through the mechanism of Community Advisory Boards (CABs) in Asian

TABLE 8.3 **Exemplar Strategies for Operationalizing CBPR Principles**

CBPR principle	Practical applications
Community is the unit of identity.	Create a CAB that represents perspectives and priorities of the community. Engage with diverse community representatives/groups/ organizations to capture different perspectives within the same community.
Leverage strengths and capacity of the community.	Supplement the deficiency-focused needs assessment with an asset assessment. Engage with community partners and CAB to identify community assets and resources. Center interventions on existing community assets and resources.
Foster collaborative, equitable partnership in all phases of research.	Include community partners as co-leads with fair budgetary allocation on grant applications. Involve community partners in decision-making throughout the research cycle (i.e., setting priorities, research conduct, dissemination, intervention development, implementation, and evaluation) – e.g., hold periodic meetings at different phases of research to solicit community partners' input.
Facilitate co-learning and capacity building for all partners.	Integrate capacity-building activities for community and academic partners within the research process – e.g., develop and conduct training in research methods and infrastructure development for community partners that is informed by partners' needs and priorities; coalition building with multisectoral partners for academic partners to facilitate practice and policy translation.
Balance knowledge generation and program/policy development to benefit for community partners.	Clarify community and academic partners' expectations at the beginning of the project.
Explore locally relevant multilevel determinants of health.	Incorporate a social determinants of health approach in CEnR. Conduct formative assessments that incorporate community partners' contextual knowledge.
Engage in systems and intervention development through a cyclical and iterative process.	Establish structured mechanisms to provide feedback at regular intervals – e.g., during periodic meetings.
Disseminate research findings to all partners and engage partners in broader dissemination.	Discuss data ownership and purpose at the beginning of the project. Develop a dissemination strategy with community partners that leverages diverse dissemination channels – e.g., academic publications disseminated through scholarly channels may be coupled with lay reports and educational materials distributed through community forums and online.

(Continued)

TABLE 8.3   *(Continued)*

CBPR principle	Practical applications
Commit to and plan for long-term sustainability	Discuss feasibility and expected challenges of sustainability with community partners at the beginning of the research project. Develop strategies for sustainability that leverage existing community infrastructure and resources. Help community partners to obtain additional funding that they will manage independently to keep the project going – e.g., grant-writing support.

Sources: Adapted from Burke et al. (2013); Kwon et al. (2018).

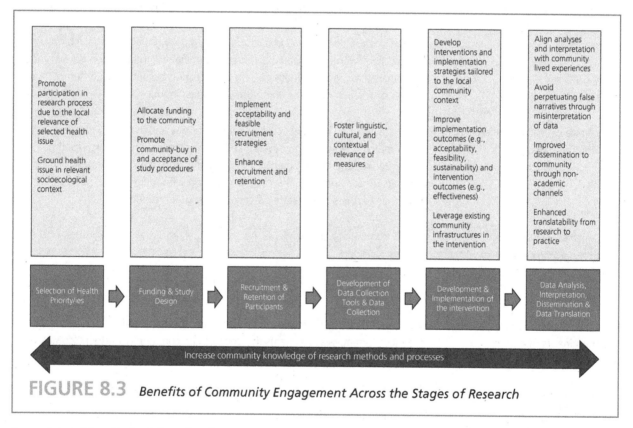

FIGURE 8.3   *Benefits of Community Engagement Across the Stages of Research*

Source: Adapted from Tandon & Kwon (2009).

ethnic communities. As CAB members, Asian Americans were adept at guiding study priorities, providing input on feasibility and cultural appropriateness of study design and methods, supporting recruitment and data collection (e.g., guidance on strategies for "hard-to-reach populations"), and contributing to intervention development, outreach, and implementation (Tandon & Kwon, 2009). These findings support the feasibility and value of implementing CBPR with Asian American communities. However, Asian American communities were less engaged in data analysis, interpretation, and dissemination, highlighting the need for greater commitment to CBPR principles across *all* research activities, particularly knowledge translation and dissemination. The benefits of CE at each stage of research are illustrated in Figure 8.3.

Participatory Action Research

Participatory action research (PAR) serves as the foundation of CBPR; in fact, CBPR falls under the rubric of PAR, and these two terms may be used interchangeably. Both approaches refute the positivist, extractive view of research and are geared toward action and social change rather than knowledge generation only (Baum et al., 2006; Townsend, 2014). Kurt Lewin, a social psychologist who was credited with coining the term *action research,* brilliantly summarized the intent driving the development of PAR: "Research which produces nothing but books will not suffice" (Lewin, 1946). Instead, he suggested that research needed to inform and be oriented toward action. To this end, PAR prioritizes democratic, equitable, liberating, and health-promoting processes (Stringer, 1999). PAR is characterized by a collaborative, community-driven, iterative process of research, reflection, and action. Interventions generated via PAR are contextually relevant and build on the community's assets and capacity, reflecting a commitment to community empowerment (Kindon et al., 2007). The CBPR approach shares these values with PAR, but the main distinctive attribute is the establishment of *principles* that guide the development and conduct of participatory research.

The PAR approach has been documented with Asian American communities, albeit less frequently than CBPR. For example, one study leveraged a Southeast Asian youth advisory board to reach a critical awareness of the impact of tobacco on participants and their community (Lee et al., 2012). The research process was cyclical and involved research activities, analysis, and reflection. Youth participants engaged in a series of trainings on research methods, tobacco policy as a social justice issue, and the political process. Participants had positive feedback on the participatory process, suggesting that PAR was an acceptable strategy with Asian American youths. Chapter 12 includes additional examples of successful applications of PAR among Asian American elders.

Patient-Centered Outcomes Research

Patient-centered outcomes research (PCOR) is the clinical equivalent to CBPR, wherein *patients* become the community. In the way that CBPR prioritizes engagement between researchers and community partners to guide and inform community-based research, PCOR integrates patients and families/caregivers as active collaborators in health service research (Domecq et al., 2014; Selby et al., 2012). *Patient-centeredness* refers to the extent to which patients' characteristics, preferences, and decision-making needs inform the research process for the purpose of increasing the relevance and translatability of research findings.

Patient engagement incorporates "lived experience" expertise and disrupts the historical patient-provider power hierarchy. Within PCOR, patients have the opportunity to articulate their own priorities and goals to inform research. Carman et al. (2013) proposed a multilevel, multidimensional framework comprising three aspects of patient engagement: (1) a patient engagement spectrum, comparable to that of CE (i.e., consultation, involvement, and shared leadership), (2) different levels at which patient engagement can occur (i.e., direct care, health care organizations, and policy), and (3) multilevel factors influencing patient engagement (i.e., patient, organizational, and societal levels) (Carman et al., 2013).

Similar to CE, achieving the highest levels of patient engagement may not be feasible or desirable in all situations. Engagement goals and strategies are best crafted collaboratively with patient input, to determine their ability and interest to participate at different stages. Research suggests that greater patient involvement in decision-making related to their care improves patient-centeredness of health outcomes. However, a systematic review revealed that patient engagement was more common in earlier (e.g., topic prioritization) than in later (e.g., implementation and dissemination) stages of research, suggesting opportunities for future PCOR (Concannon et al., 2014). For example, utilizing CBPR principles in health service research may guide genuine patient engagement throughout the research process. Table 8.4 provides examples of how to align PCOR strategies with CBPR principles (Kwon et al., 2018).

In 2010, as part of The Patient Protection and Affordable Care Act, Congress integrated PCOR into the federal health research landscape with the establishment of the Patient-Centered Outcomes Research Institute (PCORI) (Selby et al., 2012). The PCORI mission is to help "people make informed health care decisions, and improve health care delivery and outcomes, by producing and promoting high integrity, evidence-based information that comes from research guided by patients, caregivers, and the broader health care community"

TABLE 8.4   **Application of CBPR Principles in PCOR**

CBPR principle	PCOR strategy	Application in PCOR
Community is the unit of identity	Patients are participants and collaborators.	Include a patient representative or patient advocacy group as co-leads of an application. Involve patient stakeholders input fully in the decision-making, development, implementation, evaluation, and dissemination process.
Leverage strengths and capacity of the community	Use an asset-based approach to developing interventions building on assets in patient, caregivers, family, and provider settings.	Employ activation and motivational interviewing strategies for patient/ caregivers to help them feel comfortable about voicing and participating in discussions related to appropriate intervention strategies. Provide learning exchanges geared to researchers about illness and sociocultural perspectives that apply an asset-based framework.
Foster collaborative, equitable partnership in all phases of research.	Research with patients as full partners. Researcher and patient stakeholders share control equally.	Create a stakeholder board that represents different perspectives of the patient community. Develop multiple strategies for gaining input and perspectives from diverse constituents/stakeholders.
Facilitate co-learning and capacity building for all partners.	Researchers and patient stakeholders work together to help build community capacity.	Conduct learning exchanges in which both researchers and stakeholders provide expertise relevant to the research process. Examples include research methods training for stakeholders, and coalition- and consensus-building for researchers.
Balance knowledge generation and benefit for community partners.	Researchers and patient stakeholders identify at the outset their expectations goals of the research to be conducted and determine the practical benefit for patient stakeholders in engaging research.	Explore study designs that balance scientific rigor with benefits to participants and perceived community concerns of the ethics of doing research (such as depriving a group of individuals from a beneficial intervention). Examples include comparative-effectiveness trials that compare two or more relevant strategies, cross-over control, or wait-list control designs.
Explore locally relevant multilevel determinants of health.	Stakeholders identify problem or works with researcher to identify problem.	Conduct a multi-method formative assessment that includes input from these stakeholders in the design, evaluation, and interpretation of findings, and contextualizing these findings in the experiences of patients/caregivers.

Engage in systems and intervention development through a cyclical and iterative process.	Goal of the research is not only about advancing knowledge but includes a process that allows for reflection, quality improvement, and actions related to improving engagement and sustainability that includes ongoing assessments of successes and challenges.	Work with all stakeholders involved to identify measurable immediate successes and processes to identify challenges and potential solutions.
Disseminate research findings to all partners and engage partners in broader dissemination.	Data is shared, researchers and patient stakeholders decide its use and dissemination.	Disseminate findings through multiple vehicles and strategies, including patient forums, newspaper articles, policy briefs, monographs, community forums, patient education tools, provider education resources, and peer-reviewed articles.
Commit to and plan for long-term sustainability.	Sustainability is an ongoing goal to strive toward.	Place sustainability as a goal at the outset of the project and consider potential strategies for sustaining efforts throughout the life of the research.

(Patient-Centered Outcomes Research Institute, 2018). The mission is driven by PCORI engagement principles, which include reciprocal relationships, co-learning, partnerships, transparency, honesty, and trust – principles that cannot be operationalized in research studies without multi-stakeholder engagement, including patients, their families/caregivers, and other health care partners and patient advocacy groups (Concannon et al., 2012).

SUMMARY AND FUTURE DIRECTIONS

CE is at the heart of health equity research and praxis. Conducting CEnR ensures that researchers are asking the right questions (i.e., informed by community priorities and socioecological contexts), collecting the right data (i.e., focusing on the appropriate social determinants of health), and implementing the appropriate interventions to address the identified problems (i.e., feasible and acceptable interventions grounded in community capacity). CE occurs along a spectrum that begins with minimal community participation and moves toward higher levels of CE over time. Advancing along this spectrum indicates increased trust, bidirectional communication, joint ownership, and shared leadership among researchers and the communities with whom they are working. Integral elements of CEnR include asset-focused capacity building, a bidirectional learning process between community and academic partners, and coalition building to develop multi-stakeholder alliances that pool their skills and resources to address a shared health problem. CEnR represents a paradigm shift from positivist to social constructivist science, which democratizes knowledge generation and values local community knowledge. Common approaches to CEnR include CBPR, PAR, PCOR, and translational research. All of these methodologies are grounded in the principles of trust, empowerment, and the co-creation of knowledge and solutions.

Future Direction: CE Lessons from COVID-19

Historically, CE activities have been undertaken in person. For example, when launching a new research project, researchers may conduct outreach at community events, religious gatherings, and other community settings (Henry Akintobi et al., 2020). In 2020, however, researchers were forced to pivot to accommodate physical distancing mandates established in response to COVID-19. Although it might be tempting to discount CE in light of these new mandates, COVID-19 presents precisely the type of challenge that CE may prove instrumental in addressing. Given the disproportionate burden of COVID-19-related hospitalizations and deaths within underserved immigrant and racial/ethnic minority populations, and given the importance of CE to the successful design and implementation of health research in these same populations, researchers must strive to identify and develop innovative solutions to overcoming barriers to physical interactions with the communities they wish to serve.

While remote engagement strategies (e.g., online communications platforms) appear to be convenient alternatives to in-person events, unequal access to technology presents a barrier to the engagement of older adults and racial/ethnic minorities (Mitchell et al., 2018) – the same populations that are disproportionately impacted by the pandemic. For example, prior to COVID-19, CSAAH conducted a survey of its Asian American community partners across the United States and found that the majority favored in-person trainings over webinars (Kwon et al., 2012). In light of such findings, reliance on remote engagement may introduce or reinforce disparities in engagement and health by disregarding community input and generating interventions that are not responsive to local needs and contexts.

Carson and colleagues (2020) outlined some priorities for engaging with communities in COVID-19 research activities that are aligned with CBPR principles. These priorities include focusing on disenfranchised communities, seeking community input to articulate research priorities, adapting to communities' short- and long-term project goals, and including funding for community engagement (Carson et al., 2020). Creative strategies are needed to facilitate these processes during COVID-19, such as engaging community stakeholders with existing community networks and reach (e.g., community- and faith-based organizations, community groups and committees, school leaders, elected officials, representatives of housing associations (Galiatsatos et al., 2020; Gilmore et al., 2020)) and establishing feasible and accessible communications channels (e.g., *community calls,* described as large conference calls with relevant medical and community stakeholders to discuss opportunities and challenges associated with COVID-19 community responses (Galiatsatos et al., 2020)).

Ultimately, the lesson for health researchers is that existing and sustained community-academic partnerships forged through CBPR can be "repurposed" to address emergent threats (Henry Akintobi et al., 2020). These partnerships may enhance each community's capacity to swiftly respond to COVID-19 challenges by initiating research to understand key determinants and developing mitigation responses accordingly. For example, as the disproportionate toll of COVID-19 on communities of color began to emerge in local and regional datasets, NIH released the RADx Underserved Populations (RADx-UP) funding opportunity to support underserved communities *with established research infrastructures and partnerships* to examine COVID-19 testing patterns and implement responsive interventions (*RADx Programs*, 2020). In this sense, the adage, "Fortune favors the prepared," rings true. Committing to CEnR and partnership building with community entities now may be the key to enhanced community preparedness in future health emergencies or pandemics.

Future Direction: Measuring and Evaluating CE

Given the growing popularity of CBPR approaches to address health disparities, a CBPR conceptual logic model was developed in 2003 and refined in 2013 to link CBPR processes to outcomes (Belone et al., 2016; Wallerstein & Duran, 2010). The logic model integrates four overarching dimensions of collaborative participation in research: (1) context; (2) group dynamics and equitable partnerships; (3) intervention and research; and (4) outcomes. The Refined CBPR Conceptual Model stipulates that *contexts* (i.e., contextual factors) ground academic-community *group dynamics*, which, if effective within their diverse contexts, can impact and change *research and intervention designs*. The implementation of research and/or interventions in turn can contribute to *outcomes*, which include broad capacity and system changes, in addition to grant health improvements" (Belone et al., 2016). Context factors refer to community and academic capacity, history (e.g., trust and mistrust), and perceived salience of health issues on the community-academic partnerships. Group dynamics include structural (e.g., alignment with CBPR principles, power-sharing), individual (e.g., motivation for participation, academic partnership reputation within the community, cultural identity/humility), and relational factors (e.g., trust, listening, co-learning, shared decision-making). Intervention and research emphasize the local relevance of interventions (i.e., culture and capacity), as well as equal participation of community partners in intervention research, development, and evaluation. Lastly, outcomes include both health outcomes engendered by interventions and

CBPR-related capacity change at the community and academic levels. The next chapter of CBPR research must address the need for measurement of these outcomes by developing tools to operationalize and evaluate these four partnership constructs. Similar measurement challenges and opportunities exist in PCOR, with limited availability of both best practice guidance for patient engagement and measurement tools to evaluate and compare different engagement strategies (Domecq et al., 2014; Nilsen et al., 2006).

Despite the proliferation of CBPR approaches in health disparities and health equity research, formal process evaluation of partnership building efforts is rarely documented in the CBPR literature (Viswanathan et al., 2004). Relatedly, there is a lack of documentation of the time, energy, resources, funding mechanisms, tenure structures, organizational hierarchy, power-sharing arrangements, and institutional commitment required to conduct CBPR and maintain successful partnerships with communities (Faridi et al., 2007). These process data are needed to evaluate and compare different CE strategies and provide practical guidance for engaging in CBPR. For example, in a mixed-method evaluation of partnership functioning with an Asian American community coalition, VanDevanter et al. identified opportunities to re-engage with their community partners in a more equitable way (VanDevanter et al., 2011). These strategies included: (1) planning a partnership retreat to evaluate fidelity to partnership principles; (2) a commitment to align project and community partners' priorities; and (3) formalized protocols and governance documents to guide partnership functioning. Co-developing these strategies with community partners revitalized the partnership and reflected a commitment to addressing the community's concerns and priorities. Engaging in and documenting this reflective process is important not only to conform with CBPR principles but also to generate best practice examples for CBPR partnership building with underserved communities. It would be especially informative to study how community-academic partnerships were sustained and reformed during COVID-19 as a response to emergent priorities.

Future Direction: Participatory Implementation Science

Reducing health disparities will require an accelerated integration of evidence-based interventions (EBIs) into practice. As described in Chapter 8, implementation science (IS) provides frameworks and methods to guide this process. The IS frameworks emphasize contextual factors as important determinants of the success or failure of implementation of EBIs. Context can be elucidated with CE to (1) identify the determinants of a health problem, which may clarify intervention aims and facilitate the selection of EBIs best suited to achieving those aims and (2) select context-specific implementation strategies. Despite its emphasis on external validity and intervention tailoring, IS has been criticized for being one-sided, skewed toward the researchers' goals, knowledge, and preferred methods (Wallerstein & Duran, 2010). The recent move to prioritize health equity in IS research and practice presents an opportunity to introduce CE into the field (Baumann & Cabassa, 2020; Ramanadhan et al., 2018). Reflecting this new commitment, "participatory implementation science" was proposed to expand community and stakeholder engagement in the co-production of knowledge and solutions, which can improve IS translational goals (i.e., effectiveness, scalability, and sustainability) (Ramanadhan et al., 2018). Similarly, the integration of health equity into IS frameworks will require CE in all phases of implementation to improve reach and the relevance of implementation strategies (Baumann & Cabassa, 2020). This new development in IS will be an interesting one to follow in order to assess the degree to which CE may accelerate the uptake of EBIs and reduce health disparities.

DISCUSSION QUESTIONS

Consider the following scenario and answer the discussion questions below:

You are a public health researcher who received funding to conduct CEnR to examine the disproportionate burden of COVID-19 infection and mortality among the Chinese American community in your region.

1. What are some anticipated benefits and challenges of CE in this research project?

2. Write a reflexivity statement. What is your positionality relative to this community, and how might your multiple identities influence the research process?

3. What are some considerations to guide the development of a CE strategy? Who are some potential community partners? How might you foster trust and joint ownership over the course of the project?

4. Describe potential capacity-building and coalition-building activities that could be implemented with the Chinese American community to support the research project. How might these new resources prove beneficial for developing future chronic disease prevention programs with the same community?

REFERENCES

Abboud, S., Chebli, P., & Rabelais, E. (2019). The contested Whiteness of Arab identity in the United States: implications for health disparities research. *American Journal of Public Health; Washington*, *109*(11), 1580–1583. http://dx.doi.org.proxy.cc.uic.edu/10.2105/AJPH.2019.305285

Abuelezam, N. N., El-Sayed, A. M., & Galea, S. (2017). Arab American health in a racially charged U.S. *American Journal of Preventive Medicine*, *52*(6), 810–812. https://doi.org/10.1016/j.amepre.2017.02.021

Ammerman, A., Smith, T. W., & Calancie, L. (2014). Practice-Based Evidence in Public Health: Improving Reach, Relevance, and Results. *Annual Review of Public Health*, *35*(1), 47–63. https://doi.org/10.1146/annurev-publhealth-032013-182458

Artiga, S., Orgera, K., & Pham, O. (2020). *Disparities in Health and Health Care: Five Key Questions and Answers* (p. 13). Kaiser Family Foundation. https://www.careinnovations.org/wp-content/uploads/Issue-Brief-Disparities-in-Health-and-Health-Care-Five-Key-Questions-and-Answers.pdf

Balas, E. A., Weingarten, S., Garb, C. T., Blumenthal, D., Boren, S. A., & Brown, G. D. (2000). Improving preventive care by prompting physicians. *Archives of Internal Medicine*, *160*(3), 301–308. https://doi.org/10.1001/archinte.160.3.301

Baum, F., MacDougall, C., & Smith, D. (2006). Participatory action research. *Journal of Epidemiology and Community Health*, *60*(10), 854–857. https://doi.org/10.1136/jech.2004.028662

Baumann, A. A., & Cabassa, L. J. (2020). Reframing implementation science to address inequities in healthcare delivery. *BMC Health Services Research*, *20*(1), 190. https://doi.org/10.1186/s12913-020-4975-3

Belone, L., Lucero, JE., Duran, B., Tafoya, G., Baker, EA., Chan, D., Chang, C., Greene-Moton, E., Kelley, M., & Wallerstein, N. (2016). Community-based participatory research conceptual model: community partner consultation and face validity. *Qualitative Health Research*, *26*(1), 117–135. https://doi.org/10.1177/1049732314557084

Braveman, P. (2014). What are health disparities and health equity? We need to be clear. *Public Health Reports*, *129*(Suppl 2), 5–8.

Brownson, R. C., Fielding, J. E., & Green, L. W. (2018). Building capacity for evidence-based public health: reconciling the pulls of practice and the push of research. *Annual Review of Public Health*, *39*(1), 27–53. https://doi.org/10.1146/annurev-publhealth-040617-014746

Burke, J. G., Hess, S., Hoffmann, K., Guizzetti, L., Loy, E., Gielen, A., Bailey, M., Walnoha, A., Barbee, G., & Yonas, M. (2013). Translating community-based participatory research (CBPR) principles into practice: building a research agenda to reduce intimate partner violence. *Progress in Community Health Partnerships : Research, Education, and Action*, *7*(2), 115–122. https://doi.org/10.1353/cpr.2013.0025

Butterfoss, F. D., Goodman, R. M., & Wandersman, A. (1993). Community coalitions for prevention and health promotion. *Health Education Research*, *8*(3), 315–330. https://doi.org/10.1093/her/8.3.315

Carman, K. L., Dardess, P., Maurer, M., Sofaer, S., Adams, K., Bechtel, C., & Sweeney, J. (2013). Patient and family engagement: a framework for understanding the elements and developing interventions and policies. *Health Affairs*, *32*(2), 223–231. https://doi.org/10.1377/hlthaff.2012.1133

Carson, S. L., Gonzalez, C., Lopez, S., Morris, D., Mtume, N., Lucas-Wright, A., Vassar, S. D., Norris, K. C., & Brown, A. F. (2020). Reflections on the Importance of Community-Partnered Research Strategies for Health Equity in the Era of COVID-19. *Journal of Health Care for the Poor and Underserved*, *31*(4), 1515–1519. https://doi.org/10.1353/hpu.2020.0112

Concannon, T. W., Fuster, M., Saunders, T., Patel, K., Wong, J. B., Leslie, L. K., & Lau, J. (2014). A Systematic Review of Stakeholder Engagement in Comparative Effectiveness and Patient-Centered Outcomes Research. *Journal of General Internal Medicine*, *29*(12), 1692–1701. https://doi.org/10.1007/s11606-014-2878-x

Core Values, Ethics, Spectrum – The 3 Pillars of Public Participation. (n.d.). International Association for Public Participation. Retrieved November 30, 2020, from https://www.iap2.org/page/pillars

Denzin, N. K., & Lincoln, Y. S. (2017). *The SAGE Handbook of Qualitative Research*. SAGE Publications.

Domecq, J. P., Prutsky, G., Elraiyah, T., Wang, Z., Nabhan, M., Shippee, N., Brito, J. P., Boehmer, K., Hasan, R., Firwana, B., Erwin, P., Eton, D., Sloan, J., Montori, V., Asi, N., Abu Dabrh, A. M., & Murad, M. H. (2014). Patient engagement in research: A systematic review. *BMC Health Services Research*, *14*(1), 89. https://doi.org/10.1186/1472-6963-14-89

Dwyer, S. C., & Buckle, J. L. (2009). The space between: on being an insider-outsider in qualitative research. *International Journal of Qualitative Methods*, *8*(1), 54–63. https://doi.org/10.1177/160940690900800105

Faridi, Z., Grunbaum, J. A., Sajor Gray, B., Franks, A., & Simoes, E. (2007). Community-based participatory research: necessary next steps. *Preventing Chronic Disease*, *4*(3). https://www.ncbi.nlm.nih.gov/pmc/articles/PMC1955426/

Freimuth, V. S., Quinn, S. C., Thomas, S. B., Cole, G., Zook, E., & Duncan, T. (2001). African Americans' views on research and the Tuskegee Syphilis study. *Social Science & Medicine*, *52*(5), 797–808. https://doi.org/10.1016/S0277-9536(00)00178-7

Frieden, T. R. & Centers for Disease Control and Prevention (CDC). (2013). CDC health disparities and inequalities report – United States, 2013. Foreword. *MMWR Supplements*, *62*(3), 1–2.

Galiatsatos, P., Monson, K., Oluyinka, M., Negro, D., Hughes, N., Maydan, D., Golden, S. H., Teague, P., & Hale, W. D. (2020). Community calls: lessons and insights gained from a medical–religious community engagement during the COVID-19 pandemic. *Journal of Religion and Health*, *59*(5), 2256–2262. https://doi.org/10.1007/s10943-020-01057-w

Gilmore, B., Ndejjo, R., Tchetchia, A., Claro, V. de, Mago, E., Diallo, A. A., Lopes, C., & Bhattacharyya, S. (2020). Community engagement for COVID-19 prevention and control: A rapid evidence synthesis. *BMJ Global Health*, *5*(10), e003188. https://doi.org/10.1136/bmjgh-2020-003188

Glasgow, R. E., & Emmons, K. M. (2007). How can we increase translation of research into practice? types of evidence needed. *Annual Review of Public Health*, *28*(1), 413–433. https://doi.org/10.1146/annurev.publhealth.28.021406.144145

Green, L. W. (2014). Closing the chasm between research and practice: Evidence of and for change. *Health Promotion Journal of Australia*, *25*(1), 25–29. https://doi.org/10.1071/HE13101

Henry Akintobi, T., Jacobs, T., Sabbs, D., Holden, K., Braithwaite, R., Johnson, L. N., Dawes, D., & Hoffman, L. (2020). Community engagement of African Americans in the era of COVID-19: Considerations, challenges, implications, and recommendations for public health. *Preventing Chronic Disease, 17*, E83. https://doi.org/10.5888/pcd17.200255

Israel, B. A., Schulz, A. J., Parker, E. A., & Becker, A. B. (1998). Review of Community-Based Research: Assessing Partnership Approaches to Improve Public Health. *Annual Review of Public Health, 19*(1), 173–202. https://doi.org/10.1146/annurev.publhealth.19.1.173

Israel, B. A., Schulz, A. J., Parker, E. A., Becker, A. B., & Community-Campus Partnerships for Health. (2001). Community-based participatory research: Policy recommendations for promoting a partnership approach in health research. *Education for Health (Abingdon, England), 14*(2), 182–197. https://doi.org/10.1080/13576280110051055

Jewkes, R., & Murcott, A. (1996). Meanings of community. *Social Science & Medicine, 43*(4), 555–563. https://doi.org/10.1016/0277-9536(95)00439-4

Johnson, G. J., & Ambrose, P. J. (2006). Neo-tribes: The power and potential of online communities in health care. *Communications of the ACM, 49*(1), 107–113. https://doi.org/10.1145/1107458.1107463

Jun, J., & Nan, X. (2018). Determinants of cancer screening disparities among Asian Americans: A systematic review of public health surveys. *Journal of Cancer Education, 33*(4), 757–768. https://doi.org/10.1007/s13187-017-1211-x

Kerstetter, K. (2012). Insider, outsider, or somewhere between: the impact of researchers' identities on the community-based research process. *Journal of Rural Social Sciences, 27*(2). https://egrove.olemiss.edu/jrss/vol27/iss2/7

Kindon, S., Pain, R., & Kesby, M. (2007). *Participatory Action Research Approaches and Methods: Connecting People, Participation and Place.* Routledge.

Kwon, S., Rideout, C., Tseng, W., Islam, N., Cook, W. K., Ro, M., & Trinh-Shevrin, C. (2012). Developing the community empowered research training program: building research capacity for community-initiated and community-driven research. *Progress in Community Health Partnerships, 6*(1), 43–52. https://doi.org/10.1353/cpr.2012.0010

Kwon, S., Tandon, S. D., Islam, N., Riley, L., & Trinh-Shevrin, C. (2018). Applying a community-based participatory research framework to patient and family engagement in the development of patient-centered outcomes research and practice. *Translational Behavioral Medicine, 8*(5), 683–691. https://doi.org/10.1093/tbm/ibx026

Lee, J. P., Lipperman-Kreda, S., Saephan, S., & Kirkpatrick, S. (2012). Youth-led tobacco prevention: lessons learned for engaging Southeast Asian American youth. *Progress in Community Health Partnerships : Research, Education, and Action, 6*(2), 187–194. https://doi.org/10.1353/cpr.2012.0022

Lewin, K. (1946). Action research and minority problems. *Journal of Social Issues, 2*(4), 34–46. https://doi.org/10.1111/j.1540-4560.1946.tb02295.x

McCloskey, D. J., Akintobi, T. H., Bonham, A., Cook, J., & Coyne-Beasley, T. (2011). *Principles of Community Engagement (Second Edition)* (p. 197). The National Institutes of Health, The Centers for Disease Control and Prevention, The Agency for Toxic Substances and Disease Registry. https://www.atsdr.cdc.gov/communityengagement/pdf/PCE_Report_508_FINAL.pdf

McGowan, P., & Green, L. W. (1995). Arthritis self-management in native populations of British Columbia: An application of health promotion and participatory research principles in chronic disease control. *Canadian Journal on Aging / La Revue Canadienne Du Vieillissement, 14*(S1), 201–212. https://doi.org/10.1017/S0714980800005511

Mitchell, U. A., Chebli, P. G., Ruggiero, L., & Muramatsu, N. (2018). The Digital divide in health-related technology use: the significance of race/ethnicity. *The Gerontologist*, gny138–gny138. https://doi.org/10.1093/geront/gny138

Muhammad, M., Wallerstein, N., Sussman, A. L., Avila, M., Belone, L., & Duran, B. (2015). Reflections on researcher identity and power: the impact of positionality on community based participatory research (CBPR) processes and outcomes. *Critical Sociology, 41*(7–8), 1045–1063. https://doi.org/10.1177/0896920513516025

Ortiz, E., Scanlon, B., Mullens, A., & Durham, J. (2020). Effectiveness of interventions for hepatitis B and C: A systematic review of vaccination, screening, health promotion and linkage to care within higher income countries. *Journal of Community Health, 45*(1), 201–218. https://doi.org/10.1007/s10900-019-00699-6

Patient-Centered Outcomes Research Institute. (2018, October 26). *About Us.* https://www.pcori.org/about-us

Pollack, H. J., Kwon, S. C., Wang, S. H., Wyatt, L. C., Trinh-Shevrin, C., & Coalition, on behalf of the A. (2014). Chronic hepatitis B and liver cancer risks among Asian Immigrants in New York City: Results from a large, community-based screening, evaluation, and treatment program. *Cancer Epidemiology and Prevention Biomarkers, 23*(11), 2229–2239. https://doi.org/10.1158/1055-9965.EPI-14-0491

Pollack, H., Wang, S., Wyatt, L., Peng, C., Wan, K., Trinh-Shevrin, C., Chun, K., Tsang, T., & Kwon, S. (2011). A comprehensive screening and treatment model for reducing disparities in hepatitis B. *Health Affairs, 30*(10), 1974–1983. https://doi.org/10.1377/hlthaff.2011.0700

RADx Programs. (2020, June 23). National Institutes of Health (NIH). https://www.nih.gov/research-training/medical-research-initiatives/radx/radx-programs

Ramanadhan, S., Davis, M. M., Armstrong, R., Baquero, B., Ko, L. K., Leng, J. C., Salloum, R. G., Vaughn, N. A., & Brownson, R. C. (2018). Participatory implementation science to increase the impact of evidence-based cancer prevention and control. *Cancer Causes & Control : CCC, 29*(3), 363–369. https://doi.org/10.1007/s10552-018-1008-1

Reichberg, S. B., Mitra, P. P., Haghamad, A., Ramrattan, G., Crawford, J. M., Consortium, N. C. R., Berry, G. J., Davidson, K. W., Drach, A., Duong, S., Juretschko, S., Maria, N. I., Yang, Y., & Ziemba, Y. C. (2020). Rapid Emergence of SARS-CoV-2 in the Greater New York Metropolitan Area: Geolocation, demographics, positivity rates, and hospitalization for 46,793 persons tested by Northwell Health. *Clinical Infectious Diseases.* https://doi.org/10.1093/cid/ciaa922

Rhee, C. of C., & Press, via A. (2020, August 21). COVID-19's toll on people of color is worse than we knew. The Marshall Project. https://www.themarshallproject.org/2020/08/21/covid-19-s-toll-on-people-of-color-is-worse-than-we-knew

Selby, J. V., Beal, A. C., & Frank, L. (2012). The Patient-Centered Outcomes Research Institute (PCORI) national priorities for research and initial research agenda. *JAMA, 307*(15), 1583–1584. https://doi.org/10.1001/jama.2012.500

Simmons, A., Reynolds, R. C., & Swinburn, B. (2011). Defining community capacity building: Is it possible? *Preventive Medicine, 52*(3), 193–199. https://doi.org/10.1016/j.ypmed.2011.02.003

Smith, B. J., Tang, K. C., & Nutbeam, D. (2006). WHO Health Promotion Glossary: New terms. *Health Promotion International, 21*(4), 340–345. https://doi.org/10.1093/heapro/dal033

Social Determinants of Health, CDC. (2020, September 30). Centers for Disease Control and Prevention. https://www.cdc.gov/socialdetermi-nants/index.htm

Srinivasan, S., & Williams, S. D. (2014). Transitioning from health disparities to a health equity research agenda: the time is now. *Public Health Reports*, *129*(1_suppl2), 71–76. https://doi.org/10.1177/00333549141291S213

Staley, Kristina. (2009). Exploring impact: Public involvement in NHS, public health and social care research – INVOLVE. INVOLVE. https://www.invo.org.uk/posttypepublication/exploring-impact-public-involvement-in-nhs-public-health-and-social-care-research/

Tandon, S. D., & Kwon, S. (2009). Community-based participatory research. In C. Trinh-Shevrin, N. S. Islam, & M. J. Rey (Eds.), *Asian American Communities and Health: Context, Research, Policy, and Action (pp. 464–503)*. John Wiley & Sons.

Townsend, A. (2014). Weaving the threads of practice and research. In F. Rauch, A. Schuster, T. Stern, M. Pribila, & A. Townsend (Eds.), *Promoting Change through Action Research* (pp. 7–22). SensePublishers. https://doi.org/10.1007/978-94-6209-803-9_2

Translational Science Spectrum. (2015, March 12). National Center for Advancing Translational Sciences. https://ncats.nih.gov/translation/spectrum

Trinh, Q.-D., Li, H., Meyer, C. P., Hanske, J., Choueiri, T. K., Reznor, G., Lipsitz, S. R., Kibel, A. S., Han, P. K., Nguyen, P. L., Menon, M., & Sammon, J. D. (2016). Determinants of cancer screening in Asian-Americans. *Cancer Causes & Control*, *27*(8), 989–998. https://doi.org/10.1007/s10552-016-0776-8

Trinh-Shevrin, C., Islam, N. S., & Rey, M. J. (2009). *Asian American Communities and Health: Context, Research, Policy, and Action.* John Wiley & Sons.

Trinh-Shevrin, C., Nadkarni, S., Park, R., Islam, N., & Kwon, S. C. (2015). Defining an integrative approach for health promotion and disease prevention: A population health equity framework. *Journal of Health Care for the Poor and Underserved*, *26*(2 0), 146–163. https://doi.org/10.1353/hpu.2015.0067

Trinh-Shevrin, C., Pollack, H. J., Tsang, T., Park, J., Ramos, M. R., Islam, N., Wang, S., Chun, K., Sim, S.-C., Pong, P., Rey, M. J., & Kwon, S. C. (2011). The Asian American hepatitis B program: Building a coalition to address hepatitis B health disparities. *Progress in Community Health Partnerships*, *5*(3), 261–271. https://doi.org/10.1353/cpr.2011.0039

Ursua, R. A., Aguilar, D. E., Wyatt, L. C., Trinh-Shevrin, C., Gamboa, L., Valdellon, P., Perrella, E. G., Dimaporo, M. Z., Nur, P. Q., Tandon, S. D., & Islam, N. S. (2018). A community health worker intervention to improve blood pressure among Filipino Americans with hypertension: A randomized controlled trial. *Preventive Medicine Reports*, *11*, 42–48. https://doi.org/10.1016/j.pmedr.2018.05.002

VanDevanter, N., Kwon, S., Sim, S.-C., Chun, K., & Trinh-Shevrin, C. (2011). Evaluation of community–academic partnership functioning: center for the elimination of hepatitis B Health disparities. *Progress in Community Health Partnerships : Research, Education, and Action*, *5*(3), 223–233. https://doi.org/10.1353/cpr.2011.0032

Viswanathan, M., Ammerman, A., Eng, E., Garlehner, G., Lohr, K. N., Griffith, D., Rhodes, S., Samuel-Hodge, C., Maty, S., Lux, L., Webb, L., Sutton, S. F., Swinson, T., Jackman, A., & Whitener, L. (2004). Community-based participatory research: assessing the evidence: summary. *In AHRQ Evidence Report Summaries*. Agency for Healthcare Research and Quality (US). https://www.ncbi.nlm.nih.gov/sites/books/NBK11852/

Wallerstein, N., & Duran, B. (2010). Community-based participatory research contributions to intervention research: the intersection of science and practice to improve health equity. *American Journal of Public Health*, *100*(S1), S40–S46. https://doi.org/10.2105/AJPH.2009.184036

Wallerstein, N., Duran, B., Oetzel, J. G., & Minkler, M. (2017). *Community-Based Participatory Research for Health: Advancing Social and Health Equity.* John Wiley & Sons, Incorporated. http://ebookcentral.proquest.com/lib/uic/detail.action?docID=5097167

Ward, E., Jemal, A., Cokkinides, V., Singh, G. K., Cardinez, C., Ghafoor, A., & Thun, M. (2004). Cancer disparities by race/ethnicity and socioeconomic status. *CA: A Cancer Journal for Clinicians*, *54*(2), 78–93. https://doi.org/10.3322/canjclin.54.2.78

Zakocs, R. C., & Edwards, E. M. (2006). What explains community coalition effectiveness?: a review of the literature. *American Journal of Preventive Medicine*, *30*(4), 351–361. https://doi.org/10.1016/j.amepre.2005.12.004

CHAPTER

9

CLINICAL-COMMUNITY LINKAGE STRATEGIES

HAE-RA HAN

LEARNING OBJECTIVES

By the end of this chapter, readers will be able to:

- Identify linkage approaches used to promote health care and health outcomes among Asian Americans.
- Discuss innovations in linkage approaches using emerging technologies.
- Describe case examples of effective programs that facilitate linkages between health care and community settings.

Applied Population Health Approaches for Asian American Communities, First Edition. Edited by Simona C. Kwon, Chau Trinh-Shevrin, Nadia S. Islam, and Stella S. Yi.
© 2023 John Wiley & Sons, Inc. Published 2023 by John Wiley & Sons, Inc.
Companion Website: www.wiley.com/go/kwon/asianamerican

INTRODUCTION

The needs of vulnerable populations are multifold and require extensive medical and nonmedical outreach and services. Current health care service delivery does not always address the complexity of these needs. For example, following the implementation of the United States Patient Protection and Affordable Care Act – also called Obamacare or the Affordable Care Act (ACA) – the rate of uninsured individuals dropped from 17.8% in 2010 to 10% in 2016 among the non-elderly population, but starting in 2017, the coverage gains stalled (Tolbert et al., 2019). Half of adults in the United States report they or a family member delayed or skipped necessary health or dental service or relied on an alternative treatment in the past year because of the cost of care and 29% report not taking their medicines as prescribed because of the cost (Kirzinger et al., 2019). Compared with their insured counterparts, uninsured individuals are less likely to receive timely preventive care within the last year (33% versus 67% of the nonelderly with Medicaid and 74% of nonelderly individuals with employer-based insurance) or have access to appropriate follow-up care after abnormal screening results (Majerol et al., 2015). Other vulnerable groups such as older adults or persons with disabilities also have high levels of unmet health care needs. According to the State of Aging and Health in America 2013 report (Centers for Disease Control and Prevention, 2013), only about 51% of male and 53% of female older adults (65+ years) were up to date on certain preventive care measures such as flu vaccination or colorectal cancer screening.

Health disparities persist in the United States among the nation's racial/ethnic minority groups (Rodriguez-Gutierrez et al., 2019; Ng et al., 2017). People of color and low-income individuals face greater barriers to accessing care, including a higher rate of being uninsured, compared to non-Hispanic Whites (Whites) and people with higher incomes (Agency for Healthcare Research and Quality [AHRQ], 2019). Historically, Asian Americans have been both more likely to be uninsured and less likely to have access to a primary care provider compared to the general population (Artiga et al., 2020). Data also show that disparities in some health outcomes, such as cancer mortality rates among Vietnamese and type 2 diabetes (diabetes) and stroke mortality rates among Asian Indian and Filipino Americans, have increased over time (Enas et al., 2013; Hastings et al., 2015).

A linkage to care refers to a partnership between a health provider and diverse resource organizations, such as community organizations and public health agencies. The main goals of clinical-community linkages include coordinating the delivery of health care services, public health programs, and community-based activities to promote healthy behavior and forming partnerships and relationships among clinical, community, and public health organizations to fill gaps in needed health services (AHRQ, 2016). Establishing sustainable and effective linkages between clinical and community settings plays a key role in improving access to preventive services and chronic illness care, particularly among vulnerable groups of people, which, in turn, contributes to reducing and preventing disease in communities (Kim et al., 2016).

To this end, clinical-community linkages can address what Donald Berwick and colleagues described as *the Triple Aim* for improving the U.S. health care system: improving the individual experience of care; improving the health of populations; and reducing the per capita costs of care (Berwick et al., 2008). A number of linkage approaches have been used to promote health care and improve health outcomes among Asian Americans. This chapter discusses key clinical-community linkage approaches that have been used to coordinate health care service delivery, identify patients in need of additional support, and refer patients to community resources as required. In addition, the chapter addresses innovative linkage approaches using emerging technologies. Finally, case examples are provided to highlight how clinical-community linkage programs have been implemented in Asian American communities.

COMMUNITY-CLINICAL LINKAGE APPROACHES FOR ASIAN AMERICANS

Linkages to care address structural and/or behavioral barriers reported by patients. Examples of structural barriers include lack of health insurance (Tan et al., 2018; Lee & Lee, 2018; Chung et al., 2018), lack of transportation (Starbird et al., 2019), limited English proficiency (Chung et al., 2018; Jang & Kim, 2019; Sy et al., 2018) or other financial, work, and childcare constraints. Behavioral barriers include patients' lack of trust in health care providers or services (Chung et al., 2018; Fang & Stewart, 2018; Sy et al., 2018), fear of medical procedures or test results (Lee & Lee, 2018), perceived discrimination (Fang & Stewart, 2018), and lack of understanding of disease or the need for preventive care (Fang & Stewart, 2018; Lee & Lee, 2018). A number of linkage approaches have been used to address these barriers among Asian Americans. Examples include engaging community health workers (CHWs), implementing patient navigation with case management, and utilizing emerging technologies such as electronic health record (EHR)-based referrals to health or social services, the use of mobile and wireless technologies to support medical and public health objectives (mHealth), and community and clinical resource mapping using geographic information systems (GIS).

Linkages to Care Using CHWs

CHWs are frontline paraprofessionals. They are lay health workers who share the same language, ethnicity, culture, geographic community, and/or life experiences of the patients they serve. Consequently, CHWs are uniquely aware of the linguistic, ethnic, socioeconomic, cultural, and experiential factors that may influence use of health services among a specific population of interest (Giblin, 1989). These characteristics render CHWs effective in providing "linkages" between health service providers and the community via culturally appropriate health education, counseling and social support in diverse settings (e.g., community-based organizations, community clinics, or faith-based organizations), assistance in navigating the health care system, coordinating care, and facilitating access to social services (Kim et al., 2016).

CHWs are particularly effective in improving health behaviors and health outcomes among populations experiencing health inequities, including those with limited access to care. CHW interventions have demonstrated effectiveness in improving cancer and cardiovascular disparities in ethnic minority populations in the United States (Kim et al., 2016). Most CHW interventions focusing on Asian Americans addressed cancer screening behaviors such as breast and cervical cancer screening in Vietnamese (Lam et al., 2003; Mock et al., 2007; Nguyen et al., 2009; Tayler et al., 2010) and Korean American women (Fang et al., 2017; Han et al., 2017), cervical cancer screening in Chinese American women (Taylor et al., 2002), and colorectal cancer screening in Chinese (Ngyuen et al. 2017), Filipino (Maxwell et al., 2016), and Vietnamese Americans (Walsh et al., 2010). These programs were designed to reach non-native English speakers by delivering culturally-tailored interventions in the language of each population of interest.

One such program recruited bilingual CHWs who were well-versed in Korean culture to promote breast and cervical cancer screening uptake among Korean immigrant women (Han et al., 2017). In the study, Han et al. (2017) tested a CHW-led health literacy education and follow-up intervention on mammography and Papanicolaou test screening among Korean American women ($N = 560$). The odds of having received a mammogram were 18.5 (95% confidence interval [CI], 9.2–37.4) times higher in the intervention than in the control group, adjusting for covariates. Similarly, the odds of receiving a Papanicolaou test were 13.3 (95% CI, 7.9–22.3) times higher and the odds of receiving both tests were 17.4 (95% CI, 7.5–40.3) times higher in the intervention group as compared to the control group.

Other topics addressed – though not as frequently as cancer screening – include hepatitis B virus testing and vaccination in Korean (Ma et al., 2018), Hmong (Chen et al., 2013), and Cambodian American adults (Taylor et al., 2013), diabetes prevention in Korean Americans (Islam et al., 2013), and hypertension management among Filipino Americans (Ursua et al., 2018). Ma et al. (2018) conducted a cluster randomized trial involving Korean ethnic churches ($N = 32$ with 1,834 participants) to improve hepatitis B screening and vaccination among Korean Americans who were not previously screened. Bilingual community educators provided group education and patient navigation. The intervention resulted in the improvement in the hepatitis B screening and vaccination compliance rate (87% in the intervention group vs 3.8% in the control group). Likewise, Chen et al. (2013) used CHWs to promote hepatitis B testing among 260 Hmong adults through in-home education and patient navigation and Taylor et al. (2013) used CHWs to promote screening among 250 Cambodian Americans through a home visit that used in-language educational materials (e.g., educational flipchart, pamphlet, and a motivational Khmer language DVD), and follow-up phone calls. In the Chen et al. (2013) study, the CHW intervention was associated with increased self-reported hepatitis B test completion (OR 3.5; 95% CI, 1.3–9.2). In the Taylor et al. (2013) study, the difference between experimental and control participants in hepatitis B testing was significant ($p < 0.001$) in the intent-to-treat analysis using self-reported data.

Islam and colleagues (2013) pilot-tested a CHW intervention to promote diabetes prevention among Korean Americans using a randomized controlled trial design. A total of 48 Korean Americans at risk for diabetes participated in the intervention. CHWs provided six workshops on diabetes prevention, nutrition, physical activity, diabetes complications, stress and family support, and access to health care. Over 6 months, significant changes were seen in weight, waist circumference, diastolic blood pressure, physical activity nutrition, diabetes knowledge, and mental health measures. Ursua et al. (2018) assessed the efficacy of a CHW intervention to improve hypertension management among 240 Filipino Americans. Intervention participants received four educational workshops and four one-on-one visits with CHWs over a 4-month period, while control group participants received one educational workshop. At 8 months, blood pressure was controlled among a significantly greater percentage of intervention group participants compared to the control group (83.3% vs. 42.7%, $p < 0.001$). The adjusted odds of controlled blood pressure for the intervention group was 3.2 times the odds of the control group ($p < 0.001$). Individuals in the intervention group also showed significant changes in appointment keeping.

The important role for intensive outreach efforts has been demonstrated in identifying at-risk populations and keeping them in the health care system. As such, most CHW interventions have included outreach components and support services such as health system navigation, health literacy training, and provision of transportation. CHWs in these studies provided community education with (Chen et al., 2013; Fang et al., 2017; Han et al., 2017; Maxwell et al., 2016; Taylor et al., 2002) or without navigation services (Nguyen et al., 2017; Taylor et al., 2013) and culturally tailored phone counseling (Han et al., 2017; Nguyen et al., 2017; Walsh et al., 2010). Navigation services offered in these studies included clinic referral and assistance with appointment scheduling, medical interpreter services during clinic visits, and transportation assistance. For example, CHWs in the Taylor et al. (2002) study provided transportation assistance by arranging taxicabs to transport patients to and from clinic appointments.

Evidence supports CHWs as an effective linkage approach among racial/ethnic minority populations including Asian Americans. Moreover, the ACA acknowledges the essential role of CHWs in improving health behaviors and outcomes and emphasizes the need for CHWs to participate as core members of health teams in communities with a high rate of uninsured but eligible individuals with a high percentage of chronic diseases or infant mortality (Martinez et al., 2011). However, a lack of sustainable funding sources for CHWs appears to be a major barrier to the full integration and maintenance of this model within health care delivery systems (Kim et al., 2016).

Minnesota was the first state to establish a potentially sustainable funding source to maintain CHWs (Rosenthal et al., 2010) by integrating reimbursable CHW services for vulnerable populations under its state Medicaid program. To receive reimbursement, CHWs must complete a 14-credit certificate program and work under the supervision of Medicaid-approved health care professionals such as physicians, advanced practice nurses, dentists, public health nurses, or mental health providers. The Minnesota model could be ideal for adaptation and integration within other state frameworks. More systematic cost evaluations of the use of CHWs as an evidence-based linkage approach can facilitate the integration of CHWs as part of the health care system.

Patient Navigation With Case Management

Patient navigation provides individuals lacking resources with whole patient care through intensive case management. Patient navigators work "one-on-one with clients to encourage continued commitment and adherence to medical treatment, access to social services, improved communication, and prompt re-engagement in care" (Centers for Disease Control and Prevention, 2020). Communities with the highest proportions of racial/ethnic minorities are among the most vulnerable to limited health care access and quality. People with limited access to health services may benefit from individualized assistance to overcome access barriers through all phases of the disease experience.

Patient navigation has been shown to be a critical component in helping racial/ethnic minorities gain access to federally qualified health centers, as well as to other safety net facilities, which provide screening, diagnostic, and treatment services (Bernardo et al., 2019). Additionally, patient navigators may help patients gain and maintain consistent access to insurance through publicly funded programs such as Medicaid. In particular, patient navigators may advocate on behalf of patients who have experienced insurance discrimination. The ACA banned this type of discrimination, prohibiting insurance companies from excluding sicker individuals from coverage and forbidding them to charge higher premiums to these individuals (Wells et al., 2008). Among underserved populations, patient navigation services have also been shown to decrease the anxiety associated with medical treatment and increase patient satisfaction with services received (Ferrante et al., 2008). Indeed, patient navigation represents a potentially powerful tool to reduce health disparities (Liu et al., 2020).

Although the patient navigator model is widespread, there is relatively limited empirical evidence that this linkage approach is effective among Asian Americans. A comprehensive hepatitis B screening and treatment program – Bfree NYC, a New York City (NYC) pilot program – provided hepatitis B community education and awareness, free screening and vaccinations, and free or low-cost treatment primarily to immigrants from Asia, in addition to residents from other racial and ethnic minority groups (Pollack et al., 2011). Case management was offered to those participants who required vaccination or treatment. Bfree NYC reached nearly 9,000 people, and during the program, new hepatitis B cases reported annually from predominantly Asian neighborhoods in the city increased 34%. Of 3,156 hepatitis B-susceptible individuals, 2,253 people received the first vaccination and 1,652 received all three; 57% of the 1,162 patients who tested positive for hepatitis B and were evaluated by program clinical services were still in care at the end of the program.

In a randomized controlled trial, Wong and colleagues (2008) tested a comprehensive smoking cessation program, the Chinese Community Smoking Cessation Project. A total of 464 Chinese smokers were recruited from health care facilities (79%) and through Chinese language media (21%) in the San Francisco Bay area. Smokers in the intensive intervention group received physician advice and nurse counseling, with five follow-up phone contacts over 90 days. For smokers who relapsed, one repeat relapse counseling session and one additional follow-up phone call were provided. Additionally, smokers who met the criteria for nicotine dependency received nicotine replacement therapy. Smokers in the minimal intervention group received only physician advice and a self-help manual. However, this trial encountered significant challenges to enrollment and retention due to limitations within the participating health facilities. Additional work is needed to generate results that illustrate the success of this approach, but the study represents an important step toward developing tailored approaches for Asian American populations.

Kwong et al. (2013) used the primary care setting to test the effectiveness of a culturally and linguistically tailored depression care management program. Low-income Chinese Americans at a federally qualified community health center in NYC were screened for depression. A total of 57 eligible participants were randomly assigned to either enhanced physician care with care management or enhanced physician care only. The care manager coordinated depression care with physicians and reinforced physicians' treatment instructions while providing patients with educational materials, setting up patient appointments in the event of side effects, reviewing safety procedures with the patient in case of emergency, teaching self-management skills, and monitoring patient progress toward achieving self-management goals. For the physician-only arm, the physician was responsible for all aspects of the patients' treatment, including monitoring patient progress toward patient self-management goals, providing educational materials, and other patient support activities. Both groups showed significant reduction of depressive symptoms with no significant difference between the groups, which may be due, in part, to a small sample size. Employing collaborative care strategies in primary care settings may be an important approach for improving access to mental health care for Asian Americans who often experience multiple barriers that prevent them from receiving necessary treatment.

In the Chicago area, Chandrasekar and colleagues (2016) evaluated the impact of navigation to increase enrollment of Asian Americans in health insurance via "Get Covered Illinois," an initiative to expand the benefits of the ACA to underserved communities. Trained bilingual and bicultural navigators educated and assisted uninsured members of the Cambodian, Chinese, Vietnamese, Korean, and Laotian American communities. Navigators were provided by community-based organizations and had several years of prior experience working in community health. They shared the same language preference, ethnic background, socioeconomic status, and life experiences as the community members they were assigned to work with, but also rated their English language comprehension as "good" on a scale ranging from "poor" to "excellent." The navigators linked insurance enrollment activities to existing adult learning, mentoring, and family support programs. In addition, they tapped into local neighborhoods, teaming up with grocery stores and schools, and conducting outreach events at ethnic festivals and other gatherings. During the open enrollment period, navigators successfully enrolled 1,000 individuals in health insurance plans. According to evaluation surveys, prior to this initiative, more than one third (34.7%) of Asian American community members were not insured. After the navigator program was introduced, insurance coverage increased significantly from 65.3% to 77.6% ($p = 0.00$) overall. However, in subgroup analyses, the increase in coverage was significant only among Chinese and Korean Americans ($p < 0.05$), obscuring more limited gains among smaller ethnic populations.

Recently, Ma and colleagues (2019) conducted a cluster randomized trial involving 30 Korean church-based community organizations with 925 participants to promote colorectal cancer screening among Korean Americans. Key components of the intervention included patient navigation, interactive group education, physician engagement, and provision of the fecal immunochemical test kit for use at home. Patient navigation was offered based on participants' needs and included scheduling appointments with clinical partners for sigmoidoscopy or colonoscopy after a positive fecal immunochemical test result and assisting with paperwork. Participants in the intervention group were significantly more likely to receive colorectal cancer screening as compared with those in the control group (69.3% vs. 16%). The intervention was particularly effective in promoting fecal immunochemical testing among the more disadvantaged individuals in the Korean American community, including those with only a high school or lower education level, annual income of less than $40,000, low English proficiency, no health insurance, and/or no employment.

In Chicago, the Chinatown Patient Navigation Program focused on increasing cancer screening among Chinese Americans (Feinglass et al., 2019). Components included scheduling appointments, supporting communication between patients and care teams (including interpreter services), and addressing patient barriers to care such as fear, lack of transportation and lack of insurance through education, outreach, and referrals to community, local, and state resources. An analysis of claims data revealed that mammogram screening increased in the program catchment area, alongside increases in other low-income areas, demonstrating the importance of providing culturally and linguistically tailored services to underserved groups in order for all residents to attain equal access to preventive services.

As previously noted, the literature is generally limited in discussing patient navigation programs in Asian American communities. Further, available studies have yielded inconsistent findings in terms of the effectiveness of this approach. In some studies, lack of significant findings may be linked to design issues such as insufficient sample size (Kwong et al., 2013) or inadequate recruitment and poor retention of participants (Wong et al., 2008). Additionally, published reports lack rigorous evaluation of patient navigation in the Asian American population to establish strong evidence in supporting the approach; only half (Kwong et al., 2013; Ma et al., 2019; Wong et al., 2008) of the six identified used a randomized controlled trial design. Building the evidence base for the effectiveness of patient navigation among Asian American communities requires more rigorously designed trials with adequate sample sizes to provide sufficient statistical power.

Other Linkage Approaches Using Emerging Technologies

Developing and implementing novel linkage approaches to address the complex needs of vulnerable populations is an important public health goal. With the growing accessibility of health information on the internet, people are becoming more knowledgeable about their health conditions and treatment options. Electronic health records (EHRs), mHealth, and GIS are three key areas in which programs are currently being developed and evaluated for use in underserved communities, including among Asian Americans.

An EHR is an electronic system used by health care institutions to collect and store patients' health information (Ehrenstein et al., 2019). More than 8 out of 10 hospitals (86%) in the United States have at least a basic EHR, capable of recording patient demographics (e.g., age, sex/gender, race), problem lists or diagnoses, medication lists, and discharge summaries (Office of the National Coordinator for Health Information Technology, 2019). More than one-third (40%) of hospitals are equipped with a comprehensive EHR, featuring additional functions such as provider order entry (e.g., consultation requests, prescriptions) and decision support tools (e.g., clinical reminders) (Henry et al., 2016). Rapid and widespread adoption of EHRs presents an unprecedented opportunity for clinicians, public health practitioners, and research teams to develop and implement intervention programs tailored to specific populations of interest. A recent systematic review (Han et al., 2019a) revealed that EHR-based interventions may improve medication adherence, clinical decision-making, and preventive service delivery in primary care or outpatient settings. It should be noted, however, that the sample populations of the studies included in the review were comprised predominantly of White, highly educated, and highly literate patient populations, limiting the generalizability of the results. Not only did the studies lack diversity but also some studies neglected to report the race or ethnicity of the participants (Han et al., 2019a).

Using EHR-linked approaches to improve patient care and outcomes among Asian American communities is an emerging field. In fact, most studies have only recently begun to focus on diversifying their sample populations to include members of racial/ethnic minority groups. A study by Weisner and colleagues (2016) that examined the use of an EHR-linked patient portal among patients served by an outpatient alcohol and drug addiction treatment center in San Francisco provides one example. The researchers recruited patients ($N = 503$) from diverse racial and ethnic groups (60.8% White, 20.1% Hispanic, 7.4% African American, and 6.8% Asian American). Intervention participants received six group-based, manual-guided sessions on patient engagement in health care and the use of health information technology resources in the EHR. The intervention group showed an increase in the mean number of log-in days (incidence rate ratio, 1.53; 95% CI, 1.19–1.97) and patient portal use (i.e., communicating by email, viewing lab test results and information, and obtaining medical advice). Intervention participants were also more likely to talk with their physicians about addiction problems (OR, 2.30; 95% CI, 1.52–3.49).

Another example of expanding efforts to reach more diverse populations with EHR-linked interventions is the EmblemHealth Neighborhood Care program. This initiative was implemented at three locations in NYC: Central Harlem (62% Black or African American and 23% Hispanic or Latino), Cambria Heights (56% Black or African American), and Chinatown (34% Asian American, predominantly Chinese ethnicity) (Kwon et al., 2017). EmblemHealth Neighborhood Care used the EHR at those locations to communicate directly with physicians about patient care and to establish a referral system for patients, linking them to available wellness programs, community or government financial resources, and pharmacy case manager services. Preliminary analysis suggested that the linkage program was feasible and acceptable to community members, as illustrated by the large number of patients engaged in the first four years of the program ($N = 200,000+$).

Several studies are exploring the use of EHRs to provide comprehensive and tailored linkage services specifically to Asian American patients. The Diabetes Research, Education, and Action for Minorities (DREAM) Initiative is an ongoing randomized controlled trial integrating both EHR and CHW approaches to promote weight loss among South Asian patients at risk for diabetes within a network of primary care providers in NYC (Lim et al., 2019). Participating primary care providers receive technical assistance through the EHR to support clinical decision-making, including prediabetes-related registry reports, alerts, and order sets. Concurrently, CHWs provide group education sessions to enrolled patients that address diabetes prevention by focusing on weight loss and nutrition. Through use of a software platform, the study systematically tracks and monitors CHW referrals to social service organizations. The DREAM Initiative will enroll 480 South Asians at risk for diabetes into the intervention group, and an equal number will be included in a matched control group (see Case 4 in the Appendix). In a separate study, Northridge and colleagues (2018) are conducting an implementation research project to improve access to quality oral health care and to enhance oral health promotion among low-income Chinese American adults in NYC. This study is particularly noteworthy as a partnered intervention, developed by researchers in partnership with community stakeholders. The intervention will include (1) community-based dental screening of Chinese patients, whose data will be remotely entered into a customized EHR for follow-up by a dentist; (2) culturally and linguistically tailored educational materials distributed in the community and at outreach centers; (3) demonstrations of proper brushing and flossing techniques by CHWs; and (4) CHW follow-up with patients about oral health care receipt and dental hygiene behaviors.

Emerging technologies for health provide additional pathways to support patient engagement in health services and care. In particular, the World Health Organization has noted that mHealth has the "potential to transform the face of health service delivery (p. 1)" globally (Author, n.d.). One of the major strengths of mHealth programming is its ability to tailor interventions to individual needs without requiring the extensive involvement of health care providers (Anderson et al., 2019). Another strength of mHealth is facility in delivering confidential and motivational health-related messaging to recipients (Conserve et al., 2017). While much of the existing evidence addresses cardiovascular risk factor management (Delva et al., 2020), HIV testing and treatment adherence (Conserve et al., 2017; Purnomo et al., 2018), or intimate partner violence prevention (Anderson et al., 2019) among mostly Black and Hispanic populations, research has begun to investigate mHealth programs to support linkages among Asian American ethnic groups. For example, Hyun and colleagues (2020) assessed the efficacy of a mobile texting application (HepTalk) among Korean American patients who were either hepatitis B-infected or nonimmune to the hepatitis B virus ($N = 82$). HepTalk was employed for two-way communication between participants and patient navigators. On average, patient navigators sent and received 14 and 8 messages per participant, respectively, during the 6-month period. The themes of the messages included finding providers, scheduling appointments with providers, health education, and financial issues. Of the 82 participants, 78 were linked to care within 6 months – a 95% linkage rate.

Finally, mapping tools such as GIS may create searchable online community and clinical resource maps for both providers and patients, enhancing the delivery of interventions tailored to the needs of specific neighborhoods and communities. To date, GIS has been applied primarily to track and monitor health care access and disparities in health outcomes (Graves, 2008). However, GIS has been used to assess access to fresh fruit and vegetables (Gould, 2012; Fiechtner et al., 2017), public health services (Dubowitz, 2011), and resources for diabetes and related conditions (Curtis et al., 2013; Han et al., 2019b). Few controlled trials have tested GIS as a tool to promote linkage approaches, and none of these studies have focused on Asian Americans, suggesting an area for future application and research.

SUMMARY AND RECOMMENDATIONS

Linkages to care through collaborations between clinical providers, public health organizations, and community-based organizations may improve the individual experience of care and the health of populations while reducing the costs of care (Berwick et al., 2008). This chapter described both established and new linkage approaches and reviewed the evidence for the success of these approaches among Asian American populations. Assessments of CHW-led interventions have demonstrated improvements in linkages to care for cancer screening, hepatitis B testing and vaccination, and management of cardiovascular risk factors (e.g., diabetes prevention, hypertension control) among Asian Americans. Although patient navigation has also been utilized to provide support with disease screening (e.g., hepatitis B, cancer, depression), treatment, and follow-up, evidence for the effectiveness of navigation among Asian Americans is limited. Finally, given the exponential growth in the development and reach of new technologies in the health care sector and among the population at large, technology-based linkage approaches are emerging that use EHRs, mHealth, and GIS to link individuals, health services, and community resources. While research to date is limited, preliminary data look promising in terms of the utility, impact, and potential cost savings of these new technologies as compared to human resource-intensive linkage approaches.

As we consider these linkage options, it is important to recognize that linking patients to care does not automatically ensure retention in care. A successful linkage must be sustainable, reflecting more than a single encounter with the health system. As linkage approaches are introduced, evaluation strategies must be developed and implemented alongside them. For example, following an initial screening and/or treatment visit, does a patient return for follow-up visits? If not, why not? In addition to quantitative measures, eliciting feedback from providers, administrators, and beneficiaries of the linkage approaches is also essential to facilitate program evaluation and maximize retention of vulnerable populations in care.

Provisions of the ACA address four issues particularly important to reducing health disparities in the United States: prevention and early detection of disease; health care access and coordination; insurance coverage and continuity; and diversity and cultural competency (Dohan & Schrag, 2005). These issues are closely associated with key linkage functions assumed by CHWs and patient navigators. In particular, one of the benefits of using CHWs as essential linkage workers – the most established linkage approach – is the fundamental trust that exists between CHWs and patients. Yet, despite evidence demonstrating the effectiveness of this linkage approach, CHW-led interventions are plagued by uncertainty due, in large part, to inconsistent funding. Seeking CHW support from local/state governments (e.g., via Medicaid reimbursement) should be considered to maximize a CHW program's sustainability; alternatively, multiple funding sources should be pursued to ensure that programs may continue beyond the life of any single foundation grant or budget cycle. Developing standardized, rigorous training for CHWs and implementing quality monitoring systems for these programs is also strongly recommended to ensure the effectiveness and sustainability of a CHW linkage program delivery.

New technologies have the potential to catapult our progress in improving linkages to care and will play an increasingly important role in health service delivery models to maximize access to care (Purnomo et al., 2018). In working with underserved populations, integrating electronic data and surveillance systems (including GIS applications) through EHR and mobile platforms is highly recommended to better coordinate linkages to care and improve patient retention. A key component of this process will be customizing the virtual platform to ensure complete data capture for each individual. For example, EHRs have been shown to have high rates of missing data for patient demographics, including income, education, employment status, and race/ethnicity (Ehrenstein et al., 2019). Without these data, EHR-based linkage approaches cannot fulfill their promise of providing cultur-ally and linguistically appropriate services to individual patients. Developing user-friendly interfaces that include easy-to-understand instructions is also essential to ensure that diverse patient populations are able to access EHR patient portals and mHealth applications. Simultaneously, safeguarding patients' personal data is critical.

Telehealth may offer an additional solution for improving accessibility and reducing the cost of health care. Telehealth refers to the use of electronic information and telecommunication technologies to provide health care services remotely via a phone or another device connected to the internet (Health Resources & Services Administration, n.d.). The novel coronavirus (COVID-19) pandemic forced health care providers and systems to adapt to new ways of conducting our clinical, social, and business activities. Over the course of 2020, telehealth emerged as an important alternative to in-person visits through which patients were able to set up an appointment to be screened, evaluated, and treated by a health care provider, without geographic boundaries. However, we lack research on the health impact and cost-effectiveness of telehealth (Wang et al., 2020). In addition, telehealth laws and regulations across a wide range of settings and populations remain challenging (Brody et al., 2020). In the coming years, more emphasis must be placed on breaking down barriers to telehealth services for under-served populations, while still improving access to high quality and affordable in-person health care visits for high-risk individuals.

Addressing health disparities requires a complex and coordinated response that incorporates ideas and expertise from across the public health sector, health care institutions, community organizations, and community members alike. Linkage approaches – including patient education and navigation, supported by emerging tech-nologies – are critical components of this response.

DISCUSSION QUESTIONS

1. Which linkage approach is most relevant to you, and why?

2. What are some of the strategies for optimizing linkage to care for uninsured persons with limited English proficiency?

3. How can linkages between communities and health systems address health disparities in the Asian American communities?

REFERENCES

Agency for Healthcare Research and Quality (AHRQ). (2016, December). *Clinical-Community Linkages.* https://www.ahrq.gov/ncepcr/tools/com-munity/index.html

Agency for Healthcare Research and Quality. (2019, September). *2018 National Health care Quality and Disparities Report.* AHRQ Pub. No. 19-0070-EF. https://www.ahrq.gov/sites/default/files/wysiwyg/research/findings/nhqrdr/2018qdr-final.pdf

Anderson, E. J., Krause, K. C., Meyer Krause, C., Welter, A., McClelland, D. J., Garcia, D. O., Ernst, K., Lopez, E. C., & Koss, M. P. (2019). Web-based and Mhealth interventions for intimate partner violence victimization prevention: A systematic review. *Trauma, Violence, & Abuse,* 152483801988888. https://doi.org/10.1177/1524838019888889

Artiga, S., Orgera, K., & Pham, O. (2020, March). *Disparities in Health and Health Care: Five Key Questions and Answers.* http://files.kff.org/attachment/Issue-Brief-Disparities-in-Health-and-Health-Care-Five-Key-Questions-and-Answers.pdf

Bernardo, B. M., Zhang, X., Beverly Hery, C. M., Meadows, R. J., & Paskett, E. D. (2019). The efficacy and cost-effectiveness of patient navigation programs across the cancer continuum: A systematic review. *Cancer, 125*(16), 2747–2761. https://doi.org/10.1002/cncr.32147

Berwick, D. M., Nolan, T. W., & Whittington, J. (2008). The triple aim: care, health, and cost. *Health Affairs (Project Hope), 27*(3), 759–769. https://doi.org/10.1377/hlthaff.27.3.759

Brody, A. A., Sadarangani, T., Jones, T. M., Convery, K., Groom, L., Bristol, A. A., & David, D. (2020). Family- and Person-Centered Interdisciplinary Telehealth: Policy and Practice Implications Following Onset of the COVID-19 Pandemic. *Journal of Gerontological Nursing, 46*(9), 9–13. https://doi.org/10.3928/00989134-20200811-03

Centers for Disease Control and Prevention. (2013). *The State of Aging and Health in America 2013.* Centers for Disease Control and Prevention, US Dept of Health and Human Services.

Centers for Disease Control and Prevention. (2020, April 9). *Steps to care: Patient navigation.* https://www.cdc.gov/hiv/effective-interventions/treat/steps-to-care/dashboard/patient-navigation.html

Chandrasekar, E., Kim, K. E., Song, S., Paintal, R., Quinn, M. T., & Vallina, H. (2016). First Year Open Enrollment Findings: Health Insurance Coverage for Asian Americans and the Role of Navigators. *Journal of Racial and Ethnic Health Disparities, 3*(3), 537–545. https://doi.org/10.1007/s40615-015-0172-1

Chen, M. S., Jr, Fang, D. M., Stewart, S. L., Ly, M. Y., Lee, S., Dang, J. H., Nguyen, T. T., Maxwell, A. E., Bowlus, C. L., Bastani, R., & Nguyen, T. T. (2013). Increasing hepatitis B screening for hmong adults: results from a randomized controlled community-based study. *Cancer*

Epidemiology, Biomarkers & Prevention: a Publication of the American Association for Cancer Research, cosponsored by the American Society of Preventive Oncology, 22(5), 782–791. https://doi.org/10.1158/1055-9965.EPI-12-1399

Chung, J., Seo, J. Y., & Lee, J. (2018). Using the socioecological model to explore factors affecting health-seeking behaviours of older Korean immigrants. *International Journal of Older People Nursing, 13*(2), e12179. https://doi.org/10.1111/opn.12179

Conserve, D. F., Jennings, L., Aguiar, C., Shin, G., Handler, L., & Maman, S. (2017). Systematic review of mobile health behavioural interventions to improve uptake of HIV testing for vulnerable and key populations. *Journal of Telemedicine and Telecare, 23*(2), 347–359. https://doi.org/10.1177/1357633X16639186

Curtis, A. B., Kothari, C., Paul, R., & Connors, E. (2013). Using GIS and secondary data to target diabetes-related public health efforts. *Public Health Reports (Washington, D.C.: 1974), 128*(3), 212–220. https://doi.org/10.1177/003335491312800311

Delva, S., Waligora Mendez, K. J., Cajita, M., Koirala, B., Shan, R., Wongvibulsin, S., Vilarino, V., Gilmore, D. R., & Han, H. R. (2020). Efficacy of Mobile Health for Self-management of Cardiometabolic Risk Factors: A Theory-Guided Systematic Review. *The Journal of Cardiovascular Nursing*, 10.1097/JCN.0000000000000659. Advance online publication. https://doi.org/10.1097/JCN.0000000000000659

Dohan, D., & Schrag, D. (2005). Using navigators to improve care of underserved patients: current practices and approaches. *Cancer, 104*(4), 848–855. https://doi.org/10.1002/cncr.21214

Dubowitz, T., Williams, M., Steiner, E. D., Weden, M. M., Miyashiro, L., Jacobson, D., & Lurie, N. (2011). Using geographic information systems to match local health needs with public health services and programs. *American Journal of Public Health, 101*(9), 1664–1665. https://doi.org/10.2105/AJPH.2011.300195

Ehrenstein V., Kharrazi H., Lehmann H., & Taylor C.O. (2019). Chapter 4. Obtaining data from electronic health records. In Gliklich, R. E., Leavy, M. B., & Dreyer, N. A. (Eds.). *Tools and Technologies for Registry Interoperability, Registries for Evaluating Patient Outcomes: A User's Guide, 3rd Edition, Addendum 2.* Agency for Health care Research and Quality (US).

Enas, E. A., Kuruvila, A., Khanna, P., Pitchumoni, C. S., & Mohan, V. (2013). Benefits & risks of statin therapy for primary prevention of cardiovascular disease in Asian Indians - a population with the highest risk of premature coronary artery disease & diabetes. *The Indian Journal of Medical Research, 138*(4), 461–491.

Fang, C. Y., Ma, G. X., Handorf, E. A., Feng, Z., Tan, Y., Rhee, J., Miller, S. M., Kim, C., & Koh, H. S. (2017). Addressing multilevel barriers to cervical cancer screening in Korean American women: A randomized trial of a community-based intervention. *Cancer, 123*(6), 1018–1026. https://doi-org.proxy1.library.jhu.edu/10.1002/cncr.30391

Fang, D. M., & Stewart, S. L. (2018). Social-cultural, traditional beliefs, and health system barriers of hepatitis B screening among Hmong Americans: A case study. *Cancer, 124 Suppl 7*(Suppl 7), 1576–1582. https://doi.org/10.1002/cncr.31096

Feinglass, J., Cooper, J. M., Rydland, K., Tom, L. S., & Simon, M. A. (2019). Using Public Claims Data for Neighborhood Level Epidemiological Surveillance of Breast Cancer Screening: Findings from Evaluating a Patient Navigation Program in Chicago's Chinatown. *Progress in Community Health Partnerships: Research, Education, and Action, 13*(5), 95–102. https://doi.org/10.1353/cpr.2019.0042

Ferrante, J. M., Chen, P. H., & Kim, S. (2008). The effect of patient navigation on time to diagnosis, anxiety, and satisfaction in urban minority women with abnormal mammograms: a randomized controlled trial. *Journal of Urban Health: Bulletin of the New York Academy of Medicine, 85*(1), 114–124. https://doi.org/10.1007/s11524-007-9228-9

Fiechtner, L., Puente, G. C., Sharifi, M., Block, J. P., Price, S., Marshall, R., Blossom, J., Gerber, M. W., & Taveras, E. M. (2017). A Community Resource Map to Support Clinical-Community Linkages in a Randomized Controlled Trial of Childhood Obesity, Eastern Massachusetts, 2014-2016. *Preventing Chronic Disease, 14*, E53. https://doi.org/10.5888/pcd14.160577

Giblin P. T. (1989). Effective utilization and evaluation of indigenous health care workers. *Public Health Reports (Washington, DC: 1974), 104*(4), 361–368.

Gould, A. C., Apparicio, P., & Cloutier, M. S. (2012). Classifying neighbourhoods by level of access to stores selling fresh fruit and vegetables and groceries: identifying problematic areas in the city of Gatineau, Quebec. *Canadian journal of public health = Revue Canadienne de Sante Publique, 103*(6), e433–e437. https://doi.org/10.1007/BF03405633

Graves B. A. (2008). Integrative literature review: a review of literature related to geographical information systems, health care access, and health outcomes. *Perspectives in Health Information Management, 5*, 11.

Han, H. R., Gleason, K. T., Sun, C. A., Miller, H. N., Kang, S. J., Chow, S., Anderson, R., Nagy, P., & Bauer, T. (2019a). Using Patient Portals to Improve Patient Outcomes: Systematic Review. *JMIR human factors, 6*(4), e15038. https://doi.org/10.2196/15038

Han, H. R., Nkimbeng, M., Ajomagberin, O., Grunstra, K., Sharps, P., Renda, S., & Maruthur, N. (2019b). Health literacy enhanced intervention for inner-city African Americans with uncontrolled diabetes: a pilot study. *Pilot and Feasibility Studies, 5*, 99. https://doi.org/10.1186/s40814-019-0484-8

Han, H. R., Song, Y., Kim, M., Hedlin, H. K., Kim, K., Ben Lee, H., & Roter, D. (2017). Breast and Cervical Cancer Screening Literacy Among Korean American Women: A Community Health Worker-Led Intervention. *American Journal of Public Health, 107*(1), 159–165. https://doi-org.proxy1.library.jhu.edu/10.2105/AJPH.2016.303522

Hastings, K. G., Jose, P. O., Kapphahn, K. I., Frank, A. T., Goldstein, B. A., Thompson, C. A., Eggleston, K., Cullen, M. R., & Palaniappan, L. P. (2015). Leading Causes of Death among Asian American Subgroups (2003-2011). *PloS one, 10*(4), e0124341. https://doi.org/10.1371/journal.pone.0124341

Health Resources & Services Administration. (n.d.). *Understanding Telehealth.* https://telehealth.hhs.gov/patients/understanding-telehealth/

Henry, J., Pylypchuk, Y., Searcy, T., & Patel, V. (2016, May). *Adoption of Electronic Health Record Systems among US Non-Federal Acute Care Hospitals: 2008-2015.* https://dashboard.healthit.gov/evaluations/data-briefs/non-federal-acute-care-hospital-ehr-adoption-2008-2015.php

Hyun, C., McMenamin, J., Ko, O., & Kim, S. (2020). Efficacy of a Mobile Texting App (HepTalk) in Encouraging Patient Participation in Viral Hepatitis B Care: Development and Cohort Study. *JMIR mHealth and uHealth, 8*(4), e15098. https://doi.org/10.2196/15098

Islam, N. S., Zanowiak, J. M., Wyatt, L. C., Chun, K., Lee, L., Kwon, S. C., & Trinh-Shevrin, C. (2013). A randomized-controlled, pilot intervention on diabetes prevention and healthy lifestyles in the New York City Korean community. *Journal of Community Health, 38*(6), 1030–1041. https://doi.org/10.1007/s10900-013-9711-z

Jang, Y., & Kim, M. T. (2019). Limited English Proficiency and Health Service Use in Asian Americans. *Journal of Immigrant and Minority Health*, *21*(2), 264–270. https://doi.org/10.1007/s10903-018-0763-0

Kim, E. H., Linker, D. T., Coumar, A., Dean, L. S., Matsen, F. A., & Kim, Y. (2011). Factors affecting acceptance of a web-based self-referral system. *IEEE transactions on information technology in biomedicine: a publication of the IEEE Engineering in Medicine and Biology Society*, *15*(2), 344–347. https://doi.org/10.1109/TITB.2010.2088129

Kim, K., Choi, J. S., Choi, E., Nieman, C. L., Joo, J. H., Lin, F. R., Gitlin, L. N., & Han, H. R. (2016). Effects of community-based health worker interventions to improve chronic disease management and care among vulnerable populations: a systematic review. *American Journal of Public Health*, *106*(4), e3–e28. https://doi.org/10.2105/AJPH.2015.302987

Kirzinger, A., Muñana, C., Wu, B., & Brodie, M. (2019, June 11). *Data note: Americans' challenges with health care costs*. Kaiser Family Foundation. https://www.kff.org/health-costs/issue-brief/data-note-americans-challenges-health-care-costs/

Kwon, S. C., Trinh-Shevrin, C., Wauchope, K., Islam, N. S., Fifield, J., Kidd Arlotta, P., Han, H. W., & Ng, E. (2017). Innovations in Payer-Community Partnerships: The EmblemHealth Neighborhood Care Program. *International Quarterly of Community Health Education*, *38*(1), 57–64. https://doi.org/10.1177/0272684X17740694

Kwong, K., Chung, H., Cheal, K., Chou, J. C., & Chen, T. (2013). Depression care management for Chinese Americans in primary care: a feasibility pilot study. *Community Mental Health Journal*, *49*(2), 157–165. https://doi.org/10.1007/s10597-011-9459-9

Lam, T. K., McPhee, S. J., Mock, J., Wong, C., Doan, H. T., Nguyen, T., Lai, K. Q., Ha-Iaconis, T., & Luong, T. N. (2003). Encouraging Vietnamese-American women to obtain Pap tests through lay health worker outreach and media education. *Journal of General Internal Medicine*, *18*(7), 516–524. https://doi.org/10.1046/j.1525-1497.2003.21043.x

Lee, S. Y., & Lee, E. E. (2018). Access to Health Care, Beliefs, and Behaviors about Colorectal Cancer Screening among Korean Americans. *Asian Pacific Journal of Cancer Prevention*, *19*(7), 2021–2027. https://doi.org/10.22034/APJCP.2018.19.7.2021

Lim, S., Wyatt, L. C., Mammen, S., Zanowiak, J. M., Mohaimin, S., Goldfeld, K. S., Shelley, D., Gold, H. T., & Islam, N. S. (2019). The DREAM Initiative: study protocol for a randomized controlled trial testing an integrated electronic health record and community health worker intervention to promote weight loss among South Asian patients at risk for diabetes. *Trials*, *20*(1), 635. https://doi.org/10.1186/s13063-019-3711-y

Liu, D., Schuchard, H., Burston, B., Yamashita, T., & Albert, S. (2020). Interventions to Reduce Healthcare Disparities in Cancer Screening Among Minority Adults: a Systematic Review. *Journal of Racial and Ethnic Health Disparities*, 10.1007/s40615-020-00763-1. Advance online publication. https://doi.org/10.1007/s40615-020-00763-1

Ma, G. X., Lee, M. M., Tan, Y., Hanlon, A. L., Feng, Z., Shireman, T. I., Rhee, J., Wei, Z., Wong, F., Koh, H. S., Kim, C., & York, W. (2018). Efficacy of a community-based participatory and multilevel intervention to enhance hepatitis B virus screening and vaccination in underserved Korean Americans. *Cancer*, *124*(5), 973–982. https://doi.org/10.1002/cncr.31134

Ma, G. X., Lee, M., Beeber, M., Das, R., Feng, Z., Wang, M. Q., Tan, Y., Zhu, L., Navder, K., Shireman, T. I., Siu, P., Rhee, J., & Nguyen, M. T. (2019). Community-Clinical Linkage Intervention to Improve Colorectal Cancer Screening Among Underserved Korean Americans. *Cancer Health Disparities*, *3*, e1–e15.

Majerol, M., Newkirk, V., & Garfield, R. (2015, January). *The uninsured: A primer*. Kaiser Family Foundation. http://files.kff.org/attachment/the-uninsured-a-primer-key-facts-about-health-insurance-and-the-uninsured-in-america-primer

Martinez, J., Ro, M., Villa, N. W., Powell, W., & Knickman, J. R. (2011). Transforming the delivery of care in the post-health reform era: what role will community health workers play?. *American Journal of Public Health*, *101*(12), e1–e5. https://doi.org/10.2105/AJPH.2011.300335

Maxwell, A. E., Danao, L. L., Cayetano, R. T., Crespi, C. M., & Bastani, R. (2016). Implementation of an evidence-based intervention to promote colorectal cancer screening in community organizations: a cluster randomized trial. *Translational Behavioral Medicine*, *6*(2), 295–305. https://doi.org/10.1007/s13142-015-0349-5

Mock, J., McPhee, S. J., Nguyen, T., Wong, C., Doan, H., Lai, K. Q., Nguyen, K. H., Nguyen, T. T., & Bui-Tong, N. (2007). Effective lay health worker outreach and media-based education for promoting cervical cancer screening among Vietnamese American women. *American Journal of Public Health*, *97*(9), 1693–1700. https://doi.org/10.2105/AJPH.2006.086470

Ng, J. H., Tirodkar, M. A., French, J. B., Spalt, H. E., Ward, L. M., Haffer, S. C., Hewitt, N., Rey, D., & Scholle, S. H. (2017). Health Quality Measures Addressing Disparities in Culturally and Linguistically Appropriate Services: What are Current Gaps?. *Journal of Health Care for the Poor and Underserved*, *28*(3), 1012–1029. https://doi.org/10.1353/hpu.2017.0093

Nguyen, T. T., Le, G., Nguyen, T., Le, K., Lai, K., Gildengorin, G., Tsoh, J., Bui-Tong, N., & McPhee, S. J. (2009). Breast cancer screening among Vietnamese Americans: a randomized controlled trial of lay health worker outreach. *American Journal of Preventive Medicine*, *37*(4), 306–313. https://doi.org/10.1016/j.amepre.2009.06.009

Nguyen, T. T., Tsoh, J. Y., Woo, K., Stewart, S. L., Le, G. M., Burke, A., Gildengorin, G., Pasick, R. J., Wang, J., Chan, E., Fung, L. C., Jih, J., & McPhee, S. J. (2017). Colorectal Cancer Screening and Chinese Americans: Efficacy of Lay Health Worker Outreach and Print Materials. *American Journal of Preventive Medicine*, *52*(3), e67–e76. https://doi-org.proxy1.library.jhu.edu/10.1016/j.amepre.2016.10.003

Northridge, M. E., Metcalf, S. S., Yi, S., Zhang, Q., Gu, X., & Trinh-Shevrin, C. (2018). A Protocol for a Feasibility and Acceptability Study of a Participatory, Multi-Level, Dynamic Intervention in Urban Outreach Centers to Improve the Oral Health of Low-Income Chinese Americans. *Frontiers in Public Health*, *6*, 29. https://doi.org/10.3389/fpubh.2018.00029

Office of the National Coordinator for Health Information Technology. (2019, June 17). *Quick stats*. https://dashboard.healthit.gov/quickstats/quickstats.php

Pollack, H., Wang, S., Wyatt, L., Peng, C. H., Wan, K., Trinh-Shevrin, C., Chun, K., Tsang, T., & Kwon, S. (2011). A comprehensive screening and treatment model for reducing disparities in hepatitis B. *Health Affairs (Project Hope)*, *30*(10), 1974–1983. https://doi.org/10.1377/hlthaff.2011.0700

Purnomo, J., Coote, K., Mao, L., Fan, L., Gold, J., Ahmad, R., & Zhang, L. (2018). Using eHealth to engage and retain priority populations in the HIV treatment and care cascade in the Asia-Pacific region: a systematic review of literature. *BMC Infectious Diseases*, *18*(1), 82. https://doi.org/10.1186/s12879-018-2972-5

Rodriguez-Gutierrez, R., Herrin, J., Lipska, K. J., Montori, V. M., Shah, N. D., & McCoy, R. G. (2019). Racial and Ethnic Differences in 30-Day Hospital Readmissions Among US Adults With Diabetes. *JAMA Network Open*, *2*(10), e1913249. https://doi.org/10.1001/jamanetworkopen.2019.13249

Rosenthal, E. L., Brownstein, J. N., Rush, C. H., Hirsch, G. R., Willaert, A. M., Scott, J. R., Holderby, L. R., & Fox, D. J. (2010). Community health workers: part of the solution. *Health Affairs (Project Hope)*, *29*(7), 1338–1342. https://doi.org/10.1377/hlthaff.2010.0081

Starbird, L. E., DiMaina, C., Sun, C. A., & Han, H. R. (2019). A Systematic Review of Interventions to Minimize Transportation Barriers Among People with Chronic Diseases. *Journal of Community Health*, *44*(2), 400–411. https://doi.org/10.1007/s10900-018-0572-3

Sy, A. U., Lim, E., Ka'opua, L. S., Kataoka-Yahiro, M., Kinoshita, Y., & Stewart, S. L. (2018). Colorectal cancer screening prevalence and predictors among Asian American subgroups using Medical Expenditure Panel Survey National Data. *Cancer, 124 Suppl 7*(Suppl 7), 1543–1551. https://doi.org/10.1002/cncr.31098

Tan, C., Wyatt, L. C., Kranick, J. A., Kwon, S. C., & Oyebode, O. (2018). Factors Associated with Health Insurance Status in an Asian American Population in New York City: Analysis of a Community-Based Survey. *Journal of Racial and Ethnic Health Disparities*, *5*(6), 1354–1364. https://doi.org/10.1007/s40615-018-0485-y

Taylor, V. M., Hislop, T. G., Jackson, J. C., Tu, S. P., Yasui, Y., Schwartz, S. M., Teh, C., Kuniyuki, A., Acorda, E., Marchand, A., & Thompson, B. (2002). A randomized controlled trial of interventions to promote cervical cancer screening among Chinese women in North America. *Journal of the National Cancer Institute*, *94*(9), 670–677. https://doi.org/10.1093/jnci/94.9.670

Taylor, V. M., Bastani, R., Burke, N., Talbot, J., Sos, C., Liu, Q., Do, H., Jackson, J. C., & Yasui, Y. (2013). Evaluation of a hepatitis B lay health worker intervention for Cambodian Americans. *Journal of Community Health*, *38*(3), 546–553. https://doi.org/10.1007/s10900-012-9649-6

Tolbert, J., Orgera, K., Singer, N., & Damico, A. (2019, December). *Key facts about the uninsured population*. Kaiser Family Foundation Issue Brief. http://files.kff.org/attachment//fact-sheet-key-facts-about-the-uninsured-population

Ursua, R. A., Aguilar, D. E., Wyatt, L. C., Trinh-Shevrin, C., Gamboa, L., Valdellon, P., Perrella, E. G., Dimaporo, M. Z., Nur, P. Q., Tandon, S. D., & Islam, N. S. (2018). A community health worker intervention to improve blood pressure among Filipino Americans with hypertension: A randomized controlled trial. *Preventive Medicine Reports*, *11*, 42–48. https://doi.org/10.1016/j.pmedr.2018.05.002

Walsh, J. M., Salazar, R., Nguyen, T. T., Kaplan, C., Nguyen, L. K., Hwang, J., McPhee, S. J., & Pasick, R. J. (2010). Healthy colon, healthy life: a novel colorectal cancer screening intervention. *American Journal of Preventive Medicine*, *39*(1), 1–14. https://doi-org.proxy1.library.jhu.edu/10.1016/j.amepre.2010.02.020

Wang, C. J., Liu, T. T., Car, J., & Zuckerman, B. (2020). Design, Adoption, Implementation, Scalability, and Sustainability of Telehealth Programs. *Pediatric Clinics of North America*, *67*(4), 675–682. https://doi.org/10.1016/j.pcl.2020.04.011

Wells, K. J., Battaglia, T. A., Dudley, D. J., Garcia, R., Greene, A., Calhoun, E., Mandelblatt, J. S., Paskett, E. D., Raich, P. C., & Patient Navigation Research Program. (2008). Patient navigation: state of the art or is it science?. *Cancer*, *113*(8), 1999–2010. https://doi.org/10.1002/cncr.23815

Weisner, C. M., Chi, F. W., Lu, Y., Ross, T. B., Wood, S. B., Hinman, A., Pating, D., Satre, D., & Sterling, S. A. (2016). Examination of the Effects of an Intervention Aiming to Link Patients Receiving Addiction Treatment With Health Care: The LINKAGE Clinical Trial. *JAMA Psychiatry*, *73*(8), 804–814. https://doi.org/10.1001/jamapsychiatry.2016.0970

Wong, C. C., Tsoh, J. Y., Tong, E. K., Hom, F. B., Cooper, B., & Chow, E. A. (2008). The Chinese community smoking cessation project: a community sensitive intervention trial. *Journal of Community Health*, *33*(6), 363–373. https://doi.org/10.1007/s10900-008-9114-8

World Health Organization. (n.d.). *mHealth: New horizons for health through mobile technologies*. https://www.who.int/goe/publications/goe_mhealth_web.pdf

CHAPTER

10

MULTILEVEL AND MULTISECTOR APPROACHES TO HEALTH

MARGUERITE J. RO, NADINE L. CHAN

LEARNING OBJECTIVES

- Describe features of a multilevel and multisector approach that distinguish it from a single-level and single sector approach.

- Describe the historical context for use of the multilevel and multisector approach to address Asian American and Native Hawaiian and Pacific Islander (NH/PI) health.

- Describe the policy context (with regards to health care, data, and immigration) for multilevel and multisector efforts to improve Asian American and NH/PI health.

- Describe how the future work of multilevel and multisector approaches to Asian American and NH/PI health are impacted by the novel coronavirus pandemic (COVID-19) and national protests calling for anti-racist societies.

Applied Population Health Approaches for Asian American Communities, First Edition. Edited by Simona C. Kwon, Chau Trinh-Shevrin, Nadia S. Islam, and Stella S. Yi.
© 2023 John Wiley & Sons, Inc. Published 2023 by John Wiley & Sons, Inc.
Companion Website: www.wiley.com/go/kwon/asianamerican

INTRODUCTION

In 2010, Dr. Howard Koh, the Assistant Secretary for Health, announced the launch of Healthy People 2020 (U.S. Department of Health and Human Services, 2010a). For the first time, the nation's health goals included social determinants of health (U.S. Department of Health and Human Services, 2010b). The new goal of creating social and physical environments that promote good health for all called for efforts to track progress in social and economic factors, natural and built environments, and policies and programs. From the practice perspective, achieving this vision requires communities to engage in multilevel and multisector efforts that address social determinants of health. For Asian Americans and NH/PIs, multilevel and multisector approaches have been at the heart of Asian American and NH/PI efforts to address community health needs for decades. Yet there is more to be done given the health disparities that persist among Asian American and NH/PI communities and the greater need to achieve health equity for all. The need for such approaches has become more pressing as disparities have become more deeply rooted and traditional approaches to health and health care have not resulted in sustained improvements in health outcomes.

This chapter provides frameworks for multilevel and multisector approaches to health and the alignment of these approaches to the goal of achieving health equity and racial equity. We touch on challenges of designing outcomes evaluations for this type of work, which leave us with scant evidence on the impact of multilevel and multisector approaches; and we point to some of the overarching lessons learned in practice settings and share the evolution of multilevel, multisector approaches followed by examples of more recent multilevel, multisector approaches to Asian American and NH/PI health. We end with notes on the socio-political environment pre-COVID-19 and during COVID-19 that set the conditions for the development of future multilevel, multisector race- and place-based efforts.

FRAMEWORKS FOR MULTILEVEL AND MULTISECTOR APPROACHES

Multilevel approaches refers to efforts that are directed beyond working at a single level (i.e., individual level, interpersonal level, organizational level, etc.). The socio-ecological model in Figure 10.1 indicates the various levels at which services, interventions, or approaches must be considered in order to improve the health of individuals, families, and communities. Often, health interventions are directed at individuals or families with the

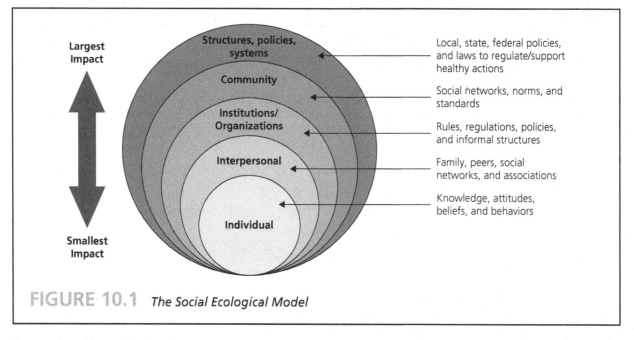

FIGURE 10.1 *The Social Ecological Model*

Source: Adapted from Frieden (2010).

goal of changing behavior within the existing environment. Alternatively, advocacy efforts are often directed at implementing policy or system changes that have broader impact which can be more difficult or time-consuming to achieve. A common multilevel approach is to do both: conduct individual/family level interventions, while also seeking policy and systems changes that will sustain and expand the interventions to have long-lasting impacts. For instance, in efforts to address hepatitis B disparities, Asian American and NH/PI health advocates have conducted health education and screening campaigns to ensure that individuals are screened (individual level), while simultaneously working to assure that hepatitis B screenings are standard medical practice (system change) and that hepatitis B screenings and treatments are included in health insurance packages (policy change) (Ma et al., 2017; Ma et al., 2018). Ultimately, success in achieving large impacts and sustained improvements results when there is alignment of policy, community support/buy-in, and practice.

There are different *multisector approaches* to health that depend on the definition of sector used and what goal is sought. For example, sectors could be defined as various stakeholder groups (e.g., government, academia, nonprofits, private) that are working in the same or related field. Another option is to define a sector as a field or type of industry (e.g., health, housing, transportation, law, or education). Both forms of multisector groups are common.

Multisector approaches to health have primarily focused on a health goal, such as collaborations between academic health institutions and community-based health organizations to develop culturally tailored diabetes programs (Lemacks et al., 2018; Lim et al., 2019; Skizim et al., 2017; Soltero et al., 2019), partnerships between providers and community-based organizations to develop effective cancer prevention strategies (Hiatt et al., 2018; Ma et al., 2018; Pyron et al., 2018; Raber et al., 2018), or cooperation between hospitals and farmers markets to promote healthy eating (Forbes et al., 2019; George et al., 2013; Kraschnewski et al., 2014; NYC Health & Hospitals, 2019). These types of partnerships tend to focus on a particular health issue or condition and involve partners who have traditionally focused on health albeit from different perspectives or lens.

More recently, there is growing interest in multisector approaches as partnerships across fields extend beyond a specific health aim to address the conditions that impact health, such as the social determinants of health. As Cooper et al. (2018) note, "Failure to address upstream factors (e.g., poverty, limited opportunities, and discrimination) that perpetuate inequities will limit the effectiveness of public health interventions among groups affected by health disparities." As an example, the authors note that working with schools to improve nutrition policies may lead to reducing obesity; however, without addressing issues of segregation and poverty, children may still experience poor health outcomes. As Figure 10.2 illustrates, cross-sector/multisector partnerships provide the opportunity to jointly tackle the conditions that result in disparities and poor quality of life across the lifespan.

As a means to an end, multilevel and multisector efforts are often directed toward achieving *health equity* and *racial equity*. Health equity, most simply put, is the opportunity for all individuals, families, and communities to attain optimal health. Health equity requires that individuals have "a fair and just opportunity to be as healthy as possible" (Braveman et al., 2019). For this opportunity to be realized, various forms of bias and discrimination that serve as barriers to optimal health must be addressed. An important corollary is the attainment of racial equity: having a fair and just opportunity, regardless of race and ethnicity, to live in health-promoting conditions and environments, which includes assuring access to basic needs such as safe and affordable housing, adequate transportation, quality childcare and education, and access to culturally and linguistically appropriate health care and social services.

Historical Context of Asian American and Native Hawaiian and Pacific Islander Approaches to Health

Multilevel and multisector approaches have been at the heart of Asian American and NH/PI efforts to address community health needs for decades. In the early 1970s, on both the East Coast and West Coast of the United States, Asian American community activists organized to meet the needs of distinct Asian American communities. Particularly in areas that were home to Asian American enclaves or large populations of Asian Americans, there was outcry at the lack of culturally and linguistically appropriate services. In 1971, community organizers held the first Chinatown Health Fair in New York City (NYC) to provide free health screenings and health education as a response to the lack of Chinese-speaking staff in hospitals. Community members also held a protest march for better health services and a more rapid opening of a new hospital in Lower Manhattan (close to

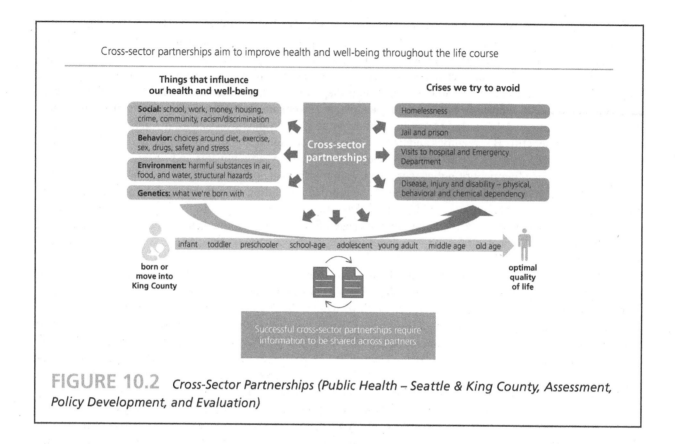

FIGURE 10.2   *Cross-Sector Partnerships (Public Health – Seattle & King County, Assessment, Policy Development, and Evaluation)*

Chinatown). They also successfully sought the establishment of a community board to provide input into the new hospital's policies (note, Gouverneur Hospital opened in 1972). The culmination of these actions included the creation of a free health clinic in NYC's Chinatown, which is today the Charles B. Wang Community Health Center.

On the West Coast, similar multilevel actions were being taken by Asian American community organizers to address the health needs of their communities. In 1974, Asian Health Services was founded as a one-room clinic in Oakland, CA. By 1978, Asian Health Services was not only providing clinical services but was also organizing patients to protest human service funding cuts from Proposition 13, an amendment regulating the assessment value on California property and a cap on annual tax increases. Further north in Seattle, during the early 1970s, community activists were working to address the conditions of Seattle's Chinatown (now known as the Chinatown/International District), including providing health care to Chinese and Filipino older adults living in Chinatown who lacked in-language health services. By 1975, the Asian Community Health Clinic was relocated to Chinatown and is now known as International Community Health Services. This was part of a larger effort around community preservation to offset the negative impacts of the nearby development of the Kingdome, a stadium designed for major league sports and other events that opened one year later.

In short, historically, Asian Americans and NH/PIs have taken a multilevel approach to make gains in assuring the health of their communities. The challenge presented by a lack of culturally and linguistically appropriate services for diverse Asian American and NH/PI groups persists today and is compounded by other issues that are described further in this chapter, such as barriers to health care; the lack of data and research on individual Asian American and NH/PI populations; and anti-immigrant policies.

Review of Evidence: Multilevel and Multisector Approaches to Health

In this section, we provide an overview of multilevel and multisector approaches that have been used in the general population – and more specifically, among Asian American and NH/PI communities. Figure 10.3 illustrates an example of the continuum from single sector, single level approaches to multisector, multilevel approaches.

Over the last decade, there has been growing attention and greater urgency to address health inequities through cross-sector efforts to achieve what more than one sector could do on its own. These efforts have resulted

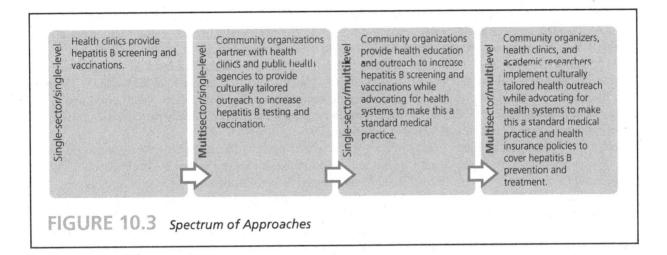

FIGURE 10.3   *Spectrum of Approaches*

in two notable approaches. The first is the "Health in All Policies" (HiAP) approach, which is a "collaborative approach to improving the health of all people by incorporating health considerations into decision-making across sectors and policy area." A five-state review by Jacobsen and Hall (2018) showed that a central feature of the HiAP approach is cross-sector collaboration. "Healthy housing" initiatives – programs designed to reduce lead exposure, injuries from fall, and asthma rates through weatherization and lead paint removal – comprise one example of a HiAP approach (Herendeen & MacDonald, 2011; Khan, 2011; Rhoads et al., 2020). In healthy housing initiatives, the focus has been on supporting housing developers to adopt healthy housing guidelines and to ensure that governing entities adopt healthy housing rules and regulations. From a health equity perspective, a HiAP approach to healthy housing in affordable housing assures that it is not only those with resources who benefit from healthy housing but also those who are most at risk for poor health outcomes. Notably, HiAP is most often centered on policy/system changes to one sector and the policies and system changes sought are not race-specific.

The second approach is the "healthy communities" approach, which stems from race- and place-based investments to address disparities and investments by national foundations in *place-making*. These initiatives have emphasized both the socio-environmental factors that impact health and structural inequities that lead to health disparities. The 2011 PolicyLink report, "Why Place and Race Matter," succinctly noted the critical intersection of race and place:

> Race is a central consideration for the healthy communities movement. Race has shaped our regions, creating places that offer profoundly unequal opportunities to their residents. In many ways, race remains our deepest divide. Effective strategies to build healthy, vibrant, sustainable communities must address both race and place, openly and authentically.

The healthy communities approach builds on the HiAP approach, focusing on the health impact of policy and system changes in a non-health sector to a broader holistic approach to health. As defined by the New York State Department of Health:

> Healthy Communities is a movement – the act of multisectoral collaborations incorporating health into decision-making across sectors and policy areas – to continuously improve the physical, social and economic environments where people live, work, play, and learn. Healthy Communities initiatives empower groups to work together in mutually supportive ways to create community-driven improvements that provide people with adequate resources and an environment that supports health-promoting behaviors. They are inclusive, accessible and available for all individuals, and aim to ensure that all people can reach their full health potential. (New York State Department of Health, n.d.)

The healthy communities approach is still relatively nascent, and while there has been some notable progress in terms of better coordination of local investments, increases in services, expansion of civic engagement, and some policy achievements, evidence for sustained population-level improvements attributable to this approach that have resulted in measurable health outcomes has yet to emerge. Analyzing 16 years of data from a large cohort of U.S. communities, Mays, Mamaril, and Timsina (2016) showed that multisector efforts implemented to support population health activities resulted in significant declines in preventable deaths due to cardiovascular disease, diabetes, and influenza. However, an evaluation of the Place Matters Initiative in the Greater Cincinnati area tracked indicators related to education, health, income, and housing over a three-year period and found inconsistent impacts by neighborhood. For some indicators, there were either no steady patterns of improvement or no improvement at all (Community Building Institute, 2019).

In some ways, the sparse and mixed evidence is not surprising. Multilevel, multisector work toward health and racial equity requires sustained efforts to develop and maintain transformative systemic changes. As the social, political, and funding contexts evolve, the specific activities and partnerships need to evolve, as well. This evolution may include changes in the level of involvement of some sectors or communities or changes in the geographies in which the work takes place. The dynamic nature of multisector initiatives presents challenges to the implementation of traditional impact evaluations. However, we are learning lessons from these experiences. Existing academic and nonacademic literature focuses primarily on the underlying components of cross-sector approaches and the principles that shape these efforts. Key themes emerge:

- *Prioritizing trust as a building block to collaboration.* Often mentioned is the importance of taking the requisite time to build trust (Elias & Moore, 2017; National Academies of Sciences, 2017; Public Health Alliance of Southern California, Communities Lifting Communities, & Hospital Association of Southern California, 2020; Scally et al., 2020).

- *Being explicit about equity as a shared value among collaborators as well as an expected outcome.* In addressing racial disparities, being explicit about racial equity as a goal as well as having an anti-racist approach to change is critical (Braveman et al., 2019; National Academies of Sciences, 2017; Public Health Alliance of Southern California et al., 2020; Scally et al., 2020)

- *Engaging affected communities as partners.* Beyond making sure that the community has a seat at the table, a recognition of the potential for achievement when a community has agency to drive the vision based on the community knowing what is best for itself. In collaborations that genuinely prioritize the community's needs and goals, community engagement is a tool for redistributing power. Lastly, for community to effectively be at the table, there is a clear need to build supporting community infrastructure (Braveman et al., 2019; Mays et al., 2016; National Academies of Sciences, 2017; Public Health Alliance of Southern California et al., 2020).

- *Focusing on social determinants and prioritizing multilevel approaches to address causes of inequities.* These include policy and systems change to address the root causes of disparities and inequities (Erickson et al., 2017; National Academies of Sciences, 2017; Scally et al., 2020).

- *Changing the narrative to illustrate the opportunities, potential, and assets of communities.* This includes moving away from a deficit-based lens (only describing how communities are behind) and bringing in a trauma-informed lens (taking into account the historical context of racial discrimination and its lasting impacts on community). See Chapter 12 for more about a trauma-informed framework. (Auerbach, 2019; National Academies of Sciences, 2017; Scally et al., 2020)

- *Using data early on and throughout collaborative efforts.* The data are important for setting the starting point, informing progress, and deepening the understanding of the interconnectedness of cross-sector work (Kania & Kramer, 2011; National Academies of Sciences, 2017; Public Health Alliance of Southern California et al., 2020).

Asian American and NH/PI Multilevel and Multisector Initiatives

As early textbooks on Asian American and NH/PI health (including the first edition of this book) have captured the research and progress of Asian American- and NH/PI-focused health efforts, this edition examines efforts from the mid-2000s forward. The mid-2000s saw the advent of two major national Asian American and NH/PI investments: Health Through Action (HTA) for Asian American, Native Hawaiian, and Pacific Islanders and the National Gender & Equity Campaign (NGEC).

The goal of HTA was to improve the health of vulnerable Asian American and NH/PI populations by simultaneously advancing a national health agenda and building community capacity to address local health needs. The seven original HTA community partners were collaboratives among local Asian American and NH/PI organizations and leaders across the country focused on effective programming and advocacy to improve the health of Asian Americans and NH/PIs. Over the five-year initiative, HTA community partners expanded programs and services, increased community health outreach and education, replicated models of patient navigation and access to care, increased provide education and training, and increased alignment of systems of care. At the local level, cross-sector partnership was a critical component for achieving notable improvements, whether the partnership involved working with local policy makers to draft legislation and discuss proposed initiatives at local policy tables or collaborating with federally qualified health centers and academic institutions to improve the collection and analysis of local data on Asian Americans and NH/PIs. A success of HTA was the increased visibility of the health needs and disparities experienced by Asian Americans and NH/PIs, both locally and nationally. However, as the community partners noted in the evaluation, more than visibility is needed to close the disparities gap and to create equitable systems of care (Inouye et al., 2012).

NGEC focused on leveraging, mobilizing, and activating philanthropic and community resources toward achieving more justice and equity for Asian American and NH/PI communities. While not a health initiative, NGEC focused on building community capacity and mobilizing communities to build a social justice movement to address the underlying causes of inequity. An example is the work conducted by NAKASEC (National Korean American Service & Education Consortium), one of the 12 lead NGEC organizations, which prioritized the issue of immigrant rights. Immigrant rights is an issue that intersects all aspects of life, from the ability to access health and social services to obtaining education and the right to work in safe conditions. To achieve policy and system changes in the area of immigrant rights, not only was a multilevel, multisector approach needed, but also it was critical to develop "strong coalition partnerships with other communities of color, Asian American and Pacific Islander populations, and immigrant groups" (Gupta & Ritoper, 2007). According to Eun Sook Lee, NAKASEC's Executive Director at that time, "The Korean American community comprises less than 1% of the population, therefore it is incumbent that they work together with other communities to build power for change" (Gupta & Ritoper, 2007).

Multilevel, Multisector Partnerships Today As we headed into the new decade, we began to see large investments by the philanthropic sector and the government sector to support multilevel, multisector partnerships through multisite demonstrations throughout the country. Notable examples where health was explicitly called out as one of the areas for focus include:

- *Building Health Communities (BHC)* is a "ten-year, $1 billion comprehensive community initiative to advance statewide policy, change the narrative, and transform 14 of California's communities most devastated by health inequities into places where all people have the opportunity to thrive" (Building Healthy Communities, n.d.). BHC is funded by The California Endowment.

- *SPARCC (Strong, Prosperous, and Resilient Communities Challenge)* is "investing in and amplifying local efforts underway in six regions to ensure that new investments reduce racial disparities, build a culture of health, and prepare for a changing climate. The initiative's long-term goal is to change the way metropolitan regions grow, invest, and build through integrated, cross-sector approaches that benefit low-income people and communities of color" (SPARCC, n.d.) SPARCC is an initiative of Enterprise Community Partners, the Low Income Investment Fund, and the Natural Resources Defense Council, with funding support from the Ford Foundation, The JPB Foundation, The Kresge Foundation, the Robert Wood Johnson Foundation, and The California Endowment.

- *The Accountable Health Communities (AHC)* model addresses a critical gap between clinical care and community services in the current health care delivery system by testing whether systematically identifying and addressing the health-related social needs of Medicare and Medicaid beneficiaries' through screening, referral, and community navigation services will impact health care costs and reduce health care utilization. AHC is funded by the Centers for Medicare & Medicaid Services (CMS, n.d.).

Extensive lists and reviews of multisector initiatives have been produced by Rethink Health, the Urban Institute, the Federal Reserve Bank of San Francisco and others (Henig et al., 2016; Kunz et al., 2017; Public Health Alliance of Southern California et al., 2020; Scally et al., 2020; Siegal et al., 2015). Unlike HTA or NGEC, most – if not all – of the multisector initiatives identified are not race- or ethnicity-specific. Rather, they are focused on place with an acknowledgement that residents in the geographic communities are experiencing poor health and well-being due to structural barriers.

While the history of Asian American and NH/PI-led health efforts is long, the published literature on multilevel efforts is short. Cases 9 and 10 take a closer look at two examples of Asian Americans and NH/PIs leading the way in multilevel, multisector efforts (see Appendix).

SOCIO-POLITICAL CONTEXT FOR MULTILEVEL AND MULTISECTOR EFFORTS TO IMPROVE ASIAN AMERICAN AND NH/PI HEALTH

Pre-COVID-19 (before 2020)

To understand the need for multilevel and multilevel approaches, we point to three major policy areas (health care, data, and immigration) that have set the national context for addressing the health and well-being of Asian American and NH/PI communities. Clearly, other critical policies and policy areas, including education, housing, and social services, also shape the local environment and must be considered within a broader assessment of the health of Asian American and NH/PI communities, but these fields are beyond the scope of this chapter. The policies listed below present either opportunities or barriers to advance the health and well-being of Asian American and NH/PI communities.

Health Care

- *Social Security Act of 1965*. Recognizing that there were vulnerable populations (i.e., older adults and low-income Americans) who needed protection against the cost of health care, this landmark legislation established *Medicare* and *Medicaid*. Then, as now, Medicare and Medicaid had eligibility requirements restricting benefits generally to U.S. citizens and certain legal immigrants. The next major expansion of health insurance came in 1997 with the *Children's Health Insurance Program* (CHIP), which expanded coverage options particularly for children of families who are near-poor (i.e., with incomes above Medicaid-eligible levels).

- *Community health center* (CHCs) demonstration program (1965). Federal investment in "modern-day" community health centers began in 1965 through a demonstration program of the Office of Economic Opportunity. CHCs were located in areas of high poverty where individuals and families struggled to meet their basic needs. The centers were designed to provide comprehensive health care, as well as training and employment services for local residents and consumers of the centers' services.

- The *Patient Protection and Affordable Care Act (ACA)* (2010). The ACA (sometimes referred to as "Obamacare") expanded access to health care for millions of Americans, though some of the key provisions were rolled back under the administration of President Donald J. Trump (2017–2021). Critical improvements included expanding data collection requirements for federally funded programs (e.g., race, ethnicity, and language); investments in diversifying the health care workforce; and expanding health research on minority health and health disparities.

Even with these policy advancements, major gaps in health care persist, including the lack of culturally and linguistically appropriate health care services for diverse populations; the lack of affordable access to quality health care for immigrant populations (particularly for nonlegal immigrants); and policy barriers such as the denial of Medicaid for COFA (Compact of Free Association) communities (i.e., the Federated States of Micronesia, The Republic of the Marshall Islands and the Republic of Palau) and the five-year waiting period for Medicaid and CHIP coverage for qualified noncitizens.

Data and Research

Data drives policy, programs, and allocation of financial and nonfinancial resources. In the movement toward health equity, there is an increasing need for data that represents hyper-local geographies and small populations. Two landmark events provide anchors for data and research on Asian American and NH/PI health:

1. *Report of the Secretary's Task Force on Black and Minority Health* (1985). This was the first national report on the health of racial and ethnic minorities. Asian American and NH/PI were called out as a separate group, with the report noting that "The Asian population within the U.S. is quite diverse and available data are often not adequate".

2. *Minority Health and Health Disparities Research and Education Act of 2000* (P.L. 106–525). This Act established the National Center for Minority Health and Health Disparities in recognition of existing disparities and major gaps in health research related to racial and ethnic minorities.

Although there is a growing body of data and research on Asian American and NH/PI health, there remains a lack of data particularly for individual Asian ethnic groups and specific PI groups (e.g., Tongans, Samoans, Chuukese, etc.). In part, this is due to the lack of disaggregated data that is collected at local, state, and national levels (see Chapter 4). Community data is fundamental to understanding the nature and extent of health inequities. Ro and Chan (2016) outlined four strategies to improve community-level data:

1. Apply community-based participatory approaches to health surveys, particularly for understanding the context of health for vulnerable populations.

2. Explore the use of multisector data to inform health interventions.

3. Collect community-level data about local policies.

4. Harness technology to gather community health data.

Immigration Policies

- *Internment of Japanese Americans* based on Executive Order 9066, during World War II, is one of the most blatant examples of racial profiling in the U.S. history. Approximately 112,000 Japanese Americans were forced into internment camps with no recourse to law nor compensation for their loss of property and personal liberty.

- *The Immigration and Nationality Act of 1965* abolished "national origins" as the basis for allocating immigration quotas to various countries, allowing for immigration from Asian countries to be on an equal footing with European immigrants for the first time in U.S. history. In the following decades, Asian American became of the fast-growing populations in the nation. As a result, two-thirds of Asian Americans and one-sixth of PIs were born outside of the United States. (AAJC website: https://www.advancingjustice-aajc.org/immigration-and-immigrant-rights). See Chapter 1 for more detail on Asian immigration flows.

- Beginning in 2017, the Trump administration sought a ban on people from *predominately Muslim countries* from entering the United States by executive orders. There have been continuous court battles over the legality of the executive orders.

- Similarly, the Trump administration faced court battles against policies and proclamations limiting or suspending entry to the United States of *immigrant visas*, including H-1B visas (Trump, 2020), which U.S. businesses use to fill positions requiring highly specialized skillsets, such as computer-related, engineering, and health care positions. In 2017, 87% of petitions for H-1B visas came from India, China, Philippines, South Korea, and Taiwan (US Citizenship and Immigration Services, 2017).

- *Public charge regulations* holds the use of certain public benefits against individuals seeking admission to the United States or who are seeking lawful permanent residence status. This complex set of rules and the fear of becoming a "public charge" prevents some immigrants from seeking needed services.

- *Deferred Action for Childhood Arrivals (DACA)*. On June 15, 2012, the Secretary of Homeland Security announced that certain people who came to the United States as children and meet several guidelines may request consideration of deferred action for a period of two years, subject to renewal. They are also eligible for work authorization.

Immigration policy remains a contentious issue, but, importantly, points to how nationality (often conflated with race/ethnicity) can be used in "othering" (i.e., treating individuals or groups of people differently).

Looking Forward: Asian American and NH/PI Health During COVID and Civil Rights Protests for Anti-Racist Systemic Changes

During the writing of this book, COVID-19 set a new stage for multilevel, multisector work with Asian American and NH/PI communities. As noted by Gee, Ro, and Rimoin (2020), "The [COVID-19] pandemic has reinvigorated old stereotypes of Chinese people, including fears of Chinese food, ranging from consumption of pets to use of monosodium glutamate (MSG)" (Gee et al., 2020). President Trump and some members of Congress continuously referred to SARS-CoV-2 as the "China virus." As soon as this pejorative terminology was adopted, Chinatowns across the nation experienced its negative effects of via a precipitous drop in business. More chilling has been the increase in anti-Asian assaults, harassments, and hate crimes that persist nationwide at the time of writing (Anti Defamation League, 2020).

More than ever, COVID-19 necessitates a multilevel, multisector approach to preventing the transmission of the virus and ensuring the safety and bolstering the resilience of Asian American and NH/PI communities. While comprehensive race/ethnicity data is lacking nationally, in states that have been tracking the COVID-19 infection rate by race/ethnicity with a separate category for NH/PI, data demonstrate that NH/PI have been disproportionately impacted by COVID-19. As of August, 2020, "nine of the states that report disaggregated NH/PI COVID cases revealed case rates that significantly exceed those of every other race and ethnicity" (Chang et al., 2020). In King County, Washington, where NH/PI COVID-19 rates have also been disproportionately high, Public Health – Seattle King County has partnered with the Pacific Islander Health Board (a group of Pacific Islander health leaders) and community organizations (including the White Center Community Development Association, Pacific Islander Community Association, Marshallese Women's Association and others) to provide culturally tailored information and support. This includes support for Marshallese Community Navigators, as the local Marshallese community has been hit particularly hard by COVID-19.

Early on in the COVID-19 pandemic, a critical step was coordination and work with elected officials, health departments, and others to use scientific nomenclature and avoid stigmatizing language. It was and continues to be critical that the language used to discuss SARS-CoV-2 be data-driven and evidence-based, so as to not fuel fear, confusion, or division. In cities such as Boston, Seattle, New York, Los Angeles, and San Francisco, collective efforts by elected officials, community-based organizations, businesses, philanthropy and others are addressing the issue of anti-Asian discrimination head-on.

As COVID-19 progressed, the nation reacted strongly to repeated examples of violence against Black, Asian, and Hispanic or Latino people. Whereas previous generations digested these events by newspaper, television, or word of mouth, today's news increasingly arrives in real-time on social media platforms through vivid images and videos from cell phone and law enforcement body or dashboard cameras. The combination of a nation on edge after being asked to stay-at-home during the pandemic and the rapid succession of social media posts documenting racist acts against Black people doing a range of activities from enjoying a park or jogging for health to being mistakenly or intentionally shot and killed by law enforcement brought the country to a tipping point. These events led to unprecedented and currently ongoing protests from multiple sectors (civilian, government, business, education, and professional sports) calling for anti-racist systemic change (Callimachi, 2020; Fausset, 2020; Fernandez & Burch, 2020; Nir, 2020). Importantly, more Americans are recognizing that if we really want to make transformational shifts in the places we live, it is important to focus on race. Supporting the Black Lives Matter movement, for example, is a critical component of equity work for all racial/ethnic minority groups and their white allies because systems of racial oppression are interconnected. As explained in a letter to the community by the Coalition of Asian American Leaders MN:

> George Floyd's death is a continuation of the long history of criminalization, dehumanization, and oppression of Black lives in this country since its founding. As immigrants and refugees to the U.S., our families may not always understand this history, but we inherited its legacy. Our communities have also benefited from Black freedom struggles that paved the way for our own fights for freedom and equal treatment in America" (Coalition of Asian American Leaders MN, 2020).

As Deepa Iyer so aptly stated in her analysis of the role of South Asian, Arab, Muslim, and Sikh immigrants in helping to shape America's multiracial future, "when Black people, who are at the bottom of America's divisive racial ladder, are free, it will be impossible for systems and policies to engage in discrimination and racism against other communities of color" (Iyer, 2015). As both the pandemic and protests continue, there will continue to be a need for tailored multilevel and multisector efforts to address the impacts of COVID-19 for Asian Americans and NH/PIs, and for all communities of color who are disproportionately and/or uniquely impacted.

SUMMARY AND RECOMMENDATIONS

In this chapter, we described how multilevel and multisector approaches can be used to both change individual behaviors as well as change policies, systems, and community conditions to sustain and expand single-level interventions for long-lasting impacts. We presented the historical and current socio-political context in which multilevel and multisector approaches are used to address Asian American and NH/PI health. We provided examples to illustrate how these approaches have been used to improve conditions to achieve Asian American and NH/PI health and racial equity; and we described lessons about key principals from the past to inform the shaping of future cross-sector initiatives. Based on the context and evidence to date, we offer the following recommendations for shaping future multilevel and multisector work:

- *Focus on the social determinants and multilevel approaches that include policy and systems change.* Learn the historical, current, and emerging social and political contexts in which the inequity is playing out in the community. How does this narrative illustrate the opportunities, potential, and assets of communities? What qualitative and quantitative data are available to help tell this holistic story? What opportunities are there to influence policy or transform systems in ways that support protective factors or get at the root of disparities and inequities for lasting change?

- *In seeking cross-sectoral partners, consider what sectors are important to represent.* Are you seeking multiple stakeholders (such as community organizers, businesses, government, etc.) in one social sector (such as education) to influence race- and place-based opportunities in one setting? Are you looking to influence multiple sectors (such as education, transportation, jobs, etc.) in a specific neighborhood or geography?

- *Be intentional about building and maintaining trust.* In entering into this work, how are you introducing your own history and connection to this community and the work? How are you including the voices of those who are meant to benefit from this work? Beyond making sure that the community has a seat at the table, how are you setting up structures that create space for the community to have agency to drive the vision based on the community knowing what is best for itself? How are you bringing people along on the journey to make collective decisions as you encounter speedbumps or unexpected roadblocks? As conflict or failures arise, how are you learning from those experiences and finding ways to heal, build, and move forward? How are you celebrating milestones and success?

- *Use data early on and often.* How is the collaborative using data to set the starting point, inform progress, and deepen the understanding of the interconnectedness of cross-sector work? How are you using qualitative data to provide context and nuance to existing quantitative data? What data assets do partners bring to the work? In considering evaluation questions, what does the collaborative want to learn by the end of each phase of the evolving work? What related measures or milestones are realistic and useful to track?

- *Be explicit about racial equity as a value and an outcome.* How is equity being integrated in the work? What does progress toward racial equity look like, and how is it measured? Why is it important to disaggregate and examine the experience of distinct Asian American and NH/PI populations?

DISCUSSION QUESTIONS

1. How can multisector work toward health equity look similar and different from multisector work toward racial equity? Describe how multilevel, multisector efforts toward racial equity can contribute to health equity for Asian Americans and NH/PIs.

2. What historical policies around health care, data, and immigration have served as barriers or opportunities to health equity for Asian American and NH/PI communities? What does the current policy and funding context look like now, and how might it influence multisector work for Asian American and NH/PI?

3. What lessons learned from past projects and initiatives can you use to develop and evaluate multilevel, multisector approaches to improving Asian American and NH/PI health?

REFERENCES

Anti Defamation League. (2020). *Reports of Anti-Asian Assaults, Harassment and Hate Crimes Rise as Coronavirus Spreads*. Retrieved from https://www.adl.org/blog/reports-of-anti-asian-assaults-harassment-and-hate-crimes-rise-as-coronavirus-spreads

Auerbach J. (2019). Social Determinants of Health Can Only Be Addressed by a Multisector Spectrum of Activities. *Journal of Public Health Management and Practice, 25*(6), 525–528. https://doi.org/10.1097/PHH.0000000000001088

Braveman, P., Gottlieb, L., Francis, D., Arkin, E., & Acker, J. (2019). *What Can the Health Care Sector Do to Advance Health Equity*. Retrieved from https://www.rwjf.org/en/library/research/2019/11/what-can-the-health-care-sector-do-to-advance-health-equity.html

Building Healthy Communities. Retrieved from https://www.buildinghealthycommunities.org/

Callimachi, R. (2020). *Breonna Taylor's life was changing.* Then the police came to her door. *The New York Times.*

Chang, R. C., Penaia, C., & Thomas, K. (2020). Count Native Hawaiian and Pacific Islanders in COVID-19 data – It's an OMB mandate. Retrieved from https://healthaffairs.org/do/10.1377/hblog20200825.671245/full/

Coalition of Asian American Leaders MN. (2020). Open letter to community: A call for unity and solidarity in the face of violence. Retrieved from https://caalmn.org/api4georgefloyd/?fbclid=IwAR2KdoEk_cikbs4HewWDYzKZ9pHclGj_y38Aoj26nGrZxgNDojtDGCmaIO0

Community Building Institute. (2019). 2018 Place Matters Year-End Report. Retrieved from https://www.xavier.edu/communitybuilding/pm_2018_year-end_report.pdf

Elias, R. R., & Moore, A. (2017). The evolution and future of the healthy communities movement. Retrieved from https://econpapers.repec.org/scripts/redir.pf?u=https%3A%2F%2Fwww.frbsf.org%2Fcommunity-development%2Ffiles%2Fevolution-and-future-of-healthy-communities-movement.pdf;h=repec:fip:fedfcr:00081

Erickson, J., Milstein, B., Schafer, L., Prtichard, K. E., Levitz, C., Miller, C., & Cheadle, A. (2017). Progress along the pathway for transforming regional health: a pulse check on multisector partnerships. Retrieved from https://www.rethinkhealth.org/wp-content/uploads/2017/03/2016-Pulse-Check-Narrative-Final.pdf

Fausset, R. (2020, June 24, 2020). What we know about the shooting death of Ahmaud Arbery. *The New York Times.*

Fernandez, M., & Burch, A. D. S. (2020). George Floyd, from "I want to touch the world" to "I can't breathe." *The New York Times.*

Forbes, J. M., Forbes, C. R., Lehman, E., & George, D. R. (2019). "Prevention produce": Integrating medical student mentorship into a fruit and vegetable prescription program for at-risk patients. *The Permanente Journal, 23*, 18–238. https://doi.org/10.7812/TPP/18-238

Frieden T. R. (2010). A framework for public health action: the health impact pyramid. *American Journal of Public Health, 100*(4), 590–595. https://doi.org/10.2105/AJPH.2009.185652

Gee, G. C., Ro, M. J., & Rimoin, A. W. (2020). Seven reasons to care about racism and COVID-19 and seven things to do to stop it. *American Journal of Public Health, 110*, 954–955.

George, D. R., Rovniak, L. S., Kraschnewski, J. L., Morrison, K. J., Dillon, J. F., & Bates, B. Y. (2013). Medical center farmers markets: a strategic partner in the patient-centered medical home. *Preventing Chronic Disease, 10*, E127. https://doi.org/10.5888/pcd10.130105

Gupta, P., & Ritoper, S. (2007). *Growing Opportunities: Will Funding Follow the Rise in Foundation Assets and Growth of AAPI Populations?* Retrieved from https://aapip.org/sites/default/files/publication/files/aapip-gopps4www.pdf

Henig, J. R., Riehl, C. J., Houston, D. M., Rebell, M. A., & Wolff, J. R. (2016). Collective impact and the new generation of cross-sector collaborations for education: a nationwide scan. Retrieved from New York, NY:

Herendeen, L. A., & MacDonald, A. (2011). Planning for the North Carolina healthy homes initiative. *Reviews on Environmental Health, 26*(3), 149–154. https://doi.org/10.1515/reveh.2011.022

Hiatt, R. A., Sibley, A., Fejerman, L., Glantz, S., Nguyen, T., Pasick, R., Palmer, N., Perkins, A., Potter, M. B., Somsouk, M., Vargas, R. A., van 't Veer, L. J., & Ashworth, A. (2018). The San Francisco Cancer Initiative: A community effort to reduce the population burden of cancer. *Health Affairs (Project Hope), 37*(1), 54–61. https://doi.org/10.1377/hlthaff.2017.1260

Inouye, T. E., Law, T., & Estrella, R. (2012). *Health Through Action for Asian American, Native Hawaiian, and Pacific Islanders: Final Evaluation Report.*

Iyer, D. (2015). *We Too Sing America.* New York, NY: The New Press.

Kania, J., & Kramer, M. (2011). Collective Impact. *Stanford Social Innovation Revew (Winter).*

Khan F. (2011). Oklahoma Healthy Homes initiative. *Public Health Reports (Washington, D.C.: 1974), 126 Suppl 1*(Suppl 1), 27–33. https://doi.org/10.1177/00333549111260S105

Kraschnewski, J. L., George, D. R., Rovniak, L. S., Monroe, D. L., Fiordalis, E., & Bates, E. (2014). Characterizing customers at medical center farmers' markets. *Journal of Community Health, 39*(4), 727–731. https://doi.org/10.1007/s10900-014-9818-x

Kunz, S., Ingram, M., Piper, R., Wu, T., Litton, N., Brady, J., & Knudson, A. (2017). Rural collaborative model for diabetes prevention and management: a case study. *Health Promotion Practice, 18*(6), 798–805. https://doi.org/10.1177/1524839917712730

Lemacks, J. L., James, R. E., Abbott, L., Choi, H., Parker, A., Bryant, A., Ralston, P. A., Rigsby, A. G., & Gilner, P. (2018). The Church Bridge Project: an academic-community perspective of a church-based weight management pilot intervention among young adult African Americans. *Progress in Community Health Partnerships: Research, Education, and Action, 12*(1S), 23–34. https://doi.org/10.1353/cpr.2018.0018

Lim, S., Wyatt, L. C., Mammen, S., Zanowiak, J. M., Mohaimin, S., Goldfeld, K. S., Shelley, D., Gold, H. T., & Islam, N. S. (2019). The DREAM Initiative: study protocol for a randomized controlled trial testing an integrated electronic health record and community health worker intervention to promote weight loss among South Asian patients at risk for diabetes. *Trials, 20*(1), 635. https://doi.org/10.1186/s13063-019-3711-y

Ma, G. X., Fang, C. Y., Seals, B., Feng, Z., Tan, Y., Siu, P., Yeh, M. C., Golub, S. A., Nguyen, M. T., Tran, T., & Wang, M. (2017). A community-based randomized trial of hepatitis B screening among high-risk Vietnamese Americans. *American Journal of Public Health, 107*(3), 433–440. https://doi.org/10.2105/AJPH.2016.303600

Ma, G. X., Lee, M. M., Tan, Y., Hanlon, A. L., Feng, Z., Shireman, T. I., Rhee, J., Wei, Z., Wong, F., Koh, H. S., Kim, C., & York, W. (2018). Efficacy of a community-based participatory and multilevel intervention to enhance hepatitis B virus screening and vaccination in underserved Korean Americans. *Cancer, 124*(5), 973–982. https://doi.org/10.1002/cncr.31134

Mays, G. P., Mamaril, C. B., & Timsina, L. R. (2016). Preventable death rates fell where communities expanded population health activities through multisector networks. *Health Affairs (Project Hope), 35*(11), 2005–2013. https://doi.org/10.1377/hlthaff.2016.0848

National Academies of Sciences and Medicine 2018. (2017). Report to Congress 2018, Washington (DC). Retrieved from https://www.nationalacademies.org/annual-report

New York State Department of Health, N. O. P. C. o. E. Healthy Communities Framework. Retrieved from https://nyopce.com/about/healthy-communities-framework/

Nguyen, T. U., Tran, J. H., Kagawa-Singer, M., & Foo, M. A. (2011). A qualitative assessment of community-based breast health navigation services for Southeast Asian women in Southern California: recommendations for developing a navigator training curriculum. *American Journal of Public Health, 101*(1), 87–93. https://doi.org/10.2105/AJPH.2009.176743

Nir, S. M. (2020, June 14). How 2 lives collided in Central Park, Rattling the Nation. *The New York Times.*

NYC Health & Hospitals. (2019). NYC Health + Hospitals to host farmers markets to help expand access to affordable, healthy food options for patients and staff [Press release]. Retrieved from https://www.nychealthandhospitals.org/pressrelease/farmers-markets-expand-access-to-affordable-healthy-food-options/

Public Health Alliance of Southern California, Communities Lifting Communities, & Hospital Association of Southern California. (2020). Innovative community investment strategies: the current state of practice and a vision for greater implementation in Southern California. Retrieved from https://communities.hasc.org/sites/main/files/file-attachments/innovative_community_investment_strategies_report_june_2020_final.pdf?1592254408

Pyron, T., Fonseka, J., Young, M., Zimmerman, L., Moore, A. R., & Hayes, N. (2018). Examining comprehensive cancer control partnerships, plans, and program interventions: successes and lessons learned from a utilization-focused evaluation. *Cancer Causes & Control, 29*(12), 1163–1171. https://doi.org/10.1007/s10552-018-1113-1

Raber, M., Huynh, T. N., Crawford, K., Kim, S., & Chandra, J. (2018). Development and feasibility of a community-based, culturally flexible colorectal cancer prevention program. *Journal of Community Health, 43*(5), 882–885. https://doi.org/10.1007/s10900-018-0497-x

Rhoads, N., Martin, S., & Zimmerman, F. J. (2020). Passing a healthy homes initiative: Using modeling to inform evidence-based policy decision making in Kansas City, Missouri. *Journal of Public Health Management and Practice, Publish Ahead of Print.* https://doi.org/10.1097/PHH.0000000000001197

Ro, M., & Chan, N. (2016). The changing practice of public health surveillance: examples from King County, *Washington.* Retrieved from https://kingcounty.gov/elected/executive/health-human-services-transformation/ach/governing-board/~/media/elected/executive/constantine/initiatives/hhs-transformation/documents/pmw/the-changing-practice.ashx

Scally, C. P., Lo, L., Pettit, K. L. S., Anoll, C., & Scott, K. (2020). Driving systems change forward. *Open Source Solutions,* 8.

Siegal, B., Winey, D., & Kornetsky, A. (2015). Pathways to system change: the design of multisite cross-sector initiatives. Retrieved from https://www.frbsf.org/community-development/files/wp2015-03.pdf

Skizim, M., Harris, N., Leonardi, C., & Scribner, R. (2017). Academic-community partnership development to enhance program outcomes in underserved communities: A case study. *Ethnicity & Disease, 27*(Suppl 1), 321. https://doi.org/10.18865/ed.27.S1.321

Soltero, E. G., Ramos, C., Williams, A. N., Hooker, E., Mendez, J., Wildy, H., Davis, K., Hernandez, V., Contreras, O. A., Silva, M., Lish, E., & Shaibi, G. Q. (2019). ¡Viva maryvale!: A multilevel, multisector model to community-based diabetes prevention. *American Journal of Preventive Medicine, 56*(1), 58–65. https://doi.org/10.1016/j.amepre.2018.07.034

SPARCC. Retrieved from https://www.sparcchub.org/communities/

Trump, D. J. (2020). Suspension of entry of immigrants who present a risk to the US labor market during the economic recovery following the 2019 coronavirus outbreak. Executive Office of the President, https://www.federalregister.gov/documents/2020/04/27/2020-09068/suspension-of-entry-of-immigrants-who-present-a-risk-to-the-united-states-labor-market-during-the.

U.S. Department of Health and Human Services. (2010a). *Healthy People 2020.* Retrieved from https://www.healthypeople.gov/sites/default/files/HP2020_brochure_with_LHI_508_FNL.pdf

U.S. Department of Health and Human Services. (2010b). HHS announces the nation's new health promotion and disease prevention agenda. Retrieved from https://www.healthypeople.gov/sites/default/files/DefaultPressRelease_1.pdf

US Citizenship and Immigration Services. (2017, June 2017). Number of H-1B Petition Filings Applications and Approvals, Country, Age, Occupation, Industry, Annual Compensation ($), and Education, FY2007 – FY2017. Retrieved from https://www.uscis.gov/sites/default/files/document/data/h-1b-2007-2017-trend-tables.pdf

Wysen, K. (2021). Listen and be ready to shift: How racial equity and community leadership launched "communities of opportunity." *Journal of Public Health Management and Practice, 27*(1), E48–E56. https://doi.org/10.1097/PHH.0000000000001048

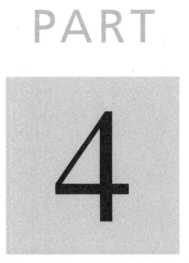

4

UNDERREPRESENTED GROUPS

CHAPTER

11

AGING, OLDER ADULTS

TINA R. SADARANGANI, SARAH M. MINER, LARISSA R. BURKA

LEARNING OBJECTIVES

By the end of this chapter, readers will be able to:

- Identify factors that underpin health disparities facing Asian American older adults.

- Describe how clinical issues commonly found in aging populations may have unique underpinnings in Asian American communities.

- Explain the role of participatory action research (PAR) in improving the health of vulnerable older Asian Americans and identify participatory action frameworks that can be applied when engaging this population.

- Implement principles of PAR within home and community-based programs serving Asian American older adults.

Applied Population Health Approaches for Asian American Communities, First Edition. Edited by Simona C. Kwon, Chau Trinh-Shevrin, Nadia S. Islam, and Stella S. Yi.
© 2023 John Wiley & Sons, Inc. Published 2023 by John Wiley & Sons, Inc.
Companion Website: www.wiley.com/go/kwon/asianamerican

INTRODUCTION

Older Asian Americans are a rapidly growing, highly vulnerable, and poorly studied subset of both the aging population and the Asian population. In 2017, there were over 2.2 million Asian Americans over the age of 65 in the United States (Administration for Community Living, 2019). This number is projected to grow to 7.9 million by 2060. During this period, the share of the older population comprised of Asian Americans will double, from 4% to 8% (Administration for Community Living, 2019). Notably, at present, Asian Americans make up 6% of all centenarians (Administration for Community Living, 2019). Yet, despite making up a growing share of the aging population, including the "oldest old," a limited body of research has focused on the heterogeneity within the older Asian American population and the role of older individuals' social and cultural context in influencing health outcomes.

Statistics on Asian Americans frequently fail to capture the unique vulnerabilities of the older subset of the population. Myths of Asian Americans as "model minorities" are based on an erroneous and incomplete picture focused on younger, educated, middle-class Asian American adults with significant earning potential and high levels of educational attainment. This misconception has obscured the reality of many Asian American older adults who are confronting poverty, limited English proficiency, and unstable housing, in addition to numerous barriers to accessing health and social services, including lack of health insurance and transportation (Weng, 2017).

There is a critical need for researchers to focus and conduct research on the unmet needs, sociocultural contexts, and health trajectories of the aging subset of the Asian American population in order to meaningfully reduce health disparities through focused, culturally relevant interventions. This chapter will present the historical and sociopolitical factors that influence health outcomes for older Asian Americans, followed by an overview of health disparities unique to older Asian Americans, and finally will offer guidance on applying principles of participatory action research (PAR) to enable community engaged participatory action research that supports improved health outcomes.

Background

In order to contextualize the needs of older Asian Americans, it is important to briefly explain their varied immigration histories. A small minority of older Asian Americans descended from the earliest generations of Asian immigrants to the United States, who arrived as laborers from China, India, Japan, Korea, and the Philippines to the west coast of the United States. Discriminatory immigration laws, passed in 1924, barred individuals from Asia who were not students from entering the United States, limiting population growth (Takaki, 1998). However, subsequent changes to immigration laws in 1965 – specifically, those contained in the Immigration and Nationality Act – have had lasting effects on the makeup of the demographic shifts seen in the Asian American aging population today.

The Immigration and Nationality Act of 1965 enabled the entry of Asian immigrants into the United States (Bhatia & Ram, 2018). This legislation admitted professionals and workers in short supply, allowed families to be reunited, and provided refugee status for those fleeing the Vietnam War. Migrants leaving their countries because of war, political, or economic instability resulted in meaningful changes to the size and composition of Asian American communities in the United States. Some of today's older Asian Americans immigrated as children with their parents following this change in immigration laws, while others came as young adults to work or pursue education and build lives in the United States. Still other older Asian Americans may have immigrated in middle adulthood or arrived as elders to be reunited with their adult children who previously immigrated under policies supporting family reunification. The period of the life course in which an immigrant arrives in the United States impacts assimilation, English language proficiency, societal integration, and in turn, affects health care needs and outcomes. Consequently, understanding the sociopolitical context and period of the life-course in which older Asian Americans arrived in the United States is fundamental to designing and conducting an effective program of research to improve their health.

Refer to Chapter 1 for a more detailed description of these immigration histories.

Sociopolitical Context of Older Asian Americans

The fact that many older Asian Americans may be first-generation immigrants may influence the disproportionate rates of poverty that affect this population and their perceptions of being marginalized by society. Older Asian American men and women earn significantly less than the average older American. For older Asian American men and women, average annual income in 2017 was $26,692 and $14,418, respectively (Administration for Community Living, 2019). The comparable figures for all older persons were $32,654 for men and $19,180 for women. The poverty rate in 2017 for Asian Americans age 65 and over was 10.8%, while the rate for all older Americans was 9.2% (Administration for Community Living, 2019). These general estimates mask the disproportionate effects of poverty within different Asian ethnic groups and among recent immigrants. For example, in 2015, 23.3% of Cambodian American adults over 65 lived in poverty compared to 7.1% of Filipino older adults (Pew Research Center, 2017).

Notably, a majority of older Asian Americans (54%) reside in three states: California, New York, and Hawaii (Administration for Community Living, 2019). While these states are home to diverse populations and offer older Asian Americans community support and opportunities for socialization, the high cost of living in these states compromises the ability of all older adults who rely on fixed incomes to age in place. Moreover, many older Asian Americans, particularly those who arrive in later life, are less likely to receive meaningful benefits from Social Security because they earned less and had fewer working years in the United States than other older adults (National Coalition for Asian Pacific American Community Development, 2016). In New York, for example, 24% of older Asian Americans live in poverty compared to 18% of all New Yorkers over the age of 65. In New York, 39% of Chinese American older adults, and 35% of Korean older adults have no Social Security income, compared to 23% of the overall aging population (Center for an Urban Future, 2013).

Among the many factors that prevent older Asian Americans from accessing necessary supports and services, the most notable are discriminatory public policies and limited English proficiency (LEP). In the majority of states, lawfully residing immigrants must wait a minimum of five years to receive Medicaid benefits (Sadarangani, Trinh-Shevrin, et al., 2019). However, even in states that do not have a waiting period for public assistance, many older Asian Americans do not take full advantage of available benefits. This reluctance to access services is partially driven by fear that accessing public assistance will jeopardize their citizenship prospects. The new Public Charge Rule, effective February 2020, codified this fear (United States Citizenship and Immigration Services, 2020). The U.S. Supreme Court found that an immigrant's receipt of public benefits for more than 12 months in a 36-month period could be deemed grounds for denying permanent resident status or citizenship to that individual. In addition, older Asian Americans experience disproportionately high rates of LEP that pose an additional access barrier. In NYC, 94% of Korean American older adults and 92% of Chinese American older adults have LEP, which severely constrains their access to much needed services (Center for an Urban Future, 2013).

The barriers older Asian Americans confront when trying to access health and social services are evidenced by their low rates of participation in these programs relative to their growing share of the aging population. In 2017, 26% of older Asian Americans had both Medicare and supplemental private health insurance (Administration for Community Living, 2019). In comparison, 46% of all older adults had both Medicare and supplemental private health insurance (Administration for Community Living, 2019). In NYC, within the Older Americans Act Home-Delivered Meals Program, less than 1% of participants are Asian, while 14% of the city's population is Asian (Sadarangani, Beasley, et al., 2020).

The cost of housing, food, transportation, and other social determinants of health, coupled with numerous barriers to accessing health and social services force older Asian Americans to compromise on essential needs, and contribute to health disparities emerging within this population.

OVERVIEW OF HEALTH DISPARITIES FACING ASIAN AMERICAN OLDER ADULTS

The five leading causes of death for Asian American men age 65 and older in 2017 were cancer, heart disease, stroke, diabetes, and chronic lower respiratory diseases. For Asian American women age 65 and older, the five leading causes of death were heart disease, cancer, stroke, Alzheimer's disease, and diabetes (Administration for Community Living, 2019). Within the limited body of research on the health care needs of older Asian Americans, most studies have focused on the most prevalent chronic diseases, including diabetes, cancer, and cardiovascular disease (Dong & Simon, 2018). Only very few studies conducted among older Asian Americans have addressed emerging issues impacting elder health, including osteoporosis, physical disability and functional decline, Alzheimer's disease and Alzheimer's disease-related dementias (ADRD), cognitive decline, depression and other mental health issues, and palliative care and end-of-life issues. Moreover, as with health research in the Asian American population more broadly, national surveys aggregate data for all older Asian Americans and Pacific Islanders (PIs). Extant data fail to capture the heterogeneity and ethnic diversity within this population as well as nuances in health outcomes across different ethnic groups. The limited studies that have disaggregated data describing older Asian Americans into separate ethnic groups are small in size, limited in geographic scope, and focused on one or two Asian ethnic groups. Nonetheless, these studies have generally found stark differences in health status among Asian populations, indicating the need for more research that explores the experiences of each ethnic group of older Asian Americans separately. We briefly highlight clinical problems that disproportionately affect older adults, including dementia, depression, functional limitations, and end-of-life issues with respect to broader Asian American populations. We also discuss how the novel coronavirus (COVID-19) pandemic has exacerbated many of these issues.

Dementia

Studies of Asian populations generally have reported prevalence and incidence rates for dementia similar to or lower than those of predominantly non-Hispanic White (White) populations. Alzheimer's disease is the most common cause of dementia, while cognitive decline – including loss of memory, language, problem-solving, and other thinking skills – characterize the onset of dementia (Alzheimer's Association, 2020). In a 14-year study of dementia incidence in Kaiser Permanente Northern California members (64 years and older), the age-standardized dementia incidence rate was 15.2 per 1,000 person-years for all Asian Americans, as compared to 19.3/1000 for Whites (Mayeda et al., 2017). Filipino Americans had the highest risk of dementia among Asian Americans while Japanese Americans had the lowest. Japanese Americans are the most extensively studied Asian American population with respect to dementia. A recent systematic review noted not only that Japanese Americans had the lowest prevalence of dementia among all ethnic groups in the United States, at 6.3%, but also that Japanese Americans may be the only Asian ethnic group with reliable data on this topic (Mehta & Yeo, 2017).

Predictors of dementia risk among older Asian Americans are poorly understood. For example, in Mayeda, Glymour, Quesenberry, & Whitmer (2017)'s northern California study, Filipino Americans had the highest levels of education among Asian American populations but also the highest dementia incidence. It is unknown whether this higher dementia risk may reflect differences in educational quality or resources available to Filipino Americans, or whether the education advantage may simply be overwhelmed by another risk factor, such as access to care. The association between higher levels of education and higher dementia incidence was also found in the Population Study of Chinese Elderly in Chicago Study (the PINE Study). The PINE Study found differences in the rates of cognitive decline among Chinese Americans by age, sex, education, and income (Li et al., 2017). Similar to Filipino Americans in the Northern California study, higher educational attainment was linked to faster rates of decline in global cognition and episodic memory in older Chinese Americans in Chicago. Higher income was associated with reduction in the rate of decline in working memory, and men had faster rates of decline in working memory than women. Ge, Wu, Bailey, & Dong (2017) highlighted a complex relationship between social support, social strain, and cognitive outcomes in the PINE Study sample, suggesting the need for further research into the complex relationships between demographic variables, cognition, and social engagement, which may be linked to acculturation and immigration factors. Higher levels of both social support and social strain were significantly associated with higher levels of cognitive outcomes (i.e., global cognitive function, episodic memory, working memory, and executive function) in this sample of older Chinese American adults, leading the researchers to hypothesize that higher social engagement of the sample may support cognitive function.

Racial and ethnic minorities with low socioeconomic status or education levels are diagnosed with dementia at more advanced disease stages and receive fewer formal services, resulting in worse health outcomes (Chodosh et al., 2018). As the U.S. population has increasingly diversified, the National Institute on Aging and the U.S. Department of Health and Human Services have called for strategies that focus on improving the health of older adults in diverse populations and, specifically, improving health outcomes for racial/ethnic minority populations by addressing factors that underpin disparities, such as access to care (National Institute on Aging, 2016). More studies specific to the Asian American population are needed to identify factors impacting access to culturally appropriate dementia care.

Depression and Mental Health Needs

Among Asian Americans, depression tends to be persistent, lasting long periods of time, and Asian Americans are less likely to seek treatment and adequate care compared to Whites (Lee et al., 2014; Kalibatseva & Leong, 2011; Lee et al, 2011). Limited data suggest that discrimination may impact depression. Self-reported discrimination was significantly and positively associated with depressive symptoms, independent of sociode-mographic characteristics, migration-related variables, and personality factors in the PINE Study's sample of older Chinese Americans in Chicago (Li & Dong, 2017). Factors linked to reporting discrimination were younger age, higher education and income, higher acculturation, longer residence in the United States, living outside Chinatown, and higher levels of neuroticism and conscientiousness. These potential predictors remain under-studied and require further investigation.

Self-neglect is an emerging area of study that is linked to suicidal ideation. A higher level of self-neglect was significantly associated with increased risk of self-reported suicidal ideation within two weeks among elderly Chinese Americans in Chicago (Dong, Xu, & Ding, 2017). Additionally, having poor personal hygiene and living in unsanitary conditions were associated with increased risk of suicidal ideation (Dong, Xu, & Ding, 2017). The PINE Study also found that greater neighborhood cohesion reduced the risk of self-neglect in this population, suggesting an avenue for future research (Hei & Dong, 2017). Low English proficiency may be associated with greater mental health needs in general. California Health Interview Survey data showed that low English proficiency was associated with the increased likelihood that an older Asian immigrant (Chinese, Filipino, or Vietnamese) would perceive a mental health need, after adjustment for health and other covariates (Nguyen, 2011). Older individuals (age 65 or older) were less likely than younger participants (age 50–64) to perceive mental health needs.

Balancing these risk factors, researchers have also identified variables that contribute to resilience in older Asian Americans and buffer symptoms of depression. For example, developing better relationships with health care providers may reduce the likelihood of depressive symptoms among older Asian Americans. Using the Trust in Physicians (TIP) scale with older Chinese Americans over two years, the PINE Study researchers found that increasing trust was associated with decreased risk of depression (Dong, Bergren, & Simon, 2017a). For Asian American grandparents, caregiving for grandchildren may reduce depressive symptoms. For Chinese American grandparents in the PINE Study, caregiving time was significantly related to having fewer depressive symptoms, but not poor quality of life (Xu et al., 2017). The association between grandparent caregiving and depressive symptoms was moderated by the perception of caregiving burden.

Intergenerational relationships may be an important area for future research related to depression among older Asian Americans. One aspect is filial expectations and care: in the PINE Study, older Chinese Americans with high filial expectations and low filial receipt had the highest risk of depressive symptoms (Dong, Li, & Hua, 2017). This work underscores the importance of conducting cultural relevant research to inform interventions for older Asian Americans, as the perception of intergenerational support would be different in other populations. In separate analyses of the PINE Study cohort, researchers found that confiding and aiding relationships with children and spouses were significantly associated with lower depressive symptom severity, while demanding and criticizing intergenerational relationships, as well as spousal criticism, predicted higher depressive symptom severity (Liu et al., 2017).

Also within the realm of intergenerational relationships, more studies are needed to explore abuse of older Asian Americans. Elder abuse is a global public health issue, but very little research has explored prevalence or incidence of elder abuse with Asian American communities. Emerging research presents some support for the hypothesis of the intergenerational transmission of violence, within which an abused child may abuse his or her abuser parent when the parent becomes elderly. Findings from the PINE Study showed that childhood abuse before 18 years old is significantly associated with increased risk of elder abuse for Chinese adult children after controlling for sociodemographic characteristics (Dong, Li, & Simon, 2017). In this study population, even though physical hurt was most prevalent among childhood abuse subitems, adult children perceived insults, threats, and screams as more serious than physical hurt. The authors suggested that this perception may be particular to Chinese culture, in which physical discipline is normalized, and indicates the importance of cultural tailoring of abuse investigations and interventions to the needs of Asian American populations. Data from the PINE Study demonstrated the incidence of overall elder abuse as 8.8% among the study population of older Chinese American adults, with 4.8% for psychological abuse, 2.9% for financial abuse, 0.5% for physical abuse, 0.1% for sexual abuse, and 1.1% for caregiver neglect (Dong & Wang, 2017).

Functional Decline, Disability, and Falls

Functional decline among older adults is an important public health issue that impacts individuals, their caregivers, and society at large (Dong, Bergren, & Simon, 2017b). Among older Asian Americans, 30% reported having at least one physical disability in 2017 (Administration for Community Living, 2019). According to American Community Survey data, older Asian Americans are less likely to report having a functional limitation or disability as compared to Whites, but this finding is poorly understood (Dallo et al., 2015). Furthermore, aggregation of data masks striking disparities among ethnic groups, with PIs, and to a lesser extent, Vietnamese Americans, having higher rates of disability than other older Asian Americans (Fuller-Thomson et al., 2011). Institutionalization of older Asian Americans with disabilities is also poorly understood, with striking disparities documented in nursing home use by ethnic group, ranging from 4.7% in South Asians to 18.8% among Koreans (Fuller-Thomson & Chi, 2012). Odds of institutionalization were higher among those who were older, unmarried, cognitively impaired, and those who spoke English at home.

The PINE Study showed that older Chinese Americans with higher education experienced a more rapid decline of physical function than those with less education (Dong, Bergren, & Simon, 2017b). However, individual yearly income and number of medical conditions were not associated with the rate of physical decline in this population – a finding that contrasts with earlier research showing that minority older adults, especially those with lower socioeconomic status, experience greater functional disability compared to their non-Hispanic white (NHW) counterparts (Mendes et al., 2005). More research is needed to understand how functional decline and disability manifest among older Asian Americans and how individuals and families cope with the changes in lifestyle new limitations demand. Functional limitations may be linked to depression, suicidal ideation and other mental health issues. In a sample of community-dwelling Koreans in Los Angeles, functional limitation had a significant contribution to suicidal ideation (Ahn & Kim, 2015).

Older Asian Americans may have lower fall risk than other ethnic groups. An analysis of CHIS data adjusting for race/ethnicity and English language proficiency found that lower English proficiency Asian Americans were significantly less likely to fall compared to Whites (Kwon et al., 2018). Within the Asian American community, less acculturated immigrants may experience fewer falls because they are healthier when they arrive in the United States, illustrating what is known as "the healthy migrant effect" (Dallo et al., 2015). Older Asian Americans are less likely to live alone and therefore may be able to request assistance from household members, thus avoiding activities that may increase their general likelihood of a fall (Kwon et al., 2018). Among older women in California, the risk of having a recent fall was substantially lower for non-Hispanic Black (Black) and Asian women when compared to White women (Geng et al., 2017). Asian women paradoxically reported more mobility limitations, but they also reported less use of assistive devices and had lower fall prevalence, which may suggest that Asian women are self-limiting certain activities based on their own perceived limitations, resulting in reduced fall risk. However, at least one systematic review cautioned that insufficient data prevent direct comparisons between racial and ethnic differences in fall rates, and that existing studies are difficult to compare due to widely variable data and methodology (Han et al., 2014).

Palliative and End-of-Life Care

Asian Americans are more likely than other groups to lack care transitions and have low rates of hospice use. Among Medicare beneficiaries who died between July and December 2011, Asian Americans were least likely to have a care transition (Wang et al., 2019). Among hospice users, White, Black, and Hispanic patients had similar length of hospice stay, which was significantly longer than that of Asian Americans. Among people with cancer, Asian Americans (and Blacks) were least likely among all ethnic groups to use hospice care (LoPresti et al., 2016). Urban geography was associated with decreased hospice use but increased referrals for Asian Americans. However, at least one Hawaii-based study found that Asian and PI cancer patients receiving palliative care consultations were more likely to be referred to hospice than White patients, in contrast to previous studies describing reduced hospice use among non-Whites (Bell et al., 2011). The association between ethnicity and hospice care was reduced after controlling for consultation intensity (i.e., plan of care versus without plan of care), indicating the importance of providing palliative care consultations for plan of care.

This finding points to the critical role of patient–provider communication in improving the health status and the health care experiences of older Asian Americans. Because the majority of older Asian Americans are foreign-born, innovative, linguistically and culturally tailored strategies are needed to engage and educate this heterogeneous population. Communicating with health care providers may be particularly difficult for older adults because of low English proficiency, low health literacy, and a lack of translators on site at health care facilities (Kim et al., 2011; Nam, 2008; Taira & Orue, 2019). Lack of communication negatively impacts all health conditions, contributing to poor chronic disease management and increased morbidity and mortality, but in the area of palliative and end-of-life care, improving patient-provider communication may be particularly critical. Limited qualitative research has highlighted the importance of involving families in end-of-life discussions for Chinese and Korean American patients (Chi et al., 2018; Kwak & Salmon, 2007) and also underscored the importance of using indirect communication approaches to assess older Chinese Americans' readiness to discuss end-of-life issues (Chi et al., 2018). These findings indicate the need for health care providers to adopt more sensitive, complex approaches to communicating with diverse older Asian Americans, and more research to inform such approaches is urgently needed. Education for older adults and their families is needed to facilitate older Asian Americans' effective participation in decision-making with health care providers. Key topics to be addressed include the aging process and the importance of long-term care. Explicit language about advance directives is essential, including clear statements about preferred medical care, including whether resuscitation is to be performed, acceptable types of treatments to sustain life, and handling of the body upon death. Yet discussions of these matters with Asian American families must be approached with cultural and linguistic sensitivity to support older Asian Americans to plan for their health and financial well-being and communicate their care preferences to loved ones – a chain of events that may contribute to better quality of care and quality of life (Chi et al., 2018). More research, education, and direct practice involving long-term care planning and advance directives among aging Asian Americans will contribute to identifying communication strategies and specific messaging for this population overall, as well as help highlight areas in which cultural tailoring for ethnic groups is most needed.

Ramifications of COVID-19

Many existing disparities facing older Asian Americans have been exacerbated by the COVID-19 pandemic. While it is established that the pandemic has disproportionately affected Black and Latino communities and ravaged frail older adults in skilled nursing facilities, the full toll of COVID-19 on communities of color, especially older Asian Americans, is unknown. A lack of accurate disaggregated data on Asian ethnicities from state and local health departments means that impacts on the health of older Asian Americans cannot be easily identified, and strategies to address COVID-19 in these communities are at best inequitable.

At the time of this writing, nearly 40% of deaths from COVID-19 have occurred among adults in skilled nursing facilities (Kamp & Mathews, 2020). Just 1.0% of adults in skilled nursing facilities identify as Asian American (Feng et al., 2011). However, older Asian Americans have been found to favor and disproportionately use community-based long-term care services, such as adult day service centers or senior centers (Sadarangani, Missaelides, et al., 2019; Sadarangani & Murali, 2018). The majority of community-based congregate settings servicing older adults have closed, either permanently or temporarily, in the wake of the pandemic. This means community-dwelling older adults from minority communities, especially Asian Americans, may lack access to nutritious meals, health monitoring, and opportunities for socialization and productive engagement (Sadarangani, 2020). As a consequence, there may be significant and underrecognized increases in cognitive and functional decline, falls, and depression. City and state-level COVID-19 response teams must implement strategies that leverage the knowledge of community-based programs serving older adults to better understand participants' needs. Engaging with these programs will help focus resources to reduce COVID-19 related disparities in these communities. In addition, cities and states must work with trusted, local stakeholders to meet the needs of marginalized older Asian Americans and ensure that the most vulnerable have sufficient access to food and housing along with culturally and linguistically appropriate materials about COVID-19.

The Role of PAR in Targeting Disparities in the Older Asian American Population

Reducing health disparities and advancing health equity in an aging population that is growing both in size and racial/ethnic diversity requires interventions that address clinical and social factors linked to poor health outcomes. It also requires meeting older adults where they are, in their communities, and working with them to eliminate barriers to participation in research, including mistrust of researchers and government agencies. A small but growing body of research suggests that PAR with older adults holds promise for helping researchers to understand and address some of the complex health and social problems faced by older adults in diverse communities, including those consisting of Asian American ethnic groups, while contributing to individual and community capacity building. PAR methodology was discussed in Chapter 8. Here, we offer examples of how that methodology may be successfully applied to elucidate the priorities and issues of older Asian Americans.

One example of PAR among community-dwelling older Asian Americans is a study by Dong et al. (2011). Dong and researchers from Rush University in Chicago, IL (2011) sought to better understand the health-related needs of Chinese older adults in Chicago's Chinatown. In partnership with community-members, the authors conducted a health needs assessment that combined epidemiological and qualitative methods to systematically identify inequalities in health and access to services among older Chinese Americans. By prioritizing community needs and stakeholder perspectives, PAR mitigates widely held perceptions that research is or needs to be driven by academic and governmental priorities (Moreno-John et al., 2004; Norris et al., 2007). The academic-community partnership between Rush University and the Chinese community emphasized core tenets of PAR – partnership and co-learning, promoting agency, and empowerment and capacity building – thereby offering participants a greater sense of control over the research process (Zimmerman, 2000). We discuss each of these tenets below:

- *Partnership and co-learning.* In order to establish an equitable *partnership* at the study onset, researchers at Rush began the PAR process by creating a community advisory board (CAB). The goal of the CAB was to engage Chinatown members, such as leaders of civic, health, social, and advocacy groups, community centers, as well as community physician and residents, and board members as key collaborators. *Co-learning* is the process by which community participants acquire research skills and competencies, such as problem-solving or data-collection skills. Community-members also contribute their own knowledge and expertise based on their nuanced understanding of their own situational context. As part of co-learning, CAB members identified a list of needs assessment topics most relevant to the Chinese community's concerns that were further incorporated into focus group topics. In later stages of research, CAB members also worked closely with investigators to review findings and reexamine study instruments to ensure cultural sensitivity and appropriateness.

- *Promoting agency.* Fundamental to PAR is the emphasis placed on the *agency* of individuals and/or communities in designing and conducting research, ensuring that research is "collaborative, equitable partnership in all phases of research" (Israel et al., 2008, p. 50). In Dong et al.'s (2011) study, *agency* took the form of working with stakeholders to identify research questions; conduct focus group interviews; identify ways to strengthen community capacity through data collection and analysis; disseminate findings; and use research findings to drive social action. Most notably, researchers engaged the Chinese American Service League, the largest social service provider for Chinese Americans in the Midwest. Potential study participants were approached after their attendance in Chinese American Service League-sponsored cultural activities such as calligraphy and tai-chi classes. Focus group interviews were guided by trained facilitators who were affiliated with the Chinese American Service League. The involvement of facilitators with the community was crucial to gaining trust and eliciting active participation based on the rationale that Asian participants would be more likely to reveal their opinions if they knew the interviewers personally (Suh et al., 2009). Sample focus group questions included, What does "healthy aging" mean to you? What do you think are some of the biggest health problems in our community? How would you describe a happy older adult in the community? What makes older adults in our community happy?

■ *Empowerment and capacity building.* By channeling community members' knowledge into rigorous research, PAR lends itself to capacity building and change at the individual, systems, and community level. This is because PAR unique builds translation of findings and community empowerment into the research process, as opposed to waiting for data collection and analysis to end before considering capacity building (Minkler & Wallerstein, 2008). Dong et al.'s approach allowed researchers to gain knowledge and cultural awareness of aging Chinese community members' health concerns and leveraged this to develop appropriate research instruments. This synergetic collaboration also increased the Chinese community's understanding of their perceived health needs, access and barriers to health care services, and knowledge of health sciences research.

PAR may hold particular promise for research with minority older adults and other marginalized groups that experience systemic mistrust that serves as a barrier to participation (Carter et al., 1991; Moreno-John et al., 2004; Norris et al., 2007). The Chinatown community had not been engaged fully in research due, in part, to anti-Chinese sentiment from the past that pervaded mainstream institutions and translated into distrust among Chinese Americans toward government and federally sponsored research projects that persists today (Lillie-Blanton & Hoffman, 1995). Barriers, including language, scientific literacy, and access to care, have further excluded the Chinese community from benefiting from progress in health sciences research (Zhan et al., 1998). Dong et al.'s approach enabled recruitment and stakeholder engagement more successfully than studies in minority groups that employ other methodologies (Carrasquillo & Chadiha, 2007; Norris et al., 2007).

To summarize, Dong et al.'s approach to PAR successfully leveraged the wisdom and insights of older adults. Stakeholder engagement, using the CAB, ensured that research questions and priority areas were relevant to communities. Co-learning ensured that culturally appropriate survey questions and other data collection tools were used and allowed participants to develop insights about their community's needs as well as about the research process. The involvement of stakeholders throughout the research process allowed for nuanced interpretation of findings that accounted for older adults' situational context, incorporated their preferences, and supported findings that strengthened programs, practices, and policies affecting vulnerable older adults (Minkler, 2005).

Case 11 (see Appendix) further illustrates key principles that underscore PAR in communities serving Asian Americans: trust between members of the community and academia that evolves over time, committed leadership, and established relationships. It also highlights the importance of engaging with trusted community-based providers of care to diverse older adults, such as adult day service centers, home health care organizations, and senior centers, in order to establish partnerships.

SUMMARY AND RECOMMENDATIONS

Asian Americans represent a rapidly growing but underresearched subset of the aging population. Asian American older adults encounter numerous barriers to health care access, including limited English proficiency, restricted access to health and social services, and low socioeconomic status that translate into meaningful health disparities. Clinical issues like dementia, falls, depression, and functional decline, which are highly prevalent across aging populations, are more complex in Asian American population due to restricted health access, delays in diagnosis, and a lack of culturally appropriate interventions. There is a critical need for researchers to hone in and conduct research on the unmet needs, sociocultural contexts, and health trajectories of the aging subset of the Asian American population in order to meaningfully reduce health disparities through focused, culturally relevant interventions.

■ One approach to engaging older Asian Americans in research partnerships is through the use of PAR. A key goal of PAR is to enhance a community's ability to address important health issues through the development of effective interventions that can be maintained over time, using a process that involves community stakeholders in all phases of the research process.

- It is vital to engage community partners serving older adults in this research in order to build collaborative partnerships that reduce disparities. These providers include adult day service centers, home health care organizations, and senior centers.

DISCUSSION QUESTIONS

1. Discuss the diverse social and cultural contexts of older Asian Americans, including examples of how context contributes to health disparities and why PAR is an important method of conducting research among older Asian Americans.

2. Although the prevalence of dementia has been found to be lower in Asian American populations, Asian American older adults may encounter barriers to diagnosis and treatment. What are these barriers, and how can PAR be used to examine and mitigate them?

3. Discuss the ways in which knowledge of available long-term care services and supports for older Asian American adults may be limited. Why might this limited awareness pose a challenge for Asian American families striving to establish and maintain healthy intergenerational relationships? How has PAR been used to address this challenge?

REFERENCES

Administration for Community Living (2019). Profiles of Asian Americans Age 65 and Over. Retrieved March 20, 2020, from https://acl.gov/sites/default/files/Aging%20and%20Disability%20in%20America/2018AsA_OAProfile.pdf.

Ahn, J., & Kim, B. J. (2015). The Relationships Between Functional Limitation, Depression, Suicidal Ideation, and Coping in Older Korean Immigrants. *Journal of Immigrant and Minority Health, 17*(6), 1643–1653. https://doi.org/10.1007/s10903-015-0204-2

Alzheimer's Association. (2020). *What is dementia?* Retrieved March 18, 2020, from https://www.alz.org/alzheimers-dementia/what-is-dementia

Bell, C. L., Kuriya, M., Fischberg, D. (2011) Hospice referrals and code status: outcomes of inpatient palliative care consultations among Asian Americans and Pacific Islanders with cancer. *Journal of Pain and Symptom Management, 42*(4), 557–564. http://doi.org/10.1016/j.jpainsymman.2011.01.010

Bhatia, S., & Ram, A. (2018). South Asian Immigration to United States: A Brief History Within the Context of Race, Politics, and Identity. In M. J. Perera & E. C. Chang (Eds.), *Biopsychosocial Approaches to Understanding Health in South Asian Americans* (pp. 15–32). Cham: Springer International Publishing.

Carter, W. B., Elward, K., Malmgren, J., Martin, M. L., & Larson, E. (1991). Participation of older adults in health programs and research: a critical review of the literature. *The Gerontologist, 31*(5), 584–592. https://doi.org/10.1093/geront/31.5.584

Carrasquillo, O., & Chadiha, L. A. (2007). Development of community-based partnerships in minority aging research. *Ethnicity & Disease, 17*(1 Suppl 1), S3–S5.

Center for an Urban Future. (2013). *The new face of New York's seniors.* Retrieved on March 18, 2020, from https://nycfuture.org/pdf/The-New-Face-of-New-Yorks-Seniors.pdf

Chi, H. L., Cataldo, J., Ho, E. Y., & Rehm, R. S. (2018). Please Ask Gently: Using Culturally Targeted Communication Strategies to Initiate End-of-Life Care Discussions With Older Chinese Americans. *The American Journal of Hospice & Palliative Care, 35*(10), 1265–1272. https://doi.org/10.1177/1049909118760310

Chodosh, J., Thorpe, L. E., & Trinh-Shevrin, C. (2018). Changing Faces of Cognitive Impairment in the U.S.: Detection Strategies for Underserved Communities. *American Journal of Preventive Medicine, 54*(6), 842–844. https://doi.org/10.1016/j.amepre.2018.02.016

Dallo, F. J., Booza, J., & Nguyen, N. D. (2015). Functional limitations and nativity status among older Arab, Asian, Black, Hispanic, and White Americans. *Journal of Immigrant and Minority Health, 17*(2), 535–542. https://doi.org/10.1007/s10903-013-9943-0

Dong, X., Bergren, S., & Simon, M. A. (2017a). Cross-sectional and longitudinal association between trust in physician and depressive symptoms among U.S. community-dwelling Chinese older adults. *The Journals of Gerontology. Series A, Biological Sciences and Medical Sciences, 72*(Suppl_1), S125–S130. http://doi.org/10.1093/gerona/glx036

Dong, X., Bergren, S. M., & Simon, M. A. (2017e). The Decline of Directly Observed Physical Function Performance Among U.S. Chinese Older Adults. *The Journals of Gerontology. Series A, Biological Sciences and Medical Sciences, 72*(suppl_1), S11–S15. https://doi.org/10.1093/gerona/glx046

Dong, X., Chang, E. S., Wong, E., Wong, B., Skarupski, K. A., & Simon, M. A. (2011). Assessing the Health Needs of Chinese Older Adults: Findings from a Community-Based Participatory Research Study in Chicago's Chinatown. *Journal of Aging Research*, 2010, 124246. https://doi.org/10.4061/2010/124246

Dong, X., Li, M., & Hua, Y. (2017). The Association Between Filial Discrepancy and Depressive Symptoms: Findings From a Community-Dwelling Chinese Aging Population. *The Journals of Gerontology. Series A, Biological Sciences and Medical Sciences, 72*(suppl_1), S63–S68. https://doi.org/10.1093/gerona/glx040

Dong, X., Li, G., & Simon, M. A. (2017). The Association Between Childhood Abuse and Elder Abuse Among Chinese Adult Children in the United States. *The Journals of Gerontology. Series A, Biological Sciences and Medical Sciences, 72*(suppl_1), S69–S75. https://doi.org/10.1093/gerona/glw205

Dong, X., & Simon, M. A. (2018). Achieving Health Equity in Asian Populations. *Gerontology & Geriatric Medicine, 4,* 2333721418778169-2333721418778169. Retrieved from https://pubmed.ncbi.nlm.nih.gov/30014006

Dong, X., & Wang, B. (2017). Incidence of Elder Abuse in a U.S. Chinese Population: Findings From the Longitudinal Cohort PINE Study. *The Journals of Gerontology. Series A, Biological Sciences and Medical Sciences, 72*(suppl_1), S95–S101. https://doi.org/10.1093/gerona/glx005

Dong, X., Xu, Y., & Ding, D. (2017). Elder Self-neglect and Suicidal Ideation in an U.S. Chinese Aging Population: Findings from the PINE Study. *The Journals of Gerontology. Series A, Biological Sciences and Medical Sciences, 72*(suppl_1), S76–S81. https://doi.org/10.1093/gerona/glw229

Feng, Z, Fennell, ML, Tyler, DA, Clark, M, & Mor, V. (2011). Growth of racial and ethnic minorities in us nursing homes driven by demographics and possible disparities in options. *Health Affairs, 30*(7), 1358–1365. https://doi.org/10.1377/hlthaff.2011.0126

Fuller-Thomson, E., Brennenstuhl, S., & Hurd, M. (2011). Comparison of disability rates among older adults in aggregated and separate Asian American/Pacific Islander subpopulations. *American Journal of Public Health, 101*(1), 94–100. https://doi.org/10.2105/AJPH.2009.176784

Fuller-Thomson, E., & Chi, M. (2012). Older Asian Americans and Pacific Islanders with Activities of Daily Living (ADL) limitations: immigration and other factors associated with institutionalization. *International Journal of Environmental Research and Public Health, 9*(9), 3264–3279. https://doi.org/10.3390/ijerph9093264

Ge, S., Wu, B., Bailey, D. E., Jr., Dong, X. (2017) Social support, social strain, and cognitive function among community-dwelling U.S. Chinese older adults. *The Journals of Gerontology. Series B, Biological Sciences and Medical Sciences, 72* (Suppl 1), S16–S21. http://doi.org/10.1093/gerona/glw221

Geng, Y., Lo, J. C., Brickner, L., Gordon, N. P. (2017) Racial-ethnic differences in fall prevalence among older women: A cross-sectional survey study. *BMC Geriatrics 17*(1), 65. http://doi.org/10.1186/s12877-017-0447-y

Han, B. H., Ferris, R., Blaum, C. (2014). Exploring ethnic and racial differences in falls among older adults. *Journal of Community Health, 39*(6),1241–1247. http://doi.org/10.1007/s10900-014-9852-8

Hei, A., & Dong, X. (2017). Association Between Neighborhood Cohesion and Self-Neglect in Chinese-American Older Adults. *Journal of the American Geriatrics Society, 65*(12), 2720–2726. https://doi.org/10.1111/jgs.15147

Israel, B. A., Schulz, A. J., Parker, E. A., Becker, A. B., Allen, A. J., III , & Guzman, J. R. (2008). *Critical issues in developing and following community based participatory research principles.* In M. Minkler , & N. Wallerstein (Eds.), Community-based participatory research for health (pp. 46 – 66). San Francisco: Jossey-Bass

Kalibatseva, Z., & Leong, F. T. (2011). Depression among Asian Americans: Review and Recommendations. *Depression Research and Treatment, 2011*, 320902. https://doi.org/10.1155/2011/320902

Kamp, J., & Mathews, A. W. (2020) *As U.S. Nursing-home Deaths Reach 50,000, States Ease Lockdowns.* Wall Street Journal. https://www.wsj.com/articles/coronavirus-deaths-in-u-s-nursing-long-term-care-facilities-top-50-000-11592306919

Kim, G., Worley, C. B., Allen, R. S., Vinson, L., Crowther, M. R., Parmelee, P., & Chiriboga, D. A. (2011). Vulnerability of older Latino and Asian immigrants with limited English proficiency. *Journal of the American Geriatrics Society, 59*(7), 1246–1252. https://doi.org/10.1111/j.1532-5415.2011.03483.x

Kwak, J., & Salmon, J. R. (2007). Attitudes and preferences of Korean-American older adults and caregivers on end-of-life care. *Journal of the American Geriatrics Society, 55*(11), 1867–1872. https://doi.org/10.1111/j.1532-5415.2007.01394.x

Kwon, S. C, Han, B. H., Kranick, J. A, Wyatt, L. C., Blaum, C. S., Yi, S. S., & Trinh-Shevrin, C. (2018). Racial and Ethnic Difference in Falls Among Older Adults: Results from the California Health Interview Survey. *Journal of Racial and Ethnic Health Disparities. 5*(2), 271–278. https://doi.org/10.1007/s40615-017-0367-8

Lee, S., Martins, S., Keyes, K., Lee, H. (2011) Mental health service use by persons of Asian ancestry with DSM-IV mental disorders in the United States. *Psychiatric Services 62*, 1180–1186. http://doi.org/10.1176/appi.ps.62.10.1180

Lee, S., Xue, Q., Spira, A,, Lee, H. (2014). Racial and ethnic differences in depressive subtypes and access to mental health care in the United States. *Journal of Affective Disorders, 155*,130–7. http://doi.org/10.1016/j.jad.2013.10.037

Li, L. W., Ding, D., Wu, B., Dong, X. (2017). Change of cognitive function in U.S. Chinese older adults: A population-based study. *The Journals of Gerontology. Series B, Biological Sciences and Medical Sciences, 72* (Suppl 1), S5–S10. http://doi.org/10.1093/gerona/glx004

Li, L. W., & Dong, X. (2017). Self-reported Discrimination and Depressive Symptoms Among Older Chinese Adults in Chicago. *The Journals of Gerontology. Series A, Biological Sciences and Medical Sciences, 72* (suppl_1), S119–S124. https://doi.org/10.1093/gerona/glw174

Lillie-Blanton, M., & Hoffman, S. C. (1995). Conducting an assessment of health needs and resources in a racial/ethnic minority community. *Health Services Research, 30*(1 Pt 2), 225–236. Retrieved from https://pubmed.ncbi.nlm.nih.gov/7721594

Liu, J., Dong, X., Nguyen, D., & Lai, D. (2017). Family Relationships and Depressive Symptoms Among Chinese Older Immigrants in the United States. *The Journals of Gerontology. Series A, Biological Sciences and Medical Sciences, 72*(suppl_1), S113–S118. https://doi.org/10.1093/gerona/glw138

LoPresti, M. A., Dement, F., & Gold, H. T. (2016). End-of-Life Care for People With Cancer From Ethnic Minority Groups: A Systematic Review. The American journal of hospice & palliative care, 33(3), 291–305. https://doi.org/10.1177/1049909114565658

Mayeda, E. R., Glymour, M. M., Quesenberry, C. P., Jr, Whitmer R. A. (2017). Heterogeneity in 14-year Dementia Incidence Between Asian American Subgroups. *Alzheimer Disease and Associated Disorders. 31*(3), 181–186. http://doi.org/10.1097/WAD.0000000000000189

Mehta, K. M., Yeo, G. W. (2017). Systematic review of dementia prevalence and incidence in United States race/ethnic populations. *Alzheimer's & Dementia: The Journal of the Alzheimer's Association. 13*(1), 72–83. http://doi.org/10.1016/j.jalz.2016.06.2360

Mendes de Leon, C. F., Barnes, L. L., Bienias, J. L., Skarupski, K. A., Evans, D. A. (2005). Racial disparities in disability: Recent evidence from self-reported and performance-based disability measures in a population-based study of older adults. *The Journals of Gerontology, Series B: Psychol Sciences and Social Sciences. 60*, S263–S271. https://doi.org/10.1093/geronb/60.5.S263

Minkler M. (2005). Community-based research partnerships: challenges and opportunities. *Journal of Urban Health: Bulletin of the New York Academy of Medicine, 82*(2 Suppl 2), ii3–ii12. https://doi.org/10.1093/jurban/jti034

Minkler, M., Roe, K. M., & Price, M. (1992). The physical and emotional health of grandmothers raising grandchildren in the crack cocaine epidemic. *The Gerontologist, 32*(6), 752–761. https://doi.org/10.1093/geront/32.6.752

Moreno-John, G., Fleming, C., Ford, M. E., Lichtenberg, P., Mangione, C. M., Pérez-Stable, E. J., Tilley, B., Washington, O. G., & Carrasquillo, O. (2007). Mentoring in community-based participatory research: the RCMAR experience. *Ethnicity & Disease, 17*(1 Suppl 1), S33–S43.

Nam, Y. (2008). Welfare reform and older immigrants' health insurance coverage. *American Journal of Public Health, 98*(11), 2029–2034. Retrieved from https://pubmed.ncbi.nlm.nih.gov/18799779

National Institute on Aging. *Aging Well in the 21st Centry: Strategic Directions for Research on Aging 2016*. Retrieved from https://www.nia.nih.gov/about/aging-well-21st-century-strategic-directions-research-aging

National Coalition for Asian Pacific American Community Development. (2016). *Findings on financial security for AAPI seniors and their families*. Retrieved on March 18, 2020, from https://www.aarp.org/content/dam/aarp/home-and-family/asian-community/2016/09/capacd-report-aarp-2016.pdf?intcmp=AE-ASIAN-COMMUNITY

Nguyen D. (2011) Acculturation and perceived mental health need among older Asian immigrants. *Journal of Behavioral Health Services and Research, 38*(4), 526–33. http://doi.org/10.1007/s11414-011-9245-z

Norris, K. C., Brusuelas, R., Jones, L., Miranda, J., Duru, O. K., & Mangione, C. M. (2007). Partnering with community-based organizations: An academic institution's evolving perspective. *Ethnicity & Disease. 17*, S27–S32.

Pew Research Center. (2017). *Cambodians in the US Fact Sheet*. Retrieved on March 18, 2020, from: https://www.pewsocialtrends.org/fact-sheet/asian-americans-cambodians-in-the-u-s/

Sadarangani, T. (2020) *How to help seniors now: Coronavirus social distancing only exacerbates some of their pressing needs*. Nydailynews.Com. Retrieved July 27, 2021, from https://www.nydailynews.com/opinion/ny-oped-how-to-help-seniors-now-20200421-osnfcmnvirfx5c3frqc4ngvwd4-story.html

Sadarangani, T., Beasley, J.M., Yi, S.S., Chodosh, J. (2020). Enriching Nutrition Programs to Better Serve the Needs of a Diversifying Aging Population. *Family and Community Health, 43*(2), 100–105. http://doi.org/10.1097/FCH.0000000000000250

Sadarangani, T, Missaelides, L, Eilertsen, E, Jaganathan, H, & Wu, B. (2019). A mixed-methods evaluation of a nurse-led community-based health home for ethnically diverse older adults with multimorbidity in the adult day health setting. *Policy, Politics, & Nursing Practice*, 20(3), 131–144. https://doi.org/10.1177/1527154419864301

Sadarangani, TR, Murali, KP. (2018). Service use, participation, experiences, and outcomes among older adult immigrants in american adult day service centers: An integrative review of the literature. Research in Gerontological Nursing, 11(6), 317–328. https://doi.org/10.3928/19404921-20180629-01

Sadarangani, T.R., Trinh-Shevrin, C., Chyun, D., Yu, G., & Kovner, C. (2019). Cardiovascular risk in middle-aged and older immigrants: Exploring residency period and health insurance coverage. *Journal of Nursing Scholarship, 51*(3), 326–336. http://doi.org/10.1111/jnu.12465

Suh, E. E., Kagan, S., & Strumpf, N. (2009). Cultural competence in qualitative interview methods with Asian immigrants. *Journal of Transcultural Nursing: Official Journal of the Transcultural Nursing Society*, 20(2), 194–201. https://doi.org/10.1177/1043659608330059

Taira, B. R., & Orue, A. (2019). Language assistance for limited English proficiency patients in a public ED: determining the unmet need. *BMC Health Services Research, 19*(1), 56. https://doi.org/10.1186/s12913-018-3823-1

Takaki, R. (1998). *Strangers from a different shore: A history of Asian Americans*. Harcourt Brace Jovanovich.

United States Citizenship and Immigration Services. (2020). *Final rule on public charge ground on inadmissibility*. Retrieved on March 18, 2020, from https://www.uscis.gov/archive/archive-news/final-rule-public-charge-ground-inadmissibility

Wang, S. Y., Hsu, S. H., Aldridge, M. D., Cherlin, E., Bradley E. (2019) Racial differences in health care transitions and hospice use at the end of life. *Journal of Palliative Medicine*. 22(6), 619–627. http://doi.org/10.1089/jpm.2018.0436

Weng, S. S. (2017). Issues of Aging: An Exploration of Asian American Families in the Southern Region of the United States from the Perspective of Community Leaders. *Journal of Cross-cultural Gerontology, 32*(4), 461–477. https://doi.org/10.1007/s10823-017-9322-8

Xu, L., Tang, F., Li, L. W., Dong, X. Q. (2017). Grandparent caregiving and psychological well-being among Chinese American older adults: The roles of caregiving burden and pressure. *The Journals of Gerontology, Series A: Biological Sciences and Medical Sciences*. 72 (suppl_1), S56–S62. http://doi.org/10.1093/gerona/glw186

Zhan, L., Cloutterbuck, J., Keshian, J., & Lombardi, L. (1998). Promoting health: perspectives from ethnic elderly women. *Journal of Community Health Nursing, 15*(1), 31–44. https://doi.org/10.1207/s15327655jchn1501_4

Zimmerman, M. A. (2000). Empowerment theory: Psychological, organizational, and community levels of analysis. In J. Rappaport & E. Seidman (Eds.), *Handbook of community psychology* (pp. 43–63). Kluwer Academic Publishers. https://doi.org/10.1007/978-1-4615-4193-6_2

CHAPTER

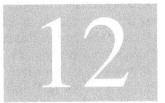

MULTIPLE MARGINALIZATION AMONG ASIAN AMERICAN POPULATIONS

SAHNAH LIM, JOHN J. CHIN, CHRISTINA Y. LEE

LEARNING OBJECTIVES

By the end of this chapter, readers will be able to:

- Understand the structural factors that shape and perpetuate multiple marginalization among Asian Americans, particularly the role of immigration and stigma as critical determinants of health inequity in Asian American populations.

- Understand the impact of multiple marginalization on the health and well-being of Asian Americans.

- Learn how an intersectional framework, community-based participatory research principles, and trauma-informed principles may enhance the impact of research when working with multiply marginalized populations.

Applied Population Health Approaches for Asian American Communities, First Edition. Edited by Simona C. Kwon, Chau Trinh-Shevrin, Nadia S. Islam, and Stella S. Yi.
© 2023 John Wiley & Sons, Inc. Published 2023 by John Wiley & Sons, Inc.
Companion Website: www.wiley.com/go/kwon/asianamerican

INTRODUCTION

As elaborated in previous chapters, despite experiencing disparities in a wide range of health outcomes, Asian Americans remain an underresearched population, comprising numerous distinct ethnic and linguistic groups whose health needs remain poorly understood. Yet even within this paradigm of marginalization, some subgroups of Asian Americans receive even less attention in terms of policy, funding, and research. These groups cross the lines of ethnic origin and include individuals that experience multiple forms of marginalization due to the fact that they not only are members of a racial minority group within the broader U.S. population but also identify with other cross-cutting minority, oppressed, or stigmatized groups, such as Asian American women, transgender Asian Americans, or Asian American sex workers. In this chapter, we specifically draw attention to the following multiply marginalized Asian American subgroups: sexual and gender minority (SGM) individuals, individuals living with HIV/AIDS, and survivors of gender-based violence (GBV). We also present a case study describing the experiences of Asian immigrant female sex workers in massage parlors. Throughout the chapter, we apply the theoretical framework of intersectionality to highlight the role of multiple marginalization in contributing to negative health consequences for these individuals.

THEORETICAL CONCEPTS

Intersectionality

Intersectionality is a valuable framework for understanding health inequity among multiply marginalized populations. The theory of intersectionality draws attention to the multiple forms of oppression and sources of resilience for those who belong to more than one marginalized social group (Bowleg, 2012; Crenshaw, 1989). To date, public health research typically has focused on exploring a single structural factor (e.g., racism) and its impact on health. Intersectionality, by contrast, simultaneously examines the full range of contextual factors that multiply marginalized populations may face (e.g., racism *and* sexism together). Intersectionality further posits that the impact of these co-occurring "-isms" are not simply additive but multiplicative. While its application has increased in recent years, intersectionality remains relatively underused within mainstream public health (Bowleg, 2012). Intersectionality has the potential to provide scholars with a critical unifying framework (both interpretive and analytical) to advance our understanding of how health inequities emerge and persist. Equally important, applying an intersectional lens to public health issues prompts scholars to examine factors driving health at multiple levels of influence.

Marginalization Within Ethnic Communities

Asian Americans who are members of additionally marginalized or oppressed groups (e.g., sexual and gender minorities, women, sex workers, people living with HIV, etc.) experience intersectional stigma as Asian Americans in combination with these other identities. Although stigmatization may have origins in society at large, multiply marginalized Asian Americans often experience marginalization most immediately within their own ethnic communities. Our exploration of this complex dynamic in this chapter is not meant to suggest that Asian American communities are more sexist, homophobic, or stigmatizing than other communities or the wider society. Rather, these communities have unique characteristics that may impact the ways Asian Americans experience multiple marginalization and, as such, they merit closer examination as we seek to characterize and better understand the diversity of Asian American health experiences.

Faced with linguistic and cultural barriers, discrimination, disrupted familial and social arrangements, and economic hardship, Asian immigrants may seek stability by turning toward their traditions and relying on their ethnic community for practical, social, and emotional support (Basch et al., 1994; Guest, 2003; Loue et al., 1999; Zhou, 1992). Immigrant community institutions, such as religious centers and social clubs, play an important role in creating places where immigrants can find resources to help them adjust to life in their new country while also reproducing many aspects of the culture and lifestyle they experienced in their countries of origin. These places, often ethnic enclaves in urban areas, serve not only immigrant residents in the immediate area but also those in outlying suburbs, who come to the immigrant neighborhood for ethnic resources, including places to worship, shop, and participate in cultural activities (Khandelwal, 2002). The traditional mores that may be seen by community members as helping to protect these enclaves and strengthen social bonds within them, may reinforce stigma, taboos, and discriminatory traditions, intensifying the marginalization experienced by some subgroups within their own racial/ethnic communities.

In this way, immigrant communities, like other social landscapes, are products of both "cultural and politico-economic" forces (Kearns & Moon, 2002, p. 610). Within immigrant communities, this intersection is mediated partly through immigrant community institutions, both as actors and more passively as gathering places. Understanding the experiences of multiply marginalized individuals within Asian American communities requires ". . .foreground[ing] the more opaque instances of exclusion, opaque, that is, from a mainstream or majority perspective, the ones which do not make the news or are taken for granted as part of the routine of daily life. These exclusionary practices are important because they are less noticed and so the ways in which control is exercised in society are concealed (Sibley, 1995, p. ix)."

Much of the immigration literature paints immigrant communities as supportive places where immigrants may be buffered from discrimination in the larger society, gain an economic foothold, and work toward attaining upward mobility for their children, if not for themselves (e.g., Zhou, 1992). Conversely, some research characterizes the immigrant community as designed to solidify the power of some subgroups over others in an exploitative ethnic economy that benefits immigrant business owners but not their co-ethnic immigrant workers (e.g., Kwong, 1987). Both functions of the immigrant community respond to and rely on the physical or social separation of immigrants from the larger society.

The maintenance of power differentials within immigrant communities may also be viewed through a feminist lens, focusing on power imbalances fundamentally based on gender even if they have economic implications. Abraham's seminal study of domestic violence in South Asian immigrant communities in the United States – which included narratives from women of Bangladeshi, Indian, and Pakistani origin – specifically pointed to the role of key community institutions in supporting traditional gender role norms, contending that religious institutions' role as protectors of the ethnic community inhibits their response to instances of domestic violence (Abraham, 2000). According to Abraham:

> . . . religious institutions are not places of prayer alone but, more important, are the arena for the construction and maintenance of values, beliefs, and customs of the immigrant community. . . . These centers of worship become the caretakers of tradition in an alien, modernistic society. The moral solidarity of the collective becomes of vital importance. (Abraham, 2000, p. 120)

In her view, religious institutions' failure to support or defend women who are targets of domestic violence is "largely a function of perceiving religion as the last bastion for the collective maintenance of traditional South Asian values (Abraham, 2000, p. 121)."

Community leaders may not explicitly link the promotion of traditional social norms to the support of a particular social, gender, or economic structure. Rather, their discourse may center on protecting cherished and immutable traditions of the ethnic group or defending moral standards in the community (Ang, 1993; Kwong, 1987; Ong, 1993). For example, the Korean church has assumed the secular function of supporting Korean immigrant small-business success by reinforcing "members' values of self-control and hard work by constantly emphasizing self-abnegation, endurance, hardship, and frugality" in religious teachings (Kim, 1987). The linking of social norms to moral or religious positions, rather than to situational and changing gender roles and economic circumstances, creates an environment where the enforcement of social norms is seen as an important goal in itself. In her classic work, *Purity and Danger*, anthropologist Mary Douglas (2002) suggested that although cultural norms and taboos are ever-changing, they may be characterized and promoted as static and primordial in order to reinforce the prevailing community structure. She wrote, "Taboo protects the local consensus on how the world is organized" (Douglas, 2002, p. xi) and that challenges to this consensus are inhibited by promoting fear of harm that may result from not adhering to norms. Change may come slowly and with difficulty since consistency protects groups that enjoy disproportionate benefits.

Intersectional Stigma

The enforcement of cultural norms can result in stigma when "elements of labeling, stereotyping, separation, status loss, and discrimination co-occur," a phenomenon that is explicitly enabled by the inequitable distribution of power across social groups (Hatzenbuehler et al., 2013). Stigma is a multidimensional construct, conceptualized as internalized, perceived, anticipated, or enacted (i.e., discriminatory acts) (Kane et al., 2019; Link & Phelan, 2001). Combining the concepts of intersectionality and stigma, intersectional stigma is defined as co-occurring forms of stigma among those holding multiply marginalized social identities. As such, stigma is gaining attention as a critical social determinant of health. In public health research, intersectional stigma has mostly been examined in the context of HIV outcomes and through the use of qualitative methods (Logie et al., 2011; Quinn et al., 2019; Rice et al., 2018) but can and should be applied more frequently when discussing health disparities among multiply marginalized Asian American populations. For example, studies have examined the role of various types of stigma in HIV prevention among Asian immigrant female sex workers but few have explicitly focused on intersectional stigma, despite their facing the convergence of multiple and intersectional stigmas including anti-Asian, anti-immigrant, anti-sex work, and HIV-related stigma. Figure 12.1 illustrates multilevel intersectional stigma affecting HIV prevention behaviors among Asian immigrant female sex workers; we elaborate on the experiences of this population in Case 13 in the Appendix.

Community-Based Participatory Research and Trauma-Informed Approaches

Operationalizing the intersectionality framework to examine the impact of immigration and stigma on multiply marginalized Asian American groups requires researchers and program planners to integrate appropriate research methodologies into their work. Community-based participatory research (CBPR) and trauma-informed care are key methodologies for this purpose. As discussed in Chapters 2 and 8, CBPR calls for equitable power sharing by researchers, community partners, and research participants (Israel et al., 2003). CBPR explicitly recognizes

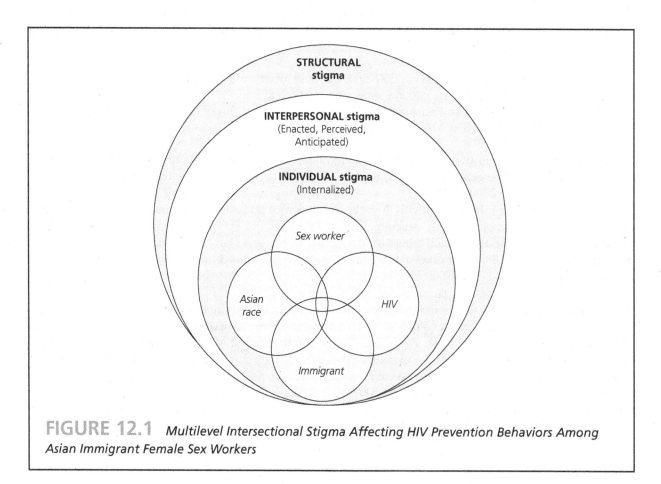

FIGURE 12.1   *Multilevel Intersectional Stigma Affecting HIV Prevention Behaviors Among Asian Immigrant Female Sex Workers*

the power imbalance between these three parties – an issue that is inherently magnified when working with multiply marginalized populations. CBPR entails co-decision-making between the researchers, community partners. and/or research participants, involving all stakeholders in each stage of research. Complementing the CBPR approach, studies may be conducted using trauma-informed approaches, which prioritize minimizing the retraumatization of participants (Elliott et al., 2005). To date, the focus of this field has been on preparing service and clinical providers to deliver care within a safe, nontriggering space through recognition of the connection between trauma and health (Miller & Najavits, 2012) as well as through empathetic interactions with clients and patients to promote resilience and empowerment (Randall & Haskell, 2013). Campbell (2019), an advocate and researcher working with survivors of GBV, recently outlined key principles of trauma-informed care adapted for research, which included referral to culturally competent trauma services and using participatory research methods (Campbell et al., 2019). Subsequent sections in this chapter will highlight the disproportionate exposure to trauma and burden of mental health disorders in specific Asian American groups – a disparity that is driven largely by the multiple marginalization and intersectional stigma that these populations face.

While valuable as independent methodologies, CBPR and trauma-informed approaches may be combined effectively to enhance the impact of health equity research. We will illustrate the value of this combined approach by presenting two real-world research examples. First, in 2019, the authors of this chapter sought to describe qualitatively the factors influencing recovery and well-being among international Asian survivors of sex trafficking in New York City (NYC) (Lim, Lee, et al., 2020). To conduct this study, we established a community-based partnership with Sanctuary for Families (Sanctuary) – one of the largest service providers for survivors of GBV in the United States with a dedicated anti-trafficking program. Sanctuary was involved in the development of the research questions and research instruments, implementation of the research, and interpretation and dissemination of results. In order to minimize re-traumatization, researchers did not make the first contact with survivors. Instead, Sanctuary staff evaluated survivors to determine whether they were emotionally prepared to participate in research. Additionally, interview guides were carefully reviewed by Sanctuary's mental health counselors; questions did not directly ask about sex trafficking unless the participant volunteered the information. In addition, a mental health counselor was available consistently on site during and after the interview in case the participant desired support.

Second, in 2020, we conducted a study to explore the prevalence of and attitudes related to sexual violence among South Asian young adults in the New York Tri-State area – a region that encompasses NYC and parts of its neighboring states (New York, New Jersey and Connecticut). The study involved an anonymous online survey conducted among nearly 400 participants who self-identified as South Asian (Lim, Mohaimin, et al., 2020). The survey development, participant recruitment, and implementation were guided by members of RAISSE (Research & Action Improving South-Asian Sexual Education), an advisory board comprised of South Asian young adult women specifically convened for the purposes of this study. In order to protect participant safety and confidentiality, an "exit" button was provided throughout the survey so that participants could exit the browser as needed. Participants were also reminded several times during the survey to clear their browsing history. A list of curated and culturally tailored resources specific to the Tri-State area were provided at the end of the survey. At the time of writing this chapter, RAISSE was spearheading a multi-pronged effort to disseminate study results to the communities of interest – a key component of CBPR that too often may be missed as researchers complete their work with community partners. The effort included development and dissemination of a community brief in plain language describing study results as well as a complete research report that included comprehensive data and findings. RAISSE was also preparing to present results at a planned community listening session on GBV targeted toward Asian American service providers, young adult leaders, and sexual violence survivors.

We now turn to describing how multiple marginalization adversely impacts the health of specific Asian American subgroups, including SGM populations, individuals living with HIV/AIDS, survivors of GBV, and immigrant female sex workers in massage parlors.

ASIAN AMERICAN SGM POPULATIONS

Sexual minority populations comprise individuals who identify as lesbian, gay, or bisexual. Gender minority populations include individuals who may identify as transgender, nonbinary, gender queer and/or nonconforming. Collectively, the term *lesbian, gay, bisexual, transgender, and queer* (LGBTQ) is commonly used, with the understanding that the term may not be exhaustive. According to estimates from the U.S. 2010 American Community Survey, there are approximately 32,931 Asian American and Pacific Islander (PI) adults in same-sex relationships living in the United States, accounting for 0.4% of all Asian American and PI households (Kastanis & Gates, 2013). Individuals in Asian American and PI same-sex households tend to live in states where there are higher numbers of Asian American and PI individuals overall, such as Hawaii, California, and New York. In addition to the lack of population size estimates, there is a general lack of research conducted with Asian American LGBTQ populations, particularly among those who identify as gender minority, intersex, and asexual individuals.

Limited research has shown that LGBTQ Asian Americans have high incidence rates of substance use, sexual risk behaviors, and mental health problems such as depression, anxiety, post-traumatic stress disorder, and suicidality (Tan et al., 2016; Choi et al., 2013; Lee & Hahm, 2012). Lifetime prevalence rates of depression are reportedly as high as 97% among LGBTQ Asian Americans (Ching et al., 2018). Data from national surveys indicate greater risk of suicidal ideation among LGB Asian Americans as compared to heterosexual Asian Americans (Cochran et al., 2007; Lytle et al., 2014). One study found that highly acculturated LGBQ South Asian men and women – including Indian, Pakistani, Bangladeshi, Sri Lankan and "Other South Asian" individuals – with higher degrees of "outness" experienced higher levels of psychological distress than those with lower degrees, a finding that is in direct contrast to results of research conducted among non-Hispanic Whites (Whites) (Sandil et al., 2015). Limited research has also identified unmet mental health care needs among lesbian and bisexual Asian American women, and limited availability of services tailored to the needs of the many diverse subgroups within this population (Hahm et al., 2016). These findings underscore the need for deeper exploration of mental health issues among LGBTQ Asian subgroups. Exposure to traumatic experiences, such as race- and sexuality-related stress, combined with the experiences of internalized stigma and maladaptive coping, have been found to be predictive of psychological distress in this population (Ching et al., 2018; Cochran et al., 2007; Szymanski & Henrichs-Beck, 2014; Szymanski & Sung, 2010).

LGBTQ Asian Americans, like other LGBTQ persons of color, are at risk of LGBTQ-specific assault and intimate partner violence (IPV) at rates higher than their White counterparts (Shim, 2018). Although IPV is highly prevalent among SGM communities, only limited research has explored IPV in the Asian American community (Kanuha, 2013; King et al., 2021).

Studies of intersectionality and minority stress, including racism toward people of color combined with heterosexism and homophobia experienced by LGBTQ people, have suggested that trends among Asian Americans may differ markedly from other ethnic groups. The higher burden of adverse health outcomes among Asian American SGM individuals have been attributed to the dual marginalization and discrimination experienced by Asian Americans who belong to both a racial/ethnic minority and a SGM group (McConnell et al., 2018; Szymanski & Sung, 2010). One internet-based study conducted among LBGTQ people of color demonstrated that, as compared to non-Hispanic Black (Black) and Latino LGBT individuals, Asian American LGBTQ individuals reported more relationship racism (e.g., being rejected by potential or current sexual partners because of their race/ethnicity) (Balsam et al., 2011).

Challenging the marginalization of LGBTQ individuals within Asian American populations would require communities to re-evaluate their core social norms – a major undertaking for any social group. If core social norms are perceived by community members as crucial for maintaining community structures, challenging them may be viewed as a threat to the very survival of the community. Even members of subgroups that might gain power from a change in social structure might be reluctant to pursue it in order to preserve order. This concept is illustrated by work examining women's gender roles within Asian communities. For example, Kibria's early qualitative research among Vietnamese immigrants in Philadelphia showed that Vietnamese women had to carefully balance two roles in their new environment: an increasingly important position as the family's primary interface with mainstream society and a subordinate role in relation to their husbands within the household, in line with their traditional family structure (Kibria, 1993). The women demonstrated an orientation toward collectivism and cooperation, which they felt were threatened by change. Thus, the women were reluctant to elevate their status in relation to men within the household, even as their status outside the home rose.

In short, more studies are needed to understand the impact of LGBTQ status on health care experiences and health disparities among Asian Americans. Directions for future study include patient, provider, and encounter-centered factors (Bi et al., 2019), as well as intrapersonal factors (such as stigma and minority stress), interpersonal factors (including verbal and nonverbal community discrimination stemming from implicit and automatic biases) and institutional factors, such as clinical policies and provider factors (Tan et al., 2016).

ASIAN AMERICANS LIVING WITH HIV/AIDS

Since the first cases of HIV emerged in 1981, the HIV/AIDS epidemic has disproportionately impacted racial/ethnic minorities and gay and bisexual men and other men who have sex with men (MSM). However, the HIV epidemic took a longer time to penetrate Asian American communities; while the absolute number of HIV/AIDS diagnoses remains relatively low in comparison to other racial groups, Asian Americans are the only racial group in the United States with a rising HIV infection rate (Kim & Aronowitz, 2019; CDC, 2019a).

Among the general U.S. population, male-to-male sexual contact remains a primary pathway for HIV transmission (CDC, 2019b, p. 110, Table 19a), underscoring another potential level of marginalization for the Asian American gay and bisexual male population. According to the most recent data available from the Centers for Disease Control (CDC), there were 14,244 reported cases of Asian Americans living with an HIV diagnosis in 2017 (CDC, 2019b, p. 107, Table 17b). In 2018, male-to-male sexual contact accounted for 683 of 766 new HIV infections among male Asian adults and adolescents in the United States. These data suggest that Asian American MSM comprise a key population of interest for HIV prevention, treatment, and support. There were 103 new infections among Asian female adults and adolescents, mostly ($n = 96$) through heterosexual contact (CDC, 2019b, p. 54, Table 3a), suggesting a need for tailored HIV prevention information and education for diverse groups of Asian American women who have sex with men. This group may include women who are at risk of contracting HIV from their husbands or boyfriends, as well as women working in the sex industry (see Case Study 13 in the Appendix). Studies have shown that Asian American women with lower perceived relationship power had higher rates of forced sex and HIV risk behaviors (Hahm et al., 2012).

One review reported that Asian Americans perceive themselves at low risk for contracting HIV and report high rates of HIV-associated stigma and depression (Kim & Aronowitz, 2019). Numerous studies have documented fear and stigma associated with HIV among Asian Americans and some have indicated that HIV-related stigma may be particularly intense among Asian immigrant communities (Chin & Kroesen, 1999; Eckholdt et al., 1997; Kang et al., 2003; Sy et al., 1998; Yoshikawa et al., 2001; Yoshioka & Schustack, 2001). Fear and stigma are related not only to HIV infection and disease but also to the association of HIV/AIDS with stigmatized behaviors, both in the larger society (Kaiser Family Foundation, 2002; Sibley, 1995) and in Asian immigrant communities (Choi et al., 1995; Takahashi, 1997). Qualitative work with Asian American immigrants living with HIV has suggested they are at high risk for depression and anxiety, job loss, excessive time spent seeking specialized HIV health care access, and disconnection from their usual social support due to HIV-related stigma (Chen et al., 2015). The high prevalence of hepatitis B and C among individuals of Asian descent may further complicate linkage and retention in care and treatment for HIV/AIDS (Russ et al., 2012).

Integrated, culturally and linguistically appropriate care is essential, but so, too, is systemic and provider awareness, which may influence an individual's decision to seek care. Availability and visibility of HIV-related services for Asian Americans must consider stigma in the planning and implementation of programs. For example, one AIDS-specific community-based organization in NYC serving Asian immigrants avoided storefront locations to safeguard the privacy of their clientele. Yet this same organization underwent a contentious debate with its HIV-positive Asian immigrant client population regarding having the word *AIDS,* which was part of the organization's name, on the door of the second-floor office. The conflict escalated to the point at which a client scratched the word from the professionally lettered sign on the door.[1] This conflict underscored the different perspectives of the organization's leadership – which aimed to elevate HIV education within the community and enhance AIDS-related service provision to Asian immigrants – and some of its clients – who continued to be fearful of being stigmatized by their diagnosis. Ultimately, the word *AIDS* was replaced and remained on the door, although a small group of clients continued to disagree with that practice.

ASIAN AMERICAN SURVIVORS OF GBV

GBV refers to harm that is perpetrated against an individual or group of individuals because of their gender and is a significant public health issue, including among Asian American and PI women. GBV takes many forms, including sexual or physical violence as well as verbal, psychological and socioeconomic violence that relies on gender-based imbalances of power. National data have shown that among adult women, nearly one in five women (18.3%) in the United States has been raped at some time during her life (Black et al., 2011). More than one-third (36%) reported lifetime prevalence of IPV (i.e., rape, physical violence, and/or stalking).

Survivors are at greater risk for chronic conditions (e.g., injuries, fibromyalgia, gastrointestinal disorders) and negative sexual and reproductive health outcomes (e.g., unsafe abortion, unplanned or unwanted pregnancy, miscarriage, sexually transmitted infections, including HIV, low birthweight). There are also extensive psychological and behavioral outcomes for Asian American survivors, such as depression and suicidality, substance use, eating disorders, post-traumatic stress disorder, and risky sexual behaviors (Buchanan et al., 2018; Hahm et al., 2017; La Flair et al., 2008). Survivors may also experience a short-term increase in risk of further violence when attempting to change their current life situation, emphasizing the need to be connected to services (Morrison et al., 2007). A unique mental health outcome within Asian Americans who experience IPV may be somatization, or the expression of mental disorders as physical symptoms. For some Asian immigrant women who have experienced IPV, they may experience symptoms such as fatigue, sleep difficulty, or chest pains, for example, which are considered manifestations of internalized victimization (Lee & Hadeed, 2009), which may pose an additional barrier in navigating health care and other resources for survivors.

According to national data, prevalence estimates of GBV among Asian American and PI populations are lower than those of other racial/ethnic groups. For example, 31.9% of Asian American and PI women have experienced other sexual violence not including rape, such as sexual coercion, unwanted sexual contact, and unwanted noncontact sexual experiences, which is lower than that of all other racial/ethnic groups (Breiding, 2014). Lifetime prevalence rates for Asian American and PI women for rape or stalking are not available due to insufficient case counts for developing reliable estimates from CDC's National Intimate Partner and Sexual Violence Survey, which is an ongoing, nationally representative telephone survey dedicated solely to monitoring intimate partner and sexual violence among adult women and men in the United States. Additionally, when available, prevalence estimates for these populations are typically presented in the aggregate, masking important disparities across Asian subgroups (Breiding, 2014). Some community-based or college-based studies that disaggregate by ethnicity or region report much higher estimates of sexual violence (KAN-WIN, 2017; Shenoy et al., 2009). In one report by a community-based organization that primarily surveyed Asian women (majority Korean, Chinese, Filipino, mixed race, other Asian ethnicities), more than half (53.5%) of the sample reported experiencing sexual violence (KAN-WIN, 2017).

Rates of GBV are likely underreported among Asian American and PI survivors. For example, limited research has shown that Asian American women report IPV at lower rates than women of other ethnicities (Crowne et al., 2012), which may be a reflection of the lack of in-language, culturally tailored, accessible services for women from diverse Asian subgroups. Among first-generation immigrants, IPV reporting rates may be especially low due to fear of deportation, low literacy, and lack of trust (Nije-Carr et al., 2019), while among children of immigrants, IPV has been linked to childhood abuse and mental health issues, such as depression and suicidal ideation (Hahm et al., 2017). Limited research within Asian subgroups underscores important differences among these communities. A study conducted among the Asian Indian Gujarati community in Detroit found that length of time in the United States did not impact patriarchal gender roles (Yoshihama et al., 2014). Because those roles were linked to IPV-supporting attitudes, risk of IPV did not decline with time in the United States. This finding differs markedly from other immigrant groups and highlights the urgent need for community-based participatory approaches to engage Asian American women of different ethnic subgroups to develop culturally appropriate approaches to this issue in their communities. See Case 13 in the Appendix for an example of such an approach.

SUMMARY AND RECOMMENDATIONS

This chapter sought to illuminate how multiple marginalization among Asian Americans is shaped and perpetuated and how it impacts health disparities. Multiply marginalized Asian Americans face a confluence of "-isms" and "-phobias," including racism, sexism, heterosexism, homophobia, and xenophobia. Health-related data for multiply marginalized Asian American communities are sorely lacking, in part due to the broader omission of Asian Americans from federally funded and other research (see Chapter 13). We highlighted the role of intersectional stigma, immigration, and cultural and community factors (e.g., community institutions) in potentiating adverse health outcomes and impacting overall well-being.

The following recommendations from the chapter's authors are not exhaustive, and we hope that they provide the foundation for more robust discussion, increased interest, and a keener imperative to work with multiply marginalized Asian American communities:

- We invite stakeholders interested in working with these communities to consider applying an intersectional framework as both an interpretative and analytic tool. In particular, policies, programs, and research – including programs or interventions that seek to reduce community-level stigma toward these groups – should seek to address intersectional stigma as a critical determinant of health.

- In recognition of the high levels of recurring exposure to trauma in multiply marginalized groups, we encourage the incorporation of trauma-informed principles in the conduct of programs and research in these populations. Further, CBPR and trauma-informed principles may complement each other to produce greater empowerment and impact in advancing health equity among multiply marginalized Asian American populations.

- Interventions and programs should focus on factors at multiple levels of influence, with particular attention to structural- and community-level factors that address the social determinants of health.

  - Social norms concerning appropriate behaviors and topics of discussion, overall and in particular venues, may be particularly potent barriers to effective public health efforts to serve multiply marginalized populations. Enlisting influential immigrant community institutions in raising awareness, combating stigma, and changing norms may be a vitally important first step that could allow subsequent direct interventions in these populations to be more effective. Understanding how proposed organizational changes are perceived by community institutions as either enhancing or threatening their roles may help to refine strategies for increasing institutional involvement and identifying their potential strengths and weaknesses to partner with public health researchers and others in this work.

DISCUSSION QUESTIONS

1. What are some culturally specific or unique forms of stigma in Asian American communities that may lead to adverse health outcomes?

2. What are some pathways by which immigration acts as a social determinant of health among Asian Americans, including among multiply marginalized Asian Americans?

3. What are some other multiply marginalized Asian American populations that have not been discussed in this chapter, and what specific types of marginalization do these populations face?

NOTE

1. This example is drawn from personal communication between the author and the executive director and program director of the organization.

REFERENCES

Abraham, M. (2000). *Speaking the Unspeakable: Marital Violence among South Asian Immigrants in the United States*. New Brunswick, NJ: Rutgers University Press.

Ang, I. (1993). To be or not to be Chinese: diaspora, culture and postmodern ethnicity. *Southeast Asian Journal of Social Science, 21*(1), 1–17.

Balsam, K. F., Molina, Y., Beadnell, B., Simoni, J., & Walters, K. (2011). Measuring multiple minority stress: the LGBT People of Color Microaggressions Scale. *Cultural Diversity and Ethnic Minority Psychology, 17*(2), 163.

Basch, L., Glick Schiller, N., & Szanton Blanc, C. (1994). *Nations Unbound: Transnational Projects, Postcolonial Predicaments, and Deterritorialized Nation-States*. Langhorne, PA: Gordon and Breach.

Bi., S., Gunter, K. E., & Lopez, F. Y. (2019). Improving shared decision making for Asian American Pacific Islander sexual and gender minorities. *Medical Care. 57*(12), 937–944. https://doi.org/10.1097/MLR.0000000000001212

Black, M., Basile, K., Breiding, M., Smith, S., Walters, M., Merrick, M., Chen, J., & Stevens, M. (2011). National intimate partner and sexual violence survey: 2010 summary report.

Bowleg, L. (2012). The problem with the phrase women and minorities: intersectionality-an important theoretical framework for public health. *Am J Public Health, 102*(7), 1267–1273. doi:10.2105/AJPH.2012.300750

Breiding, M. J. (2014). Prevalence and characteristics of sexual violence, stalking, and intimate partner violence victimization – National Intimate Partner and Sexual Violence Survey, United States, 2011. *Morbidity and Mortality Weekly Report.* Surveillance summaries (Washington, DC: 2002), *63*(8), 1.

Buchanan, N. T., Settles, I. H., Wu, I. H., & Hayashino, D. S. (2018). Sexual harassment, racial harassment, and well-being among Asian American women: An intersectional approach. *Women & Therapy, 41*(3–4), 261–280.

Campbell, R., Goodman-Williams, R., & Javorka, M. (2019). A Trauma-Informed Approach to Sexual Violence Research Ethics and Open Science. *J Interpers Violence, 34*(23–24), 4765–4793. doi:10.1177/0886260519871530

Centers for Disease Control and Prevention (CDC). (2019). *CDC HIV* Prevention Progress Report, 2019. Retrieved from https://www.cdc.gov/hiv/pdf/policies/progressreports/cdc-hiv-preventionprogressreport.pdf. Accessed February 21, 2020.

Centers for Disease Control and Prevention. (2019). HIV Surveillance Report, 2018 (Preliminary). Retrieved from Atlanta: http://www.cdc.gov/hiv/library/reports/hiv-surveillance.html

Chen, W. T., Guthrie, B., Shiu, C. S., Wang, L., Weng, Z., Li, C. S., Lee, T. S., Kamitani, E., Fukuda, Y., & Luu, B. V. (2015). Revising the American dream: How Asian immigrants adjust after an HIV diagnosis. *Journal of Advanced Nursing, 71*(8), 1914–1925. https://doi.org/10.1111/jan.12645

Chin, D., & Kroesen, K. W. (1999). Disclosure of HIV infection among Asian/Pacific Islander American women: Cultural stigma and social support. *Cultural Diversity and Ethnic Minority Psychology, 5*(3), 222–235.

Ching, T. H., Lee, S. Y., Chen, J., So, R. P., & Williams, M. T. (2018). A model of intersectional stress and trauma in Asian American sexual and gender minorities. *Psychology of Violence, 8*(6), 657.

Choi, K. H., Coates, T. J., Catania, J. A., Lew, S., & Chow, P. (1995). High HIV risk among gay Asian and Pacific Islander men in San Francisco. *AIDS, 9*(3), 306–308.

Choi, K. H., Paul, J., Ayala, G., Boylan, R., & Gregorich, S. E. (2013). Experiences of discrimination and their impact on the mental health among African American, Asian and Pacific Islander, and Latino men who have sex with men. *American Journal of Public Health, 103*(5), 868–874. https://doi.org/10.2105/AJPH.2012.301052

Cochran, S. D., Mays, V. M., Alegria, M., Ortega, A. N., & Takeuchi, D. (2007). Mental health and substance use disorders among Latino and Asian American lesbian, gay, and bisexual adults. *Journal of Consulting and Clinical Psychology, 75*(5), 785. Retrieved from https://www.ncbi.nlm.nih.gov/pmc/articles/PMC2676845/pdf/nihms106337.pdf

Crenshaw, K. (1989). Demarginalization the Intersection of Race and Sex: A Black Feminist Critique of Antidiscrimination Doctrine, *Feminist Theory and Antiracist Politics.* Retrieved from https://chicagounbound.uchicago.edu/cgi/viewcontent.cgi?article=1052&context=uclf

Crowne, S. S., Juon, H. S., Ensminger, M., Bair-Merritt, M. H., & Duggan, A. (2012). Risk factors for intimate partner violence initiation and persistence among high psychosocial risk Asian and Pacific Islander women in intact relationships. *Women's Health Issues,* official publication of the Jacobs Institute of Women's Health, *22*(2), e181–e188. https://doi.org/10.1016/j.whi.2011.08.006

Douglas, M. (2002). *Purity and Danger.* London: Routledge.

Eckholdt, H. M., Chin, J. J., Manzon-Santos, J. A., & Kim, D. D. (1997). The needs of Asians and Pacific Islanders living with HIV in New York City. *AIDS Education & Prevention, 9*(6), 493–504.

Elliott, D. E., Bjelajac, P., Fallot, R. D., Markoff, L. S., & Reed, B. G. (2005). Trauma-informed or trauma-denied: Principles and implementation of trauma-informed services for women. *Journal of Community Psychology, 33*(4), 461–477.

Guest, K. J. (2003). *God in Chinatown: Religion and Survival in New York's Evolving Immigrant Community.* New York: New York University Press.

Hahm, H. C., Augsberger, A., Feranil, M., Jang, J., & Tagerman, M. (2017). The associations between forced sex and severe mental health, substance use, and HIV risk behaviors among Asian American women. *Violence Against Women, 23*(6), 671–691.

Hahm, H. C., Lee, J., Chiao, C., Valentine, A., & Lê Cook, B. (2016). Use of Mental Health Care and Unmet Needs for Health Care Among Lesbian and Bisexual Chinese-, Korean-, and Vietnamese-American Women. *Psychiatric Services* (Washington, DC), *67*(12), 1380–1383. https://doi.org/10.1176/appi.ps.201500356

Hahm, H. C., Lee, J., Rough, K., & Strathdee, S. A. (2012). Gender power control, sexual experiences, safer sex practices, and potential HIV risk behaviors among young Asian-American women. *AIDS Behav, 16*(1), 179–188. doi:10.1007/s10461-011-9885-2

Hatzenbuehler, M. L., Phelan, J. C., & Link, B. G. (2013). Stigma as a fundamental cause of population health inequalities. *Am J Public Health, 103*(5), 813–821. doi:10.2105/AJPH.2012.301069

Israel, B. A., Schulz, A. J., Parker, E. A., Becker, A. B., Allen, A. J., & Guzman, J. R. (2003). Critical issues in developing and following community-based participatory research principles. In M. Minkler & N. Wallerstein (Eds.), *Community-Based Participatory Research for Health* (pp. 53–76). San Francisco: Jossey-Bass.

Kaiser Family Foundation. (2002). Policy brief: Critical policy challenges in the third decade of the HIV/AIDS epidemic. Retrieved from Menlo Park, CA:

KAN-WIN. (2017). Community Survey Report On Sexual Violence in the Asian American/Immigrant Community. Retrieved from http://www.kanwin.org/downloads/sareport.pdf

Kane, J. C., Elafros, M. A., Murray, S. M., Mitchell, E. M. H., Augustinavicius, J. L., Causevic, S., & Baral, S. D. (2019). A scoping review of health-related stigma outcomes for high-burden diseases in low- and middle-income countries. *BMC Med, 17*(1), 17. doi:10.1186/s12916-019-1250-8

Kang, E., Rapkin, B. D., Springer, C., & Kim, J. H. (2003). The "Demon Plague" and access to care among Asian undocumented immigrants living with HIV disease in New York City. *Journal of Immigrant Health, 5*(2), 49–58.

Kanuha, V. K. (2013). "Relationships so loving and so hurtful": the constructed duality of sexual and racial/ethnic intimacy in the context of violence in Asian and Pacific Islander lesbian and queer women's relationships. *Violence Against Women, 19*(9), 1175–1196. https://doi.org/10.1177/1077801213501897

Kastanis, A., & Gates, G. J. (2013). LGBT Asian and Pacific Islander individuals and same-sex couples: Williams Institute, UCLA School of Law.

Kearns, R., & Moon, G. (2002). From medical to health geography: novelty, place and theory after a decade of change. *Progress in Human Geography, 26*(5), 605–625.

Khandelwal, M. S. (2002). *Becoming American, Being Indian: An Immigrant Community in New York City*. Ithaca: Cornell University Press.

Kibria, N. (1993). *Family Tightrope: The Changing Lives of Vietnamese Americans*. Princeton, NJ: Princeton University Press.

Kim, I. (1987). The Koreans: small business in an urban frontier. In N. Foner (Ed.), *New Immigrants in New York*. New York: Columbia University Press.

Kim, B., & Aronowitz, T. (2019). Invisible Minority: HIV Prevention Health Policy for the Asian American Population. *Policy, Politics, & Nursing Practice, 20*(1), 41–49. https://doi.org/10.1177/1527154419828843

King, W. M., Restar, A., & Operario, D. (2021). Exploring multiple forms of intimate partner violence in a gender and racially/ethnically diverse sample of transgender adults. *Journal of Interpersonal Violence, 36*(19–20). Advance online publication. https://doi.org/10.1177/0886260519876024

Kwong, P. (1987). *The New Chinatown*. New York: The Noonday Press.

La Flair, L. N., Franko, D. L., & Herzog, D. B. (2008). Sexual assault and disordered eating in Asian women. *Harvard Review of Psychiatry, 16*(4), 248–257.

Lee, Y.-S., & Hadeed, L. (2009). Intimate partner violence among Asian immigrant communities: Health/mental health consequences, help-seeking behaviors, and service utilization. *Trauma, Violence, & Abuse, 10*(2), 143–170.

Lee. J., & Hahm, H. C. (2012) HIV risk, substance use, and suicidal behaviors among Asian American lesbian and bisexual women. *AIDS Education and Prevention, 24*(6), 549–563. https://doi.org/10.1521/aeap.2012.24.6.549

Lim, S., Lee, S., Cohen, L., Chin, J. J., Trinh-Shevrin, C., & Islam, N. S. (2020). Understanding the multi-level factors that influence recovery and well-being for Asian survivors of international criminal sex trafficking in an urban U.S. city. [Under Review at *Journal of Interpersonal Violence*].

Lim, S., Mohaimin, S., Dhar, R., Chowdhury, L., Rahman, F., Islam, T., . . . Trinh-Shevrin, C. (2020). Prevalence, attitudes, and correlates of sexual violence among South Asian young adults in the New York City area. [Under preparation].

Link, B. G., & Phelan, J. C. (2001). Conceptualizing Stigma. *Annual Review of Sociology, 27*, 363–385.

Logie, C. H., James, L., Tharao, W., & Loutfy, M. R. (2011). HIV, gender, race, sexual orientation, and sex work: a qualitative study of intersectional stigma experienced by HIV-positive women in Ontario, Canada. *PLoS Med, 8*(11), e1001124. doi:10.1371/journal.pmed.1001124

Loue, S., Lane, S. D., Lloyd, L. S., & Loh, L. (1999). Integrating Buddhism and HIV Prevention in U.S. Southeast Asian Communities. *Journal of Health Care for the Poor and Underserved, 10*(1), 100–121.

Lytle, M. C., De Luca, S. M., & Blosnich, J. R. (2014). The influence of intersecting identities on self-harm, suicidal behaviors, and depression among lesbian, gay, and bisexual individuals. *Suicide and Life-Threatening Behavior, 44*(4), 384–391.

McConnell, E. A., Janulis, P., Phillips II, G., Truong, R., & Birkett, M. (2018). Multiple minority stress and LGBT community resilience among sexual minority men. *Psychology of Sexual Orientation and Gender Diversity, 5*(1), 1.

Miller, N. A., & Najavits, L. M. (2012). Creating trauma-informed correctional care: a balance of goals and environment. Eur J Psychotraumatol, 3. doi:10.3402/ejpt.v3i0.17246

Morrison, A., Ellsberg, M., & Bott, S. (2007). Addressing gender-based violence: a critical review of interventions. *The World Bank Research Observer, 22*(1), 25–51.

Nije-Carr, V. P. S., Sabri, B., Messing, J. T., Ward-Lasher, A., Johnson-Agbakwu, C. E., McKinley, C., Campion, N., Childress, S., Arscott, J., & Campbell, J. (2019). Methodological and ethical considerations in research with immigrant and refugee survivors of intimate partner violence. Journal of Interpersonal Violence. 886260519877951. https://doi.org/10.1177/0886260519877951

Ong, A. (1993). On the edge of empires: flexible citizenship among Chinese in diaspora. *Positions, 1*(3), 745–778.

Quinn, K., Bowleg, L., & Dickson-Gomez, J. (2019). "The fear of being Black plus the fear of being gay": The effects of intersectional stigma on PrEP use among young Black gay, bisexual, and other men who have sex with men. Soc Sci Med, 232, 86–93. doi:10.1016/j.socscimed.2019.04.042

Randall, M., & Haskell, L. (2013). Trauma-informed approaches to law: why restorative justice must understand trauma and psychological coping restorative justice. *Dalhousie Law Journal, 36*, 501–533. Retrieved from https://heinonline.org/HOL/P?h=hein.journals/dalholwj36&i=287

Rice, W. S., Logie, C. H., Napoles, T. M., Walcott, M., Batchelder, A. W., Kempf, M. C., Wingood, G. M., Konkle-Parker, D. J., Turan, B., Wilson, T. E., Johnson, M. O., Wiser, S. D., & Turan, J. M. (2018). Perceptions of intersectional stigma among diverse women living with HIV in the United States. Soc Sci Med, 208, 9–17. doi:10.1016/j.socscimed.2018.05.001

Russ, L. W., Meyer, A. C., Takahashi, L. M., Ou, S., Tran, J., Cruz, P., Magalong, M., & Candelario, J. (2012). Examining barriers to care: provider and client perspectives on the stigmatization of HIV-positive Asian Americans with and without viral hepatitis co-infection. *AIDS Care, 24*(10), 1302–1307. https://doi.org/10.1080/09540121.2012.658756

Sandil, R., Robinson, M., Brewster, M. E., Wong, S., & Geiger, E. (2015). Negotiating multiple marginalizations: experiences of South Asian LGBQ individuals. Cultural Diversity & *Ethnic Minority Psychology, 21*(1), 76–88. https://doi.org/10.1037/a0037070

Shenoy, D. P., Neranartkomol, R., Ashok, M., Chiang, A., Lam, A. G., & Trieu, S. L. (2009). Breaking Down the Silence. *Californian Journal of Health Promotion, 7*(2), 78–91.

Shim, H. S., Stacy; Kang, Esther; Kang, Eugene; Kim, Jean; Cho, Molly. (2018). With You: Queer & Trans Koreans Survive Violence. A Community-based Research Report. Retrieved from https://www.api-gbv.org/resources/with-you-queer-and-trans-koreans-surviving-violence-2018/

Sibley, D. (1995). *Geographies of Exclusion: Society and Difference in the West*. London and New York: Routledge.

Sy, F. S., Chng, C. L., Choi, S. T., & Wong, F. Y. (1998). Epidemiology of HIV and AIDS among Asian and Pacific Islander Americans. *AIDS Education & Prevention*, 10(3 Suppl), 4-18.

Szymanski, D. M., & Henrichs-Beck, C. (2014). Exploring sexual minority women's experiences of external and internalized heterosexism and sexism and their links to coping and distress. *Sex Roles, 70*(1–2), 28–42.

Szymanski, D. M., & Sung, M. R. (2010). Minority stress and psychological distress among Asian American sexual minority persons. *The Counseling Psychologist, 38*(6), 848–872. https://doi.org/10.1177/0011000010366167

Takahashi, L. M. (1997). Stigmatization, HIV/AIDS, and communities of color: exploring response to human service facilities. *Health Place, 3*(3), 187–199. Retrieved from http://www.ncbi.nlm.nih.gov/entrez/query.fcgi?cmd=Retrieve&db=PubMed&dopt=Citation&list_uids=10670970

Tan, J. Y., Xu, L. J., Lopez, F. Y., Jia, J. L., Pho, M. T., Kim, K. E., & Chin, M. H. (2016). Shared decision making among clinicians and Asian American and Pacific Islander sexual and gender minorities: An intersectional approach to address a critical care gap. *LGBT Health, 3*(5):327–334. https://doi.org/10.1089/lgbt.2015.0143

Yoshihama, M., Blazevski, J., & Bybee, D. (2014). Enculturation and attitudes toward intimate partner violence and gender roles in an Asian Indian population: Implications for community-based prevention. *American Journal of Community Psychology, 53*(3–4), 249–260. https://doi.org/10.1007/s10464-014-9627-5

Yoshikawa, H., Wilson, P., Hsueh, J., Rosman, E. A., Chin, J., & Kim, J. H. (2001). What front-line NGO staff can tell us about culturally anchored theories of change in HIV prevention for Asian/Pacific Islanders in the U.S. *American Journal of Community Psychology, 32*(1–2), 143–158.

Yoshioka, M. R., & Schustack, A. (2001). Disclosure of HIV status: cultural issues of Asian patients. *AIDS Patient Care & Standards, 15*(2), 77–82.

Zhou, M. (1992). *Chinatown: the Socioeconomic Potential of an Urban Enclave*. Philadelphia: Temple University Press.

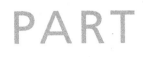

PART

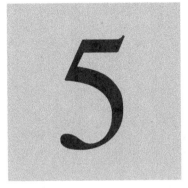

5

POLICY

CHAPTER

13

FEDERAL LANDSCAPE FOR HEALTH RESEARCH

LAN N. ĐOÀN, CHANDAK GHOSH, KATHY KO CHIN, JULIET K. CHOI

LEARNING OBJECTIVES

By the end of this chapter, readers will be able to:

- Describe the overall state of federal funding for health research in Asian American communities.
- Understand the challenges and opportunities for funding Asian American health research.
- Describe the role of funding opportunities in building capacity and infrastructure that may impact the health status and health outcomes of Asian American communities.

Applied Population Health Approaches for Asian American Communities, First Edition. Edited by Simona C. Kwon, Chau Trinh-Shevrin, Nadia S. Islam, and Stella S. Yi.
© 2023 John Wiley & Sons, Inc. Published 2023 by John Wiley & Sons, Inc.
Companion Website: www.wiley.com/go/kwon/asianamerican

INTRODUCTION

Understanding the impact of the federal landscape on Asian American health research must begin with recognizing diversity that exists within and across Asian ethnic subgroups and assessing the consequences of the model minority stereotype on the national health agenda. Asian Americans constitute the fastest-growing minority population in the United States and comprise over 50 unique ethnic groups, speaking more than 65 languages, with varying levels of English language proficiency, socioeconomic status, and migration experiences. Six subgroups – Asian Indian, Chinese, Filipino, Japanese, Korean, and Vietnamese – comprise 85% of the Asian American population. However, smaller subgroups, like the Bhutanese population, are increasing rapidly (Budiman et al., 2019). Asian Americans currently constitute 5.7% of the U.S. population and are overlooked frequently due to their small population relative to other racial/ethnic minority groups, including non-Hispanic Black (Black) and Hispanic/Latinx individuals (Vespa et al., 2020). However, the Asian American population is projected to double in the coming decades, with its proportion estimated to reach 9.1% of the U.S. population by 2060. Alongside this rapid population growth, existing economic and social disparities are expected to widen.

Historically, the model minority myth has perpetuated a narrative that Asian Americans have achieved greater economic and academic success as compared to other racial/ethnic minority groups, resulting in the pervasive assumption that Asian Americans do not experience health disparities or inequities (Yi, 2020; Yi et al., 2016). The persistence of this stereotype may be seen in the aggregation of Asian American data, which obscures important health differences among Asian American subgroups and results in the repeated omission of Asian Americans from clinical trial and epidemiologic study samples (Holland & Palaniappan, 2012). Given the current overall deficiency of racial/ethnic data for Asian American subgroups, inequities in health outcomes experienced by Asian Americans as a whole, and particularly among emerging Asian subgroups, likely will continue to be overlooked at the federal level, even as the proportion of Asian Americans within the broader U.S. population grows.

The definitions of federal policy priorities, allocation of federal resources, and development of federal programs are linked inextricably to social determinants of health, such as substandard educational opportunities, residential segregation, and insufficient access to language concordant health care resources. The misrepresentation and underrepresentation of Asian Americans in federal data collection efforts related to describing the social determinants of health have contributed to inaccurate definitions of secular trends in health status and other factors among this population. The incomplete picture of the Asian American experience in the United States, in turn, has impacted decisions made related to federal funding and resource allocation and constrained the capacity of governmental agencies to direct resources to the Asian American communities experiencing the greatest disparities. These decisions have reinforced the invisibility of the Asian American population, ignoring the unique needs faced by diverse groups of Asian Americans. This chapter describes the current state of federal funding and policy related to Asian American health research and discusses challenges and opportunities that will influence the federal landscape in the coming years.

CURRENT STATE OF ASIAN AMERICAN HEALTH RESEARCH FUNDING

The National Institutes of Health (NIH) is the largest funder of health research in the United States and globally, contributing $26 billion to health research in 2013 as compared to an annual expenditure of $1 billion from the U.S. Department of Defense and $582 million from the Centers for Disease Control (CDC) (Viergever & Hendriks, 2016). Thus, our review will focus on NIH funding.

Previously, Ghosh (2003, 2010) posited that to improve the health of Asian American populations, a more complete baseline picture of Asian American health is needed to identify health disparities within individual Asian ethnic groups through collection of disaggregated racial/ethnic data. More recently, there has been a shift to move beyond the identification of disparities toward a health equity agenda, through which data analyses intersect with advocacy and action to achieve the highest attainment of health for all. From both perspectives, baseline data are required to understand trajectories of health and illness over time, particularly because the demographic makeup of the Asian American population continues to change, and current data may not be generalizable to emerging populations.

Trends in Federal Funding for Clinical Research Among Asian American Populations

Federal investment supporting research on health disparities increased overall during the last decades (Institute of Medicine, 2006). Đoàn and colleagues (2019), however, uncovered a striking trend of disproportionately low long-term investments by NIH to eliminate health disparities among Asian American and Native Hawaiian and Pacific Islander (NH/PI) communities. Đoàn et al. queried the NIH Research Portfolio Online Reporting Tools Expenditures and Results (RePORTER) system for investigator-initiated grants (i.e., research project grants, centers, research career awards, and training fellowships) that included any mention of 23 Asian American and NH/PI countries of origin. Between 1992 and 2018, NIH funded only 529 clinical research studies that included Asian American and NH/PI participants (Figure 13.1), with funding for these studies comprising a mere 0.17% of overall NIH research expenditures over the course of those 26 years (Figure 13.2). After 2000, funding for Asian American- and NH/PI-related research nominally increased from 0.12% to 0.18%, but funding remains substantially less than 1% of the total NIH research budget – a disproportionately low figure, given that Asian Americans comprise nearly 6% of the total U.S. population.

Table 13.1 shows the top 10 of the total 17 NIH Institutes and Centers that contributed the largest dollar amounts toward Asian American and NH/PI clinical research. More than 50% of funds were awarded by the National Cancer Institute, National Institute on Aging, and National Heart, Lung, and Blood Institute. Over 60% (331 out of 529) of projects were conducted in only five states – California, Hawaii, New York, Washington, and Illinois – with about 40% of the total funding allocated to California alone. About half of the funded projects that included Asian American and NH/PI participants also included other racial/ethnic minority groups (e.g., Hispanic, Black). Among projects that included only Asian American or NH/PI participants, over 75% of projects focused on a single ethnic subgroup. Most research focused on one or more of the six largest Asian American subgroups (i.e., Chinese, Korean, Vietnamese, Filipino, Asian Indian). The few studies that included NH/PIs focused mainly on Native Hawaiians.

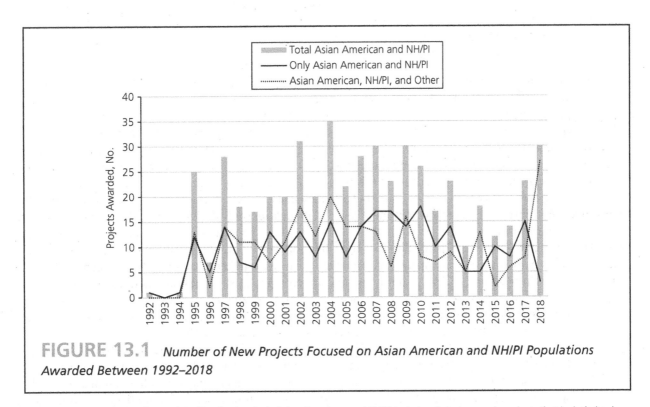

FIGURE 13.1   *Number of New Projects Focused on Asian American and NH/PI Populations Awarded Between 1992–2018*

Note: NH/PI = Native Hawaiian and Pacific Islander. *Only Asian American and NH/PI* includes clinical research projects that included only Asian American and NH/PI participants. *Asian American, NH/PI, and Other* includes clinical research projects that included Asian American, NH/PI and other racial/ethnic groups. *Total Asian American and NH/PI* is the sum of *Only Asian American and NH/PI* and *Asian American, NH/PI, and Other*.

Source: Adapted from Đoàn et al. (2019).

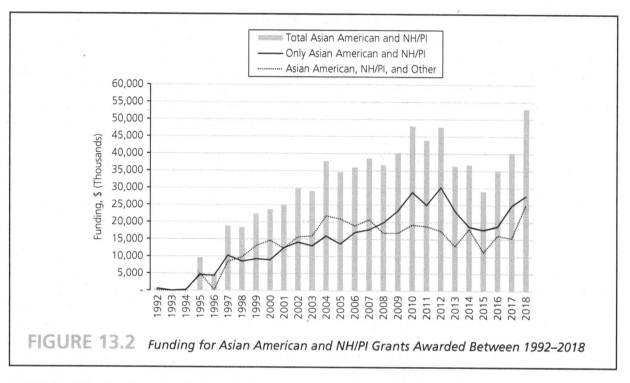

FIGURE 13.2 *Funding for Asian American and NH/PI Grants Awarded Between 1992–2018*

Note: NH/PI = Native Hawaiian and Pacific Islander. *Only Asian American and NH/PI* includes clinical research projects that included only Asian American and NH/PI participants. *Asian American, NH/PI, and Other* includes clinical research projects that included Asian American, NH/PI and other racial/ethnic groups. *Total Asian American and NH/PI* is the sum of *Only Asian American and NH/PI* and *Asian American, NH/PI, and Other.*
Source: Adapted from Đoàn et al. (2019).

In contrast to the dearth of federal funding earmarked for Asian American- and NH/PI-focused research via research project grants, NIH awarded 39 fellowships and 41 research career development funding to researchers focused on expanding research within Asian American and NH/PI populations between 1992–2008. NIH offers two main types of support to individual researchers: research career development awards (K awards), intended for senior postdoctoral fellows and faculty-level candidates, and fellowships (F awards), designated for predoctoral and postdoctoral students. This trend in grantmaking at the federal level signals the emergence of a new generation of researchers who are broadening the health research agenda to include an underrepresented population that, to date, has been rendered nearly invisible to policy makers due to lack of data. These researchers will be instrumental in developing more complex, nuanced, and thoughtful study designs, data collection methodologies, and analytical techniques to advance health research in small populations, in general, and in individual Asian American ethnic groups, in particular. Extant studies conducted have struggled both to recruit and retain Asian American participants and to analyze the data collected. Researchers that come from Asian American communities may prove more adept at tailoring participant recruitment strategies and inclusion criteria to the unique needs of ethnic subgroups. This would be achieved by recognizing and addressing systemic barriers to clinical research recruitment among Asian American populations, including limited availability of in-language outreach and education about clinical trials (George et al., 2013; S. Lee et al., 2010).

Although the designation of these NIH career development awards for Asian American and NH/PI researchers represents an important and promising step toward developing a diverse workforce for the coming decades, systemic barriers persist for investigators conducting health disparities and minority health research at all levels (Ginther et al., 2011, 2018; Hoppe et al., 2019). For example, Black researchers are more likely to investigate health disparities-related research topics than non-Hispanic White (White) researchers and, in parallel, health disparities topics have lower NIH award rates overall. The intersection of these trends accounts for 21% of the funding gap between Black and White researchers (Hoppe et al., 2019). Health disparities span research topics,

TABLE 13.1 Top 10 National Institutes of Health Institutes and Centers Funders for Asian American and NH/PI Clinical Research

Institutes and centers	Awards, no. (%)	Total funding amount, $
National Cancer Institute (NCI)	132 (25.0)	231,584,664
National Institute on Aging (NIA)	57 (10.8)	108,365,124
National Heart, Lung, and Blood Institute (NHLBI)	31 (5.9)	67,232,910
National Institute on Minority Health and Health Disparities (NIMHD)	34 (6.4)	62,982,901
National Institute on Mental Health (NIMH)	62 (11.7)	60,072,779
Eunice Kennedy Shriver National Institute of Child Health and Human Development (NICHD)	48 (9.1)	48,992,219
National Institute on Drug Abuse (NIDA)	33 (6.2)	37,276,683
National Institute of Diabetes and Digestive and Kidney Diseases (NIDDK)	26 (4.9)	31,638,678
National Center for Research Resources (NCRR)	17 (3.2)	30,236,345
National Institute of Nursing Research (NINR)	37 (7.0)	22,691,061

Note: The National Institutes of Health Institutes and Centers are ordered by descending total funding amount.
Source: Adapted from Đoàn et al. (2019).

and the goal of eliminating health disparities requires the prioritization of research studies that focus on minority health and health disparities. The federal government has a key role to play in evaluating diversity, inclusion, and equity efforts at all levels and in designing and implementing strategies to expand diversity where needed, starting with the prioritization and reallocation of taxpayer dollars to address health disparities (Carnethon et al., 2020).

Federal funding for health research in Asian American populations remains insufficient to address existing and emerging health disparities, particularly among rapidly growing Asian American subgroups. The NIH investment of less than 0.5% of its total budget for Asian American–focused research represents a glaring injustice for a population that not only comprises nearly 6% of the current U.S. population but also is projected to grow 101% between 2016 and 2060 (Vespa et al., 2020). Collecting more granular data and improving data quality for Asian ethnic groups and for Asian Americans, as a whole, are imperative. Key barriers to address include lack of enforcement of existing federal data collection standards and inconsistent data collection at the state and local levels; need for even more granular data collection, analysis, reporting, and dissemination standards; small sample sizes and innovation in sample construction methodologies (e.g., pooled geographically or over time); inconsistent definitions of the term *Asian American*; limited survey administration in Asian languages; and a lack of geographic diversity in study samples (Islam et al., 2010). These issues were addressed in Chapter 4.

Establishment of a Federally Designated Comprehensive Center of Excellence

In 1993, as part of federal efforts to expand research to investigate health disparities among racial/ethnic minority populations, NIH established an Office of Research on Minority Health (ORMH) (National Institutes of Health

Revitalization Act of 1993, 1993). ORMH was expanded in 2000 to become the National Center on Minority Health and Health Disparities (NCMHD) (Minority Health and Health Disparities Research and Education Act of 2000, 2000) and, in 2010, was redesignated as the National Institute on Minority Health and Health Disparities (NIMHD) (The Patient Protection and Affordable Care Act, 2010). In 2020, NIMHD celebrated its first decade as a fully developed and funded NIH institute, providing a noteworthy example of the NIH's commitment to advancing minority health and addressing health disparities in racial/ethnic minority populations nationwide.

As part of these efforts, in 2002, NIMHD launched the Excellence in Partnership Outreach Reach and Training (EXPORT) program. The NYU Center for the Study of Asian American Health (CSAAH) at NYU Grossman School of Medicine (NYUGSOM) was established in 2003 as a NIMHD EXPORT Center (Trinh-Shevrin et al., 2015) and was renewed as a Specialized Center of Excellence in 2007, 2012, and 2017. As one of the 12 Specialized Centers of Excellence programs focused on minority health and health disparities populations, CSAAH focuses specifically on understanding, addressing, and reducing Asian American health disparities through community-engaged research, training, and national partnerships. CSAAH conducts research in five scientific tracks: cardiovascular disease and diabetes disparities, cancer prevention disparities, mental health, healthy aging, and gender equity. Additionally, CSAAH's innovative pilot project research focuses on emerging communities and health disparities research topic areas. CSAAH integrates research comprehensively with the social determinants of health, utilizes community-based participatory research approaches, supports practice and policy translation, and is actively engaged in community and scientific dissemination. The pilot project program extends CSAAH's reach to train the next generation of researchers through mentorship and career development opportunities around minority health and health disparities. To accomplish this work, CSAAH operationalizes a population health equity framework described in detail in Chapter 2.

NYUGSOM received joint recognition with the City University of New York (CUNY) as a CDC Prevention Research Center (PRC) in 2009. The PRCs are 25 U.S. academic research centers that conduct applied public health prevention research, with an emphasis on developing, testing, and evaluating public health interventions for wide dissemination, particularly in underserved communities. Within NYUGSOM, CSAAH is the coordinating group for this award. NYU Langone, which includes NYUGSOM, is one of few academic medical centers in the United States to hold designations as NIH and CDC Centers of Excellence, as well as a CDC PRC. The focus of the NYUGSOM-CUNY PRC is to implement, evaluate, and disseminate community-clinical linkage interventions to reduce cardiovascular disease disparities in ethnically diverse NYC communities. IMPACT (Implementing Million Hearts for Provider and Community Transformation) was the first core research project implemented under the PRC. Funded in 2014, the IMPACT study is a randomized-controlled trial designed to evaluate the feasibility, adoption, and effectiveness of an integrated community health worker (CHW)-led and provider-level electronic health record (EHR)-based intervention to improve blood pressure control among South Asian patients receiving care in small primary care practices (PCPs) in New York City (NYC) (Lopez et al., 2019). CHWs are frontline health workers who understand the nuances of the communities they represent, providing them with the ability to deliver programming efforts to socially and linguistically isolated communities. The CHW intervention component demonstrates that a culturally adapted CHW-led intervention among hypertensive South Asians delivered in small primary care settings can achieve significant improvements in blood pressure control after six months. Explicit funding streams to health systems that predominantly serve Asian American communities are an example of how funding at the organizational level can improve health status for Asian American individuals through better clinical care and the provision of nonclinical services addressing the social determinants of health. See Case 4 in the Appendix for more detail about how Project IMPACT has improved clinical-community linkages for South Asians in NYC.

Over the last decade, by operationalizing a population health equity framework and a community-engaged research approach, CSAAH has made important progress toward reducing health disparities among Asian American communities. A key example is the implementation of two waves of Community Health Resource and Needs Assessments (CHRNA) data collection in partnership with community organizations serving diverse Asian subgroups. CHRNA is a groundbreaking, large-scale health needs assessment conducted among diverse, low-income Asian American communities in NYC that has used a community-engaged and community venue-based approach to assess existing health issues, available resources, and best approaches to meet community needs. The success of this initiative led to the development and funding of two new CHRNA cycles for implementation in 2020, one of which will update the regional CHRNA process while the other will focus specifically on older adults. Additionally, during 2012–2014 and again in 2020, CSAAH and the Asian & Pacific Islander American Health Forum (APIAHF) co-led the CDC Strategies to Reach and Implement the Vision of Health Equity (STRIVE) Program to implement evidence-based, policy, systems, and environmental strategies to increase healthy behaviors among Asian American and NH/PI communities. In 2018, CSAAH launched a new scientific track to address healthy aging and Alzheimer's disease and related dementias (ADRD). Several NIHMD supplemental awards under this healthy aging track included scoping reviews related to ADRD prevalence, risk factors, and screening tools for use among Asian American populations (Lim, Chong, et al., 2020; Lim, Mohaimin, et al., 2020); the Delphi study, which is described in Case 5 in the Appendix; the cultural and linguistic adaptation of the Kickstart-Assess-Evaluate-Refer Toolkit (KAER), created by the Gerontological Society of America, that primary care providers use in community settings to diagnose cognitive impairment and early dementia (discussed in Chapter 6); and the Systems to Understand Nutrition, Diet, and Active Living Opportunities in Adults 50+ Years (SUNDIAL) project focused on improving lifestyle behaviors that prevent or slow cognitive decline in older adults. In another successful collaboration, CSAAH co-led the Assessment of Policies through Prediction of Long-term Effects on Cardiovascular Disease Using Simulation (APPLE CDS) Project, in partnership with the New York Academy of Medicine. Funded by the National Heart, Lung, and Blood Institute (NHLBI), the goal of APPLE CDS is to assess the effects of dietary policies and programs on cardiovascular disease risk factors, outcomes and associated health care costs in the NYC adult population utilizing agent-based modeling. Agent-based modeling simulates population health trajectories, engages community members and stakeholders with data visualization around health outcomes, evaluates intervention programs, and establishes evidence for future implementation of programs to improve population health. APPLE CDS demonstrates that agent-based modeling can be used by local health departments to facilitate and inform evidence-based decision-making (Li et al., 2015) and as a population health management tool to compare the short- and long-term impacts of different healthy lifestyle programs (Li et al., 2014). More detail about agent-based modeling and other innovative systems science methods employed by CSAAH can be found in Chapter 6.

These projects and programs build on CSAAH's breadth of scientific expertise in community-engaged health disparities research and have been successful due to the dedication and commitment of community and university partners. CSAAH's multiple NIH and CDC designations and its strong track record of securing federal and private funding to support its work provide striking evidence of CSAAH's abilities in successfully conducting research informed by a population health equity framework and in collaboration with community partners. CSAAH has received several prestigious awards recognizing its achievements, including the CDC National Community Committee Award for Best Practices in Community-based Participatory Research to the NYU Langone PRC (2013), Agency for Healthcare Research and Quality (AHRQ) Innovation Exchange Profile (2014), and the Founder's Award from NYC's Chinatown YMCA Spirit Awards (2019). These awards, and the diversity of the awarding organizations, underscore CSAAH's impact as a research center addressing health disparities in Asian American communities at multiple levels. More broadly, CSAAH's successes highlight the important role of long-term federal investments to support the growth and development of research centers dedicated to investigating and addressing health disparities among Asian American communities.

Designation of the Asian Resource Center for Minority Aging Research

Launched in 1997 by the NIH National Institute on Aging (NIA), the Resource Centers for Minority Aging Research (RCMARs) are designed to diversify the workforce in aging research through mentorship of promising early scientists from underrepresented groups and build infrastructure necessary to support expansion of health disparities research among racial/ethnic minority elders (Harawa et al., 2017). The traditional RCMAR priority areas include social, behavioral, and economic research on aging. In 2018, these areas were expanded to include research centers focused on social and behavioral research related to Alzheimer's Disease. RCMAR-supported scholars have roles that extend beyond academia and encompass individuals who also serve in leadership roles in other sectors including public health, philanthropy, nonprofit research organizations, and research-related organizations (e.g., NIH) (Harawa et al., 2017).

The Asian RCMAR was established in 2018 as part of a new allocation of $4 million in funding to expand RCMAR research through new awards and renewals of existing grants nationwide (National Institutes of Health, 2017). As part of that funding cycle, the Rutgers Asian RCMAR became one of 10 centers focused on the traditional RCMAR priority areas, working to develop research infrastructure and capacity to address needs of the rapidly growing Asian American older adult population in the United States (Dong, 2019). The Asian RCMAR includes four core areas: administration, research and education, measurement and analysis, and community liaison and recruitment. During its first three years of operation (2018–2020), the Asian RCMAR supported over 20 early-career researchers conducting pilot projects related to trauma, resilience, and health outcomes among Asian older adults. Given the alignment of RCMARs with the overall NIA mission and NIA Strategic Directions for 2020–2025, investment in the Asian RCMAR provides a unique opportunity to expand health-related research primarily focused on Asian American older adults and to train the next generation of researchers focused on aging to address the unique needs of racial/ethnic minority populations.

Impact of the Healthy People initiative

The "Healthy People" federal initiative is intended to guide national health promotion and disease prevention efforts. As such, data collected through Healthy People remain instrumental in guiding the allocation of federal resources where they are most needed. Healthy People has been released every decade since 1980 by the U.S. Department of Health and Human Services (HHS). Data collection and analysis related to the Healthy People are a collaborative federal effort led by HHS Office of the Assistant Secretary of Health (OASH), AHRQ, CDC, Health Resources and Services Administration (HRSA), and NIH. These agencies contribute to identifying priority national health indicators each decade. Healthy People 2030, released in August 2020, is the fifth iteration of this initiative and was developed based on findings from the Healthy People 2020 process. These data inform our current understanding of progress toward national health priorities, including identifying racially based health disparities. Often, the lack of data disaggregated by racial/ethnic category has hindered the understanding of Asian American health needs and, in turn, contributed to the insufficient allocation of resources to address health disparities in Asian American communities.

In Healthy People 2020, 26 leading health indicators were established under 12 health domains. Table 13.2 displays these indicators, noting where data are reported for the Asian American racial/ethnic group alone as opposed to aggregating data for Asian Americans with NH/PIs. Establishing a clear distinction between Asian American and NH/PI groups remains an unresolved issue even now, more than 20 years after the 1997 Office of Management and Budget (OMB) updated standards for the collection of racial and ethnic data by federal agencies and mandated the separation of Asian Americans from NH/PI groups (Office of Management and Budget, 1997). Although data for the Asian American population were available for the majority of indicators, six indicators (25%) combined Asian American and NH/PI data.

Assessing any longitudinal trends of improvement or worsening of the health indicators is not possible without baseline data or large sample sizes. Therefore, it is notable that for six indicators (25%), no baseline data were available for Asian Americans, precluding assessment of progress toward the Healthy People goals for this population. For example, due to discrepancies in statistical reliability, unreliable data quality, or confidentiality reasons, data were not reported for Asian American individuals with diagnosed diabetes whose hemoglobin A1c value was greater than 9% (D-5.1). This lack of data may perpetuate the notion that Asian Americans are not at risk for diabetes or do not require diabetes prevention programming, even though studies have found that Asians are more likely to develop type 2 diabetes than their White counterparts (Lee et al., 2011; Oza-Frank et al., 2009). Furthermore, collecting data for the Asian American population as a whole is not sufficient to develop a complete picture of the health status of this diverse population. Among major Asian ethnic groups, Asian Indians and Filipino have the highest prevalence of type 2 diabetes (Lee et al., 2011; Ye et al., 2009). Yet with persistent issues of inadequate data collection and small sample sizes of Asian American populations, disaggregating Asian ethnic groups remains out of reach for Healthy People. Chapter 4 provides a deeper exploration of opportunities and challenges related to federal data collection standards and population-based studies for Asian American communities.

Healthy People 2020 is a collaborative effort implemented by multiple federal agencies and stakeholders, reflecting a decade-long national health agenda and producing data that impact the development and implementation of the Healthy People 2030 agenda and beyond. Therefore, if Asian American data continue to be collected and reported in aggregate with NH/PI data, or not reported at all, the health status of Asian Americans will remain unknown. The invisibility of Asian Americans within current federal data sets allows federal agencies to

TABLE 13.2   Healthy People 2020 Leading Health Indicators

Health domain	Leading health indicator	Asian American only	Asian or Pacific Islander
Access to health services	Persons with medical insurance (AHS-1.1)	+	
	Persons with a usual primary care provider (AHS-3)	+	
Clinical preventative services	Adults receiving colorectal cancer screening based on the most recent guidelines (C-16)	+	
	Adults with hypertension whose blood pressure is under control (HDS-12)	✓	
	Persons with diagnosed diabetes whose A1c value is greater than 9% (D-5.1)	✓ (not reported)	
	Children receiving the recommended doses of DTaP, polio, MMR, Hib, HepB, varicella and PCV vaccines by age 19–35 months (IID-8)	+	
Environmental quality	Air Quality Index >100 (EH-1)		
	Children exposed to secondhand smoke (TU-11.1)	✓	
Injury and violence	Injury deaths (IVP-1.1)		–
	Homicides (IVP-29)		+
Maternal, infant, and child health	All Infant deaths (MICH-1.3)		–
	Total preterm live births (MICH-9.1)		–
Mental health	Suicide (MHMD-1)		–
	Adolescents with a major depressive episode in the past 12 months (MHMD-4.1)	–	
Nutrition, physical activity, and obesity	Adults meeting aerobic physical activity and muscle-strengthening objectives (PA-2.4)	+	
	Obesity among adults (NWS-9)	✓	
	Obesity among children and adolescents (NWS-10.4)	✓	

(Continued)

TABLE 13.2　(Continued)

Health domain	Leading health indicator	Asian American only	Asian or Pacific Islander
	Mean daily intake of total vegetables (NWS-15.1)	✓	
Oral health	Children, adolescents, and adults who visited the dentist in the past year (OH-7)	+	
Reproductive and sexual health	Sexually active females receiving reproductive health services (FP-7.1)		
	Knowledge of serostatus among HIV-positive persons (HIV-13)	+	
Social determinants of health	Students graduating from high school within 4 years of starting 9th grade (AH-5.1)		+
Substance abuse	Adolescents using alcohol or illicit drugs in past 30 days (SA-13.1)	−	
	Binge drinking in past month – Adults (SA-14.3)	−	
Tobacco	Adult cigarette smoking (TU-1.1)	+	
	Adolescent cigarette smoking in past 30 days (TU-2.2)	+	

Notes: + = improved over time; − = decreased over time; ✓ = Asian field was available but there were no baseline data for comparison or data were not reported because the data did not meet the criteria for statistical reliability, data quality, or confidentiality.

disregard the needs of this diverse population. With insufficient federal attention and resources allocated to Asian Americans, racially based health disparities will continue to widen, preventing progress toward health equity for all Americans.

Philanthropic Support for Asian American Research

The lack of attention and resources directed toward the Asian American population within the federal funding landscape is reflected in foundation grantmaking, as well. Currently, the federal government remains the largest funder of health research, but the role of foundations in supporting health research is expanding nationally (Research!America, 2019). Philanthropic giving includes both public charities, which are funded typically by donations from the general public, and private foundations, which are supported primarily by a family, corporation, or individual. The term, *foundation* may refer to either of these types of philanthropic organizations. Both types are registered not-for-profit 501(c)3 corporations. As foundations become an increasingly important source of funding for health research nationally, more attention must be given to combat the persistence of the model minority myth and invisibility of Asian Americans within this sphere.

Philanthropic funding for Asian American communities remains less than 1% of total giving, a proportion that has not increased meaningfully over time. In 2004, a report on philanthropic giving estimated that support from the top 20 foundations to Asian American and NH/PI communities comprised only 0.4% of total grant dollars disbursed that year (Gupta & Ritoper, 2007). Ten years later, in 2014, the Philanthropic Initiative for Racial

Equity reported that while a total of 7.4% ($2 billion) of all philanthropic giving was disbursed to communities of color as a whole, only 0.26% of all charitable dollars was awarded to Asian American and NH/PI communities (Philanthropic Initiative for Racial Equity, 2017; Ramkrishnan et al., 2020).

More recent data on philanthropic giving demonstrates misperceptions among philanthropic leaders and staff related to trends in giving to Asian American and NH/PI communities. AAPI Data and Asian Americans/ Pacific Islanders in Philanthropy (AAPIP) conducted a survey of philanthropic staff and leadership and found that 11% of those surveyed considered Asian Americans a high priority for their foundation (defined as causes to which the foundation should allocate more than 25% of grant dollars) and 30% reported there had been an increase in funding for Asian Americans over the last five years (Ramkrishnan et al., 2020) – perceptions that are not reflected in the actual dollar amounts disbursed by foundations to Asian American communities. The AAPIP survey also found a misalignment between foundations' giving priorities versus perceived priorities of the Asian American community. For example, even though 68% of foundations perceived immigrant rights to be top priority for the Asian American community, this area was only a top priority for 18% of foundations (Ramkrishnan et al., 2020). These data indicate, at a minimum, the need for training and education among philanthropic staff and leadership to remedy this disconnect documented between intentions and actions vis à vis Asian American- and NH/PI-focused initiatives.

Given the large portfolio of innovative projects funded by philanthropic organizations, foundations have the potential to transform environments and create positive downstream impacts on the health of communities. Furthermore, as compared to federal funding opportunities, philanthropic giving has a more flexible administrative structure, rendering foundation funding more accessible to less established researchers and organizations. These features position foundations to be critical partners for Asian American communities in the years to come. By evaluating their portfolios critically for investments in communities of color, particularly Black, Indigenous, and People of Color (BIPOC)-led organizations and entities, and increasing their commitments meaningfully to Asian American-focused initiatives, foundations may prove to be pivotal community and research partners, helping advancement toward achieving health equity.

FEDERAL LEGISLATION IMPACTING ASIAN AMERICAN HEALTH

While legislation at all levels has tremendous impact on physical and social environments where individuals live, learn, work, and play, a federal legislative landscape focused on advancing health equity is foundational to developing health-promoting policies at the state and local levels. Advancing the agenda for Asian American health at the federal level requires focusing an equity and racial justice lens on the development of legislation across sectors. For example, the "Health in All Policies" (HiAP) approach, discussed in Chapter 10, is a key methodology to ensure this cross-sectoral approach to advancing health equity. HiAP provides a collaborative framework to improving the health of all people by incorporating health considerations into policymaking in all sectors, guiding decision-making toward creating healthier communities. Legislation directly impacts how resources are distributed and the conditions that determine whether individuals and communities have fair and just opportunities to attain the fullest health possible. With HiAP in place at the federal level, the development of health-promoting legislation at lower levels of governance may be more easily developed, passed, and integrated into communities. In the following sections, we present key aspects of the federal legislative landscape that currently affect the health of Asian Americans and that promise to influence the health status of this diverse and growing population in the decades ahead.

Affordable Care Act

The Patient Protection and Affordable Care Act (The Patient Protection and Affordable Care Act, 2010), also known as the Affordable Care Act (ACA) or Obamacare, was enacted in March 2010 and fully implemented in January 2014. The ACA stands as the most significant health care legislation to have passed in the over 45 years since Medicare and Medicaid were created in 1965 (Oberlander, 2010), providing near-universal health coverage options and reforming the health care delivery system (Blumenthal et al., 2015; Rosenbaum, 2011). Briefly, the ACA increased the availability of affordable health insurance for Americans by instituting federal subsidies for individuals and families who need them, expanding Medicaid eligibility to include adults with incomes at or below 138% of the federal poverty level, requiring insurers to offer coverage to children of employees until they are 26 years of age, and preventing insurance companies from discriminating against people with preexisting conditions and those who become ill (Blumenthal et al., 2015).

The ACA has been instrumental in expanding health care access for Asian Americans. During 2009–2013, prior to the full implementation of the ACA, a national study reported that 18.8% of Asian Americans and NH/PIs were uninsured as compared to 15.1% of Whites. The highest uninsurance rates were among Korean (29.9%), Vietnamese (25.4%), and Other Asian (24.4%) adults (Park et al., 2018). As the ACA neared full implementation, in 2013, 13.9% of Asian Americans were uninsured as compared to a 14.5% uninsurance rate among the total U.S. population. The highest rates of uninsurance were among Pakistani (20.9%), Korean (20.5%), Cambodian (18.9%), Vietnamese (18.5%), and Bangladeshi (18.2%) adults (National Council of Asian Pacific Islander Physicians, 2015). Compared to other racial and ethnic minority groups, uninsured Asian Americans were more likely to have limited English proficiency, be foreign-born, and have less than a high school education (National Council of Asian Pacific Islander Physicians, 2015).

In subsequent years, the expansion of the ACA has contributed to higher rates of insurance across all racial/ethnic groups, including Asian Americans, and helped to narrow the insurance gap among Asian populations. Figures 13.3 shows trends in uninsurance over the years 2010–2018, using American Community Survey data (Gunja et al., 2020).

The ACA eliminated the insurance coverage gap between Asian Americans and Whites. By 2017–2018, Asian Americans had the lowest uninsured rate of any racial or ethnic group in the United States, with 7.9% of Asian Americans uninsured as compared to 8.5% of Whites (Gunja et al., 2020; Park et al., 2018). Importantly, Asian subgroups that have had difficulty historically in accessing and affording health care and experienced lower quality of care due to limited English proficiency, immigration status, and other factors (*2018 National Healthcare Quality and Disparities Report*, 2019) gained coverage as states expanded Medicaid access and provided subsidies to individuals and families through state-managed private insurance markets (Gunja et al., 2020). The narrowing of the insurance coverage gap between individual Asian American populations as well as between Asian Americans as a whole and other racial/ethnic groups is also attributable to efforts from community-based organizations, federally qualified health centers, and national coalitions like *Action for Health Justice* that engage low-income, immigrant, and limited English-proficient Asian Americans and NH/PIs through culturally and linguistically-appropriate outreach, education and enrollment activities (Action for Health Justice, 2014).

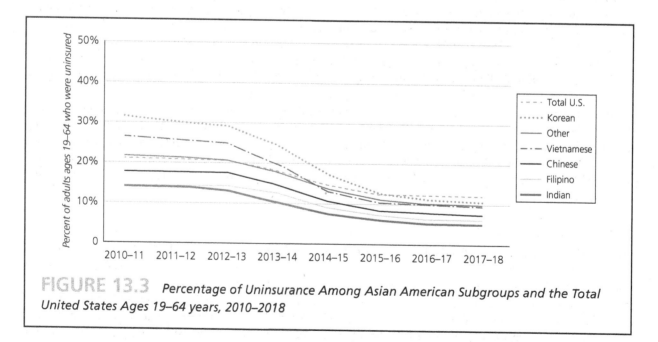

FIGURE 13.3 *Percentage of Uninsurance Among Asian American Subgroups and the Total United States Ages 19–64 years, 2010–2018*

Source: Adapted from Gunja et al. (2020).

The ACA has several provisions focused on eliminating health disparities. An example is "Section 4302 Understanding Health Disparities: data collection and analysis," which focuses on improving data standards for race, ethnicity, sex, primary language and disability status (Dorsey et al., 2014). These updated standards require improving the collection and reporting of data in national population health surveys and federally support programming and alignment with Healthy People 2020 goals to understand and address health care disparities. To date, there remain inconsistent use and enforcement, methodological challenges, and challenges to collection of these data categories (Ponce et al., 2016). Data-related issues and challenges for federal surveys are discussed in Chapter 4.

Opponents have mounted repeated legal challenges to cut key provisions of the ACA or repeal the legislation altogether. While the ACA remains in place, these challenges impact the implementation of the ACA on a state-by-state basis and influence public perceptions of individual rights to health care insurance and access. These difficult realities may be especially true for Asian Americans, who are disproportionately impacted by policy changes like the expanded public charge rule under the Trump Administration, discussed in the next section (Artiga et al., 2019). Moving forward, researchers will need to assess whether the gains achieved to date in expanding health insurance coverage and health care access for Asian Americans will be maintained. Exploring the impact of expanded coverage and access on health care outcomes for Asian populations will also be critical to developing the evidence base for the importance of federal legislation in improving the health status of Asian Americans.

Public Charge

The administration of President Donald J. Trump (2017–2021) oversaw a substantial expansion of criteria used to bar immigrants from legal residence in the United States under the Immigration and Nationality Act of 1952. One of the most significant policy changes for immigrants seeking health care is the expanded scope of the Public Charge Rule. While devastating to all immigrant communities, this change in criteria disproportionately impacted the Asian American population, of which nearly 60% of individuals are foreign-born (Budiman et al., 2019). The Public Charge grounds for inadmissibility have existed for more than a century (U.S. Citizenship and Immigration Services, 2020), defining reasons why foreign-born individuals may be denied legal residency in the United States (Quinn & Kinoshita, 2020). Until 2018, Public Charge criteria were limited to new immigrants receiving federal cash benefits like Supplemental Security Income (SSI) and Temporary Assistance for Needy Families (TANF). However, in October 2018, enhancements to these criteria began to take shape, and, in August 2019, the U.S. Department of Homeland Security released revisions to the Immigration and Nationality Act of 1952, titled the "Inadmissibility on Public Charge Grounds final rule."

Adopted in February 2020, the new Public Charge Rule identified numerous additional criteria that could be used to deny lawful permanent residency status to legal immigrants. These criteria included age, education level, English proficiency, and an assessment, at the discretion of a federal U.S. Citizenship and Immigration Services (USCIS) officer, of whether an applicant is likely to apply to receive noncash federal benefits. These benefits include Medicaid, Federal Public Housing or Section 8 Housing Assistance, or Supplemental Nutrition Assistance Program (SNAP) support (One Nation Commission Report, 2019; One Nation AAPI, 2020). The expanded criteria were extolled by the Trump administration as important tools for blocking immigrants from taking advantage of systems supported by American taxpayers. The exclusion of children, older adults, low-income individuals, people with low English proficiency, and individuals with chronic medical conditions or disabilities from a pathway to legal residency was presented as a protective mechanism, integral to ensuring government support remains available for U.S. citizens.

Guidance for the application of these criteria, however, has remained unclear, leading to confusion and fear among immigrants and their families. In 2019, prior to the adoption of the new rule, a nationally representative internet-based survey found that one in seven adults in immigrant families (15.6%) avoided accessing government benefits such as Medicaid, Children's Health Insurance Program (CHIP), SNAP, or housing subsidies for fear of jeopardizing their legal residency status. Additionally, more than one in four adults in low-income immigrant families (26.2%) reported experiencing negative consequences due to avoiding use of these services (Berstein et al., 2020). The coronavirus disease 2019 (COVID-19) pandemic temporarily delayed implementation of the new Public Charge Rule on grounds of a national public health emergency. However, the Public

Charge Rule was reinstated in September 2020. Given evidence of its chilling effect on immigrant families even prior to its implementation, the Public Charge Rule is likely to have negative short- and long-term consequences on the social determinants of health and the health of all immigrants.

Beginning in 2018, Asian Americans and NH/PI communities joined together to speak out against the expansion of Public Charge criteria and continue to organize against the implementation of the new Public Charge Rule. The One Nation Commission, led by a panel of experts including economists, health care providers, philanthropists, academics, and community leaders, was formed to mobilize Asian Americans and NH/PI communities against the administration's assault against immigrants. In parallel, the One Nation Asian American and Pacific Islander (AAPI) Movement was formed to mobilize over 100 community partners. In October 2019, through One Nation Campaign, more than 23,000 public comments (8.6% of total comments) were submitted against the Public Charge Rule. The Campaign also held public rallies and organized civic engagement activities. One Nation Campaign mobilized support for H.R.3222, the "No Funds for Public Charge Act," introduced into Congress in June 2019 by Congresswoman Barbara Lee (CA-13), Congresswoman Judy Chu (CA-27), the Congressional Tri-Caucus (Congressional Asian Pacific American Caucus [CAPAC], Congressional Hispanic Caucus [CHC], and Congressional Black Caucus [CBC]), and the Congressional Progressive Caucus (CPC) (One Nation Commission Report, 2019). Although the legislation stalled, the bill was a critical statement by a broad coalition of communities of color against the use of federal funds to implement, administer, enforce or carry out the new Public Charge Rule (Chu, 2020).

The effects of Public Charge on immigrant health and well-being will be important to track, particularly since the new rule was released during the chaos of the COVID-19 pandemic and a long-overdue national reckoning with the devastating consequences of racism and racially based health disparities (Clark et al., 2020). In March 2021, President Joe Biden ended enforcement of the Trump administration's Public Charge restrictions following a federal court order blocking them.

PERVASIVE CHALLENGES TO ACHIEVING ASIAN AMERICAN HEALTH EQUITY

Advocacy for Asian American Health Research at the Federal Level

Consistent, multisectoral advocacy is essential to increasing the visibility of Asian Americans at the federal level and garnering the attention and resources necessary to address the unique health and social needs of this diverse population. Under the administration of President Barack Obama (2009–2017), a key mechanism to allow for this type of advocacy was created with the signing of Executive Order 13515 in October 2009. (EO 13515: Increasing Participation of Asian Americans and Pacific Islanders in Federal Programs, 2009). This executive action reestablished the 1999 White House Initiative on Asian Americans and Pacific Islanders (WHIAAPI) and, as its guiding body, the President's Advisory Commission on Asian Americans and Pacific Islanders. The purpose of the initiative was to "improve the quality of life and opportunities for this population through increased access to and participation in federal programs in which they may be underserved." The President's Advisory Commission was tasked with providing advice to the president and his administration about specific ways to achieve that goal by informing federal efforts to increase access to programs and services for Asian Americans and NH/PIs and encouraging community involvement to improve the well-being of Asian Americans and NH/PIs (White House Initiative on Asian Americans and Pacific Islanders, 2014).

The President's Advisory Commission was comprised of 20 representatives from the business, philanthropic, and nonprofit sectors. They brought a broad spectrum of experience in working with the government. During its first four years, WHIAPPI, led by the Commission, organized over 200 events, including national and regional interagency working groups, that successfully engaged over 30,000 people in over 50 cities and 25 states in the United States and the U.S.-affiliated Pacific Islands. The Commission acted as a liaison between the federal government and Asian American and NH/PI communities by providing education about federal resources and offering a forum for emerging Asian American and NH/PI communities to share their concerns and policy recommendations for federal programs. The Commission engaged an HiAP approach to work with federal agencies responsible for designing and implementing programs related to education, economic development, housing, community development, and health and human services by offering policy recommendations that could impact health and influence social determinants of health across sectors. The Commission also held the federal agencies accountable for integrating those recommendations and making progress toward the initiative's goals through regular and periodic agency reports. An important priority for WHIAAPI was to provide information to help Asian Americans and NH/PIs navigate and access federal funding and programs for which they qualify, such as health care programs for veterans and their families and food and housing resources for low-income individuals. One important product was the *Guide to Federal Agency Resources* and another was a series of capacity building workshops held across the country and delivered by the APIAHF, under contract with WHIAAPI, on how to apply for federal funding for community-based organizations (White House Initiative on Asian Americans and Pacific Islanders, 2011).

The Commission identified four priority areas for federal departments and agencies: (1) building the capacity of Asian American and NH/PI communities to engage with them; (2) improving data collection and analyses of disaggregated Asian American and NH/PI groups; (3) ensuring language access for individuals with limited English proficiency; and (4) increasing federal workforce opportunities for Asian Americans and NH/PIs. The Commission worked across 23 federal agencies to design and implement initiatives to support these priority areas. Examples included working with the Department of Education to release a Request for Proposals (RFP) for states that wished to disaggregate their education data further and partnering with HHS to conduct health-related outreach and education to Asian Americans and NH/PIs. The collaboration with HHS included webinars and roundtables on ACA implementation, mental health and disabilities, training nail salon owners and workers about health risks and safety measures regarding chemical exposure, and developing and disseminating a culturally tailored Let's Move Program, adapted for NH/PI communities from First Lady Michelle Obama's national health education and physical activity initiative to lower rates of overweight and obesity (LaBreche et al., 2016).

In 2014, the Commission identified two key recommendations to advance health equity (White House Initiative on Asian Americans and Pacific Islanders, 2014):

1. Catapult efforts to disaggregate data collection and analyses for Asian American and NH/PI subgroups in federal surveys.

2. Increase funding for health research on Asian Americans and NH/PIs and for services related to prevention and alleviation of the disease conditions prevalent among Asian Americans and NH/PIs.

Additionally, the Commission recommended creating a task force to address hate crimes impacting Asian Americans and NH/PIs (under the Civil Rights and Civil Liberties Focus) and ensuring that the nation's immigration enforcement objectives align with U.S. values (under the Commonsense Immigration Reform and Immigrant Integration Focus). The goals of the President's Advisory Commission were indicative of an overall responsiveness by the Obama administration to calls for moving the needle toward health equity for Asian American and NH/PI communities.

However, shortly after the Trump administration took office, in February 2017, 16 of the 20 commissioners resigned, a clear sign of the drastic shift in the political climate (Nguyen et al., 2017). The resigning commissioners cited reasons for their departure as being President Trump's immediate actions upon taking office to cut federal resources to sanctuary cities, ban refugees from predominately Muslim countries, increase border and immigrant enforcement, and attempt to repeal the ACA. Collectively, these changes threatened the civil rights and civil liberties of Asian American, NH/PI, and other communities of color.

In May 2019, the WHIAAPI was revived in the Department of Commerce, shifting its focus away from health equity toward business and economic issues. Without explicit strategic planning for a national health agenda, the prioritization of business and economy could result in worsening health outcomes and widening disparities for Asian Americans.

OPPORTUNITIES AND CHALLENGES FOR ASIAN AMERICAN HEALTH RESEARCH

As described in the previous sections, establishing dedicated funding streams for Asian American health research have shown success in meeting the needs of Asian American communities with sustainable and scalable federal health research initiatives. In the sections below, we describe opportunities and challenges to improving knowledge about Asian American health disparities and eliminating these disparities by addressing social determinants of health.

All of Us Research Program

The Precision Medicine Initiative (PMI) was launched by President Obama in 2015, invigorating a research era focused on identifying better treatments and disease interventions based on individual differences in genes, environments, and lifestyle factors (Collins & Varmus, 2015). The All of Us research program is a direct product of the PMI and was allocated $1.02 billion by Congress in 2015, with an additional $1.14 billion allocated through 2026 (All of Us Research Program Investigators et al., 2019). This study aims to enroll over one million adults, from over 340 recruitment sites, to understand relationships among lifestyle, environment, and genetic factors, with the overarching goal of accelerating precision diagnosis, prevention, and treatment (All of Us Research Program Investigators et al., 2019). The research program collects participant data from a variety of sources, including EHRs, self-reported health surveys, biospecimens, physical measures, and digital health information. The All of Us program launched in May 2018 and enrolled over 175,000 participants who provided biospecimens by July 2019.

In efforts to engage more participants underrepresented in biomedical research, All of Us has community engagement partners and champions tasked with increasing awareness about the research program and encouraging their respective communities to participate in precision medicine research. Awarded community partners and champions focused on Asian American populations include the Asian Health Coalition (Chicago, Illinois), Arab Community Center for Economic and Social Services (Dearborn, Michigan), Asian Pacific Community in Action in (Phoenix, Arizona), Filipino American Community Health Initiative of Chicago (Chicago, Illinois), and Healthy Asian Americans Project (Ypsilanti, Michigan). Because All of Us community partners and champions bridge the gap between researchers and research participants, selecting organizations serving Asian American populations may promote the recruitment and retention of Asian American participants. The data collected from this longitudinal cohort study has the potential to advance current knowledge about Asian American health and influence the trajectory of future research priorities.

Census 2020

The U.S. Constitution mandates that a census is conducted every decade for an accurate count of the population, including individuals who are citizens, non-citizens, and undocumented immigrants, living in the United States and U.S. territories (Puerto Rico, American Samoa, the Commonwealth of the Northern Mariana Islands, Guam, and the U.S. Virgin Islands). The Census Bureau collected 2020 Census information from households online, by mail, or by phone. Several logistical elements of the 2020 Census threaten the accuracy of the census population count. For example, as compared to the 2010 Census, the 2020 Census had a budget shortfall for planning and administration, which affected such vital components as piloting the internet survey and conducting community outreach and education. Additionally, Census 2020 had a shorter implementation timetable compared to the 2010 Census. These changes could result in inaccurate population counts, particularly for communities of color and immigrants who experience barriers to participation such as limited English proficiency and housing insecurity. Such inaccuracies have serious long-term consequences. Census results determine how many seats each state is given in the House of Representatives and influence the drawing of congressional and state legislative districts. Census data also directly affect how hundreds of billions of federal funding dollars will be allocated to U.S. communities to support large projects such as highway construction as well as for public assistance programs (e.g., Medicaid, Section 8 housing, SNAP), hospitals, and fire departments. Census 2020 will affect whether Asian American communities gain access to resources to improve the conditions in which individuals and families are born, live, work, and age over a decade. Advocacy efforts to inform politicians and other health stakeholders about possible inaccuracies in official Census numbers will be critical. Additionally, Asian American communities and their advocates must develop innovative strategies to mitigate challenges that could result from such inaccuracies, while simultaneously acknowledging that these data are essential to guiding funding decisions for research among the Asian American population as a whole.

Lessons Learned from COVID-19

With the lessons learned from the COVID-19 pandemic and a change in the political landscape, potential areas of focus have become clearer. For example, the omission of Asian Americans from research study samples remains critical, particularly as clinical trials conducted to date to develop vaccines for COVID-19 and identify therapies to treat COVID-19 have excluded Asian American participants (Jackson et al., 2020). Furthermore, the

COVID-19 pandemic underscored the importance of disaggregated data, highlighting the need for greater transparency in the collection of race/ethnicity data and for more precision in the methodologies employed to analyze these data. However, in a September 30, 2020, NIH press release, Asian Americans were omitted from the list of underserved and racial and ethnic minority communities to be prioritized by the Rapid Acceleration of Diagnostics for Underserved Populations (RadX-UP) initiative. RadX-UP, which is dedicated to exploring ways to accommodate cultural, ethnic, geographic, and community-based differences in the development of COVID-19-related technologies and treatments, disseminated nearly $283 million in its first two rounds of awards, but only two of the funded projects included outreach to Filipino Americans and one focused on Chinese, Vietnamese, and Hmong Americans – together representing only four of more than 40 ethnic subgroups within the Asian American population (National Institutes of Health, 2021). The persistent omission of the Asian American population from funding consideration is striking given data demonstrating the disproportionate impact of COVID-19 on Asian American communities (Yan et al., 2020).

Overlooking Asian Americans will only exacerbate health disparities and worsen health status in this diverse and rapidly growing population. Advocates must prioritize the recommendations of the Commission to address cross-cutting challenges and develop an inclusive national health agenda for Asian Americans. The lack of disaggregated data for Asian American subpopulations remains a key challenge, perpetuating the invisibility of this population at the federal level (Ponce et al., 2016). Without detailed data describing the health status of Asian Americans, federal policies and resource allocation will continue to perpetuate false generalizations about the population as a whole and overlook the needs of the Asian subgroups most vulnerable to worse health outcomes. Researchers have identified best practices for use in collecting, analyzing, and disaggregating data for small populations (Rubin et al., 2018). These innovative methodologies should be incorporated into federal survey design, administration, analysis, and reporting. Additionally, improving and enforcing existing policies to improve the collection of race and ethnicity data must be prioritized at the local, state, and federal levels. Examples of progress are found in the passage of state-level legislation supporting disaggregation of Asian American and NH/PI data in California (Assembly Bill No. 1726) and New York (Assembly Bill A7352). Chapter 4 further describes best practices on working toward more meaningful and representative data collection and analyses.

Despite persistent underfunding of Asian American–focused health research and the invisibility of health disparities in Asian American communities, this chapter has highlighted several examples of successful efforts to explore and address health disparities using a population health equity framework and leveraging multisectoral collaborations and partnerships. Building on these successes, federal resource allocation and legislative efforts, as well as philanthropic funding streams, must prioritize research topics that reflect the current and emerging needs of culturally, linguistically, and socioeconomically heterogeneous Asian American communities. Asian Americans are the fastest-growing racial/ethnic population in the United States, with the majority of growth attributed to high international migration (Vespa et al., 2020). Although inclusion of Asian Americans in research studies has increased slightly over time (Đoàn et al., 2019), there remains a persistent need to disaggregate data for Asian Americans and focus research efforts on growing immigrant subgroups in emerging geographic locations with high densities of Asian Americans.

SUMMARY AND RECOMMENDATIONS

The examples provided in this chapter underscore the many social and political influences that influence the health status of Asian Americans. The persistent invisibility of Asian Americans within the federal landscape must be addressed in order to ensure research is adequately funded and directed toward the health needs of this growing and diversifying population. Decreasing health disparities experienced by Asian Americans – and advancing health equity for all Americans – remains dependent on increasing federal investment and expanding legislation addressing the needs of Asian American communities. The following recommendations are offered to advance a National Asian American Health Agenda:

- *Establish an accountability system of federal programming and enforce reporting standards for maintaining, collecting, analyzing, and presenting data on race and ethnicity at all governmental levels.* At a minimum, there should be consistent definitions for race and ethnicity and mandatory racial/ethnic data collection across all federal agencies and with state and local governments. Asian American data should be reported separately from the NH/PI category, in accordance with the OMB Statistical Policy Directive No. 15, released in 1997. Collecting and presenting granular data on Asian American subgroups must be encouraged to promote data transparency so that Asian American individuals from all subgroups have access to data to advocate for their health.

■ *Increase funding opportunities for Asian American health research.* Federal funding must intentionally focus health research on the Asian American community, particularly among the fastest growing Asian American subpopulations, such as Asian American older adults, certain Asian ethnic subgroups, and multiracial Asian Americans. Funding is linked typically to short-term projects. Multiyear investments and sustained engagement with Asian American communities and research organizations are required to eliminate health disparities, particularly because of the heterogeneity of the population. The health equity framework needs to be embedded in all policies and funding announcements. Furthermore, funding opportunities for Asian American health research should not be limited to the silo of minority health research.

■ *Advocacy and mobilizing.* The slow progression toward data disaggregation and adequate investments to address health disparities requires continued linkages across multiple sectors (e.g., community-based organizations, academic institutions, health plans, providers, industry, advocacy groups) to align national, local, and individual priorities to best address the health needs of the community.

■ *Dedicated funding opportunities for community-based participatory research.* Community-based participatory research (CBPR), discussed in more detail in Chapter 8, has proved itself a successful methodology in creating systemic change for health equity research and for fostering sustainable partnerships and research capacity and infrastructure among the racial/ethnic minority populations typically deemed "hard-to-reach." The CBPR framework addresses these barriers through engagement of small populations via multisectoral collaborations. Efforts like community outreach and in-language programming are model practices that improve study recruitment, ensuring that Asian Americans are engaged throughout the research process. Funding opportunities must be intentional in directing resources toward less established and local organizations. Philanthropic organizations have a key role to play in this regard.

■ *Support the diversification of the health workforce.* The changing demographics of the Asian American community require a diverse multi-sectoral workforce attuned to the linguistic and cultural needs of this increasingly aging and growing population. Training students and researchers to focus on minority health issues is key to ensuring that Asian American health is addressed in federally funded health research. Training and education should begin early, with programs for secondary school students, and continue through graduate programs. Support must also continue beyond graduation, to bolster the careers of Asian American–focused health researchers. Within the clinical and community-based workforce, Asian American CHWs could be particularly effective in improving care for underserved Asian subgroups. As described in Chapter 9, given that evidence documenting the effectiveness and cost efficiency of the CHW model has been published, policy efforts should support the integration of CHWs into clinic-based settings through multiyear, sustainable funding streams.

DISCUSSION QUESTIONS

1. What is the impact of federal funding on improving or exacerbating gaps in Asian American health research?

2. What proportion of federal funding should be allocated to Asian American populations and what should the research priorities be?

3. What other recommendations should be offered to advance a National Asian American Health Agenda?

REFERENCES

2018 National Healthcare Quality and Disparities Report (AHRQ Pub. No. 19-0070-EF). (2019). Agency for Healthcare Research and Quality. https://www.ahrq.gov/sites/default/files/wysiwyg/research/findings/nhqrdr/2018qdr-final.pdf

Action for Health Justice. (2014). Improving the Road to ACA Coverage: Lessons Learned on Outreach, Education, and Enrollment for Asian American, Native Hawaiian, and Pacific Islander Communities. https://www.apiahf.org/wp-content/uploads/2014/10/2014.10.14_Improving-the-Road-to-ACA-Coverage_National-Report-1.pdf

All of Us Research Program Investigators, Denny, J. C., Rutter, J. L., Goldstein, D. B., Philippakis, A., Smoller, J. W., Jenkins, G., & Dishman, E. (2019). The "All of Us" Research Program. *The New England Journal of Medicine*, *381*(7), 668–676. https://doi.org/10.1056/NEJMsr1809937

Artiga, S., Garfield, R., & Damico, A. (2019). *Estimated Impacts of Final Public Charge Inadmissibility Rule on Immigrants and Medicaid Coverage* (p. 13). Henry J. Kaiser Family Foundation. http://files.kff.org/attachment/Issue-Brief-Estimated-Impacts-of-Final-Public-Charge-Inadmissibility-Rule-on-Immigrants-and-Medicaid-Coverage

EO 13515: Increasing Participation of Asian Americans and Pacific Islanders in Federal Programs, Executive Order 13515, United States. Office of the Federal Register, 74 53635 (2009). https://www.hsdl.org/?view&did=799535

Berstein, H., Gonzalez, D., Karpman, M., & Zuckerman, S. (2020). *Amid Confusion over the Public Charge Rule, Immigrant Families Continued Avoiding Public Benefits in 2019*. Urban Institute. https://www.urban.org/sites/default/files/publication/102221/amid-confusion-over-the-public-charge-rule-immigrant-families-continued-avoiding-public-benefits-in-2019_2.pdf

Blumenthal, Abrams, M., & Nuzum, R. (2015). The Affordable Care Act at 5 Years. *The New England Journal of Medicine*, 8.

Budiman, A., Cilluffo, A., & Ruiz, N. G. (2019). *Key facts about Asian origin groups in the U.S.* Pew Research Center.

Carnethon, M. R., Kershaw, K. N., & Kandula, N. R. (2020). Disparities Research, Disparities Researchers, and Health Equity. *JAMA*, *323*(3), 211–212. https://doi.org/10.1001/jama.2019.19329

Chu, J. sponsor. (2020). *H.R. 3222—116th Congress: No Federal Funds for Public Charge Act of 2019*, (2020). https://www.govtrack.us/congress/bills/116/hr3222

Clark, E., Fredricks, K., Woc-Colburn, L., Bottazzi, M. E., & Weatherhead, J. (2020). Disproportionate impact of the COVID-19 pandemic on immigrant communities in the United States. *PLoS Neglected Tropical Diseases*, *14*(7). https://doi.org/10.1371/journal.pntd.0008484

Collins, F. S., & Varmus, H. (2015). A new initiative on precision medicine. *New England Journal of Medicine*, *372*(9), 793–795.

Đoàn, L. N., Takata, Y., Sakuma, K.-L. K., & Irvin, V. L. (2019). Trends in clinical research including Asian American, Native Hawaiian, and Pacific Islander participants funded by the US National Institutes of Health, 1992 to 2018. *JAMA Network Open*, *2*(7), e197432. https://doi.org/10.1001/jamanetworkopen.2019.7432

Dong, X. (2019). Advancing Asian Health Equity: Multimodal approach to translate research into practice and policy. *Journal of the American Geriatrics Society*, *67*(Suppl 3), S476–S478. https://doi.org/10.1111/jgs.16110

Dorsey, R., Graham, G., Glied, S., Meyers, D., Clancy, C., & Koh, H. (2014). Implementing health reform: Improved data collection and the monitoring of health disparities. *Annual Review of Public Health*, *35*, 123–138. https://doi.org/10.1146/annurev-publhealth-032013-182423

George, S., Duran, N., & Norris, K. (2013). A Systematic Review of Barriers and Facilitators to Minority Research Participation Among African Americans, Latinos, Asian Americans, and Pacific Islanders. *American Journal of Public Health*, *104*(2), e16–e31. https://doi.org/10.2105/AJPH.2013.301706

Ghosh, C. (2003). Healthy People 2010 and Asian Americans/Pacific Islanders: Defining a baseline of information. *American Journal of Public Health*, *93*(12), 2093–2098.

Ghosh, C. (2010). A national health agenda for Asian Americans and Pacific Islanders. *Jama*, *304*(12), 1381–1382.

Ginther, D. K., Basner, J., Jensen, U., Schnell, J., Kington, R., & Schaffer, W. T. (2018). Publications as predictors of racial and ethnic differences in NIH research awards. *PLOS ONE*, *13*(11), e0205929. https://doi.org/10.1371/journal.pone.0205929

Ginther, D. K., Schaffer, W. T., Schnell, J., Masimore, B., Liu, F., Haak, L. L., & Kington, R. (2011). Race, Ethnicity, and NIH Research Awards. *Science*, *333*(6045), 1015–1019. https://doi.org/10.1126/science.1196783

Gunja, M. Z., Baumgartner, J. C., Shah, A., Radley, D. C., & Collins, S. R. (2020). *Gap Closed: The Affordable Care Act's Impact on Asian Americans' Health Coverage* [Data Brief]. The Commonwealth Fund. https://www.commonwealthfund.org/sites/default/files/2020-07/Gunja_gap_closed_ACA_impact_asian_americans_coverage_db.pdf

Gupta, P., & Ritoper, S. (2007). *Growing Opportunities. Will Funding Follow the Rise in Foundation Assets and Growth of AAPI Populations?* Asian Americans/Pacific Islanders in Philanthropy. https://www.aapip.org/sites/default/files/publication/files/aapip-gopps4www.pdf

Harawa, N. T., Manson, S. M., Mangione, C. M., Penner, L. A., Norris, K. C., DeCarli, C., Scarinci, I. C., Zissimopoulos, J., Buchwald, D. S., Hinton, L., & Pérez-Stable, E. J. (2017). Strategies for enhancing research in aging health disparities by mentoring diverse investigators. *Journal of Clinical and Translational Science*, *1*(3), 167–175. https://doi.org/10.1017/cts.2016.23

Holland, A. T., & Palaniappan, L. P. (2012). Problems With the Collection and Interpretation of Asian-American Health Data: Omission, Aggregation, and Extrapolation. *Annals of Epidemiology*, *22*(6), 397–405. https://doi.org/10.1016/j.annepidem.2012.04.001

Hoppe, T. A., Litovitz, A., Willis, K. A., Meseroll, R. A., Perkins, M. J., Hutchins, B. I., Davis, A. F., Lauer, M. S., Valantine, H. A., Anderson, J. M., & Santangelo, G. M. (2019). Topic choice contributes to the lower rate of NIH awards to African-American/Black scientists. *Science Advances*, *5*(10), eaaw7238. https://doi.org/10.1126/sciadv.aaw7238

Institute of Medicine (US) Committee on the Review and Assessment of the NIH's Strategic Research Plan and Budget to Reduce and Ultimately Eliminate Health Disparities, Thomson, G. E., Mitchell, F., & Williams, M. B. (2006). Overview of Health Disparities. *In Examining the Health Disparities Research Plan of the National Institutes of Health: Unfinished Business*. National Academies Press (US). https://www.ncbi.nlm.nih.gov/books/NBK57034/

Islam, N., Khan, S., Kwon, S., Jang, D., Ro, M., & Trinh-Shevrin, C. (2010). Methodological Issues in the Collection, Analysis, and Reporting of Granular Data in Asian American Populations: Historical Challenges and Potential Solutions. *Journal of Health Care for the Poor and Underserved*, *21*(4), 1354–1381. https://doi.org/10.1353/hpu.2010.0939

Jackson, L. A., Anderson, E. J., Rouphael, N. G., Roberts, P. C., Makhene, M., Coler, R. N., McCullough, M. P., Chappell, J. D., Denison, M. R., Stevens, L. J., Pruijssers, A. J., McDermott, A., Flach, B., Doria-Rose, N. A., Corbett, K. S., Morabito, K. M., O'Dell, S., Schmidt, S. D., Swanson, P. A., . . . Beigel, J. H. (2020). An mRNA Vaccine against SARS-CoV-2—Preliminary Report. *New England Journal of Medicine*. https://doi.org/10.1056/NEJMoa2022483

LaBreche, M., Cheri, A., Custodio, H., Fex, C. C., Foo, M. A., Lepule, J. T., May, V. T., Orne, A., Pang, J. K., Pang, V. K., Sablan-Santos, L., Schmidt-Vaivao, D., Surani, Z., Talavou, M. F., Toilolo, T., Palmer, P. H., & Tanjasiri, S. P. (2016). Let's Move for Pacific Islander Communities: An Evidence-Based Intervention to Increase Physical Activity. *Journal of Cancer Education : The Official Journal of the American Association for Cancer Education*, *31*(2), 261–267. https://doi.org/10.1007/s13187-015-0875-3

Lee, J. W. R., Brancati, F. L., & Yeh, H.-C. (2011). Trends in the prevalence of type 2 diabetes in Asians versus Whites: Results from the United States National Health Interview Survey, 1997–2008. *Diabetes Care*, *34*(2), 353–357. https://doi.org/10.2337/dc10-0746

Lee, S., Martinez, G., Ma, G. X., Hsu, C. E., Robinson, E. S., Bawa, J., & Juon, H.-S. (2010). Barriers to Health Care Access in 13 Asian American Communities. *American Journal of Health Behavior, 34*(1), 21–30.

Li, Y., Kong, N., Lawley, M. A., & Pagán, J. A. (2014). Using systems science for population health management in primary care. *Journal of Primary Care & Community Health, 5*(4), 242–246. https://doi.org/10.1177/2150131914536400

Li, Y., Kong, N., Lawley, M., Weiss, L., & Pagán, J. A. (2015). Advancing the use of evidence-based decision-making in local health departments with systems science methodologies. *American Journal of Public Health, 105 Suppl 2*, S217–222. https://doi.org/10.2105/AJPH.2014.302077

Lim, S., Chong, S., Min, D., Mohaimin, S., Roberts, T., Trinh-Shevrin, C., & Kwon, S. C. (2020). Alzheimer's Disease Screening Tools for Asian Americans: A Scoping Review. *Journal of Applied Gerontology: The Official Journal of the Southern Gerontological Society, 40*. https://doi.org/10.1177/0733464820967594

Lim, S., Mohaimin, S., Min, D., Roberts, T., Sohn, Y.-J., Wong, J., Sivanesathurai, R., Kwon, S. C., & Trinh-Shevrin, C. (2020). Alzheimer's disease and its related dementias among Asian Americans, Native Hawaiians, and Pacific Islanders: a scoping review. *Journal of Alzheimer's Disease: JAD, 77*(2), 523–537. https://doi.org/10.3233/JAD-200509

Lopez, P. M., Divney, A., Goldfeld, K., Zanowiak, J., Gore, R., Kumar, R., Laughlin, P., Sanchez, R., Beane, S., Trinh-Shevrin, C., Thorpe, L., & Islam, N. (2019). Feasibility and outcomes of an electronic health record intervention to improve hypertension management in immigrant-serving primary care practices. *Medical Care, 57*(Suppl 6 2), S164–S171. https://doi.org/10.1097/MLR.0000000000000994

Minority Health and Health Disparities Research and Education Act of 2000, no. P.L. 106–525, 2507 (2000).

National Council of Asian Pacific Islander Physicians. (2015). *The Impact of the Affordable Care Act on Asian Indian, Chinese, Filipino, Korean, Pakistani, and Vietnamese Americans* [Policy Brief]. https://www.searac.org/wp-content/uploads/2018/04/2015_ACA_policy_brief_v13_final.pdf

National Institutes of Health. (2017). *Resource Centers for Minority Aging Research (RCMAR) (P30)*. Department of Health and Human Services. https://grants.nih.gov/grants/guide/rfa-files/RFA-AG-18-003.html

National Institutes of Health. (2021, July 2). Rapid Acceleration of Diagnostics (RADx). https://www.nih.gov/research-training/medical-research-initiatives/radx

National Institutes of Health Revitalization Act of 1993, no. PL 103-43 (1993).

Nguyen, T. T., Okada, M., Byun, M., Ko Chin, K., Fitisemanu, J., Kwok, D., Mailer, D. J., Pancholy, M., Phan, L., & Pradhan, S. (2017, February 15). Letter to President Trump from 10 Members of the President's Advisory Commission on Asian Americans and Pacific Islanders. https://www.scribd.com/document/339498786/Letter-to-President-Trump-from-10-Members-of-the-President-s-Advisory-Commission-on-Asian-Americans-and-Pacific-Islanders

Oberlander, J. (2010). Long time coming: why health reform finally passed. *Health Affairs, 29*(6), 1112–1116. https://doi.org/10.1377/hlthaff.2010.0447

Office of Management and Budget. (1997). *Revisions to the Standards for the Classification of Federal Data on Race and Ethnicity* (Notice Federal Register 62FR58781–58790; pp. 58782–58790). https://www.govinfo.gov/content/pkg/FR-1997-10-30/pdf/97-28653.pdf

One Nation AAPI. (2020). Public charge rule changes FAQ for community members. https://static1.squarespace.com/static/5b155efb5b409be6e602534c/t/5e471c819f51720ffbdc0090/1581718657864/Public+Charge+Final+Rule+FAQ+2-13-2020.pdf

One Nation Commission Report. (2019). *One Nation Built on the Strength of Immigrants*. https://static1.squarespace.com/static/5b155efb5b409be6e602534c/t/5e50824a976c87268cd204ec/1582334543015/OneNationCommisionReport_web.pdf

Oza-Frank, R., Ali, M. K., Vaccarino, V., & Narayan, K. M. V. (2009). Asian Americans: diabetes prevalence across U.S. and World Health Organization weight classifications. *Diabetes Care, 32*(9), 1644–1646. https://doi.org/10.2337/dc09-0573

Park, J. J., Humble, S., Sommers, B. D., Colditz, G. A., Epstein, A. M., & Koh, H. K. (2018). Health insurance for Asian Americans, Native Hawaiians, and Pacific Islanders under the Affordable Care Act. *JAMA Internal Medicine, 178*(8), 1128–1129. https://doi.org/10.1001/jamainternmed.2018.1476

Philanthropic Initiative for Racial Equity. (2017). What does philanthropy need to know to prioritize racial justice? [Infographic]. https://racial-equity.org/wp-content/uploads/2018/12/PRE-Infographic.pdf

Ponce, N., Scheitler, A., & Shimkhada, R. (2016). *Understanding the culture of health for Asian American, Native Hawaiian and Pacific Islanders* (AANHPIs): What do population-based health surveys across the nation tell us about the state of data disaggregation for AANHPIs? Robert Wood Johnson Foundation. http://www.policylink.org/sites/default/files/AANHPI-draft-Report-9-262016.pdf

Quinn, E., & Kinoshita, S. (2020). An overview of public charge and benefits. Immigrant Legal Resource Center. https://www.ilrc.org/sites/default/files/resources/overview_of_public_charge_and_benefits-march2020-v3.pdf

Ramkrishnan, K. S., Do, M., Shao, S., Eng, P., Hadi, B., & Kan, L. M. (2020). State of Philanthropy among Asian Americans and Pacific Islanders: Findings and Recommendations to Strengthen Visibility and Impact (p. 16). AAPI Data.

Research!America. (2019). U.S. Investments in Medical and Health Research and Development 2013–2018. https://www.researchamerica.org/sites/default/files/Publications/InvestmentReport2019_Fnl.pdf

Rosenbaum, S. (2011). The Patient Protection and Affordable Care Act: Implications for public health policy and practice. *Public Health Reports, 126*(1), 130–135.

Rubin, V., Ngo, D., Ross, A., Butler, D., & Balaram, N. (2018). Counting a diverse nation: disaggregating data on race and ethnicity to advance a culture of health. PolicyLink. https://www.policylink.org/sites/default/files/Counting_a_Diverse_Nation_08_15_18.pdf

The Patient Protection and Affordable Care Act, no. H.R.3590, 124 119 (2010). https://www.congress.gov/111/plaws/publ148/PLAW-111publ148.pdf

Trinh-Shevrin, C., Kwon, S. C., Park, R., Nadkarni, S. K., & Islam, N. S. (2015). Moving the dial to Advance Population Health Equity in New York City Asian American Populations. *American Journal of Public Health, 105*(Suppl 3), e16–e25. https://doi.org/10.2105/AJPH.2015.302626

U.S. Citizenship and Immigration Services. (2020, September 22). *Public Charge Fact Sheet*. https://www.uscis.gov/news/public-charge-fact-sheet

Vespa, J., Medina, L., & Armstrong, D. M. (2020). Demographic turning points for the United States: Population projections for 2020 to 2060 (Current Population Report). https://www.census.gov/content/dam/Census/library/publications/2020/demo/p25-1144.pdf

Viergever, R. F., & Hendriks, T. C. C. (2016). The 10 largest public and philanthropic funders of health research in the world: What they fund and how they distribute their funds. *Health Research Policy and Systems, 14*(1). https://doi.org/10.1186/s12961-015-0074-z

White House Initiative on Asian Americans and Pacific Islanders. (2011). *Guide to Federal Agency Resources.* Washington, D.C. https://obamawhitehouse.archives.gov/sites/default/files/whiaapi_accomplishment_highlights.pdf

White House Initiative on Asian Americans and Pacific Islanders. (2014). *Building the American Mosaic: Report from the President's Advisory Commission on Asian Americans and Pacific Islanders.* U.S. Department of Education. https://obamawhitehouse.archives.gov/sites/default/files/docs/american-mosaic_digital.pdf

Yan, B., Ng, F., Chu, J., Tsoh, J., & Nguyen, T. (2020, July 13). *Asian Americans Facing High COVID-19 Case Fatality.* Health Affairs Blog. https://doi.org/10.1377/hblog20200708.894552

Ye, J., Rust, G., Baltrus, P., & Daniels, E. (2009). Cardiovascular Risk Factors among Asian Americans: Results from a National Health Survey. *Annals of Epidemiology, 19*(10), 718–723. https://doi.org/10.1016/j.annepidem.2009.03.022

Yi, S. S. (2020). Taking Action to Improve Asian American Health. *American Journal of Public Health, 110*(4), 435–437.

Yi, S. S., Kwon, S. C., Sacks, R., & Trinh-Shevrin, C. (2016). Commentary: persistence and health-related consequences of the model minority stereotype for Asian Americans. *Ethnicity & Disease, 26*(1), 133–138. https://doi.org/10.18865/ed.26.1.133

AFTERWORD: WHERE TO NEXT?

SHOBHA SRINIVASAN, RINA DAS

"There comes a point where we need to stop just pulling people out of the river. We need to go upstream and find out why they're falling in." Desmond Tutu

The readers of this book will note that research with Asian American communities has significantly increased in the last 25 years, with a growing number of researchers interested in exploring this area of health research. This expansion has led to a deeper understanding of the challenges in and opportunities for advancing health care and public health research with Asian American communities. In this final section, we highlight key avenues for further research and future directions with Asian American and Native Hawaiian and Pacific Islander (NH/PI) communities over the next decade.

AN ETHICAL QUESTION: TO COMBINE OR NOT TO COMBINE?

Appropriate data collection and use remains a significant obstacle to researchers focused on Asian Americans and NH/PIs. While this population is growing in the United States, conducting research among the smaller racial sub-populations that comprise this population remains challenging. Small-population research requires a deep understanding of the unique context in which people live so that appropriate studies may be developed and implemented with communities. In larger studies, the lack of sufficient data on Asian Americans and NH/PI has resulted in either the exclusion of this population from analyses entirely or the collapsing or aggregating of all subpopulations into one amorphous whole – a methodological approach that masks within-group differences and indirectly contributes to the exacerbation of health disparities and inequities for smaller racial/ethnic populations.

Aggregating data for all Asian Americans and NH/PI for purposes of expediency without regard to variability in the social determinants of health, immigration experiences, environmental or genetic variances, and other factors among various Asian Americans and NH/PI subpopulations is inappropriate and ethically questionable. When designing a study, health researchers must evaluate whether data aggregation is feasible and ethically informed for that particular project or whether the situation demands that aggregation be avoided and the population kept "small."

For that matter, when is it appropriate to combine data from all racial/ethnic groups or groups based on factors such as geographic location or social conditions? Sociodemographic factors are not mere nuances of research design. Understanding the unique circumstances in which populations of interest live will be critical to promoting research about Asian Americans and NH/PI health, especially for smaller, marginalized subpopulations. A recent National Institutes of Health (NIH) workshop, *Identifying Research Opportunities for Asian Americans, Native Hawaiians, and Pacific Islanders (NHPI) Health*, found the lack of data and limited disaggregated data regarding disease prevalence, incidence, natural history, risk factors, and health outcomes, especially for specific sub-populations, indicated major gaps in the field, hampering progress toward achieving equity for all. To address these gaps, researchers need to identify new ways to leverage and enhance existing data sources through greater inclusion and more systematic identification of Asian Americans and NH/PI subgroups (https://www.nhlbi.nih.gov/events/2021/identifying-research-opportunities-asian-american-native-hawaiian-and-pacific-islander).

Applied Population Health Approaches for Asian American Communities, First Edition. Edited by Simona C. Kwon, Chau Trinh-Shevrin, Nadia S. Islam, and Stella S. Yi.
© 2023 John Wiley & Sons, Inc. Published 2023 by John Wiley & Sons, Inc.
Companion Website: www.wiley.com/go/kwon/asianamerican

Achieving health equity may require partnerships for research with various other underserved populations. Working with groups that face similar challenges will help inform and build advocacy to address ongoing disparities in health.

ETIOLOGY STUDIES

Future research among Asian American and NH/PI subpopulations must also prioritize investment in multidisciplinary etiology studies – those that can delineate the social histories, processes of immigration (including discrimination and exclusion), and genetic and phenotypical characteristics. As this book has shown, we are investing in our communities now to understand and address current disparities in health – but this investment will only serve as a Band-Aid until we can explore the underlying social determinants of health, including the interplay of structural, social, cultural, environmental, and neighborhood factors. Only by developing a better understanding of the complex causes of these disparities can we address them effectively.

Etiological and epidemiological multisite prospective cohort studies that go beyond individual-level studies will help us identify areas for future research and develop interventions that are multifactorial and multilevel, providing a step forward in eradicating disparities and promoting health equity. Future research will also need to examine the intersection of heath and disease with race/ethnicity, culture, socioeconomic position, gender, geography, and co-morbidities to improve health outcomes.

MULTISITE CENTERS FOR ASIAN AMERICAN HEALTH

Research and advocacy at the community, local, state, and national levels have been critical to improving Asian American health. Much of this research has taken place because there have been centers to promote research on Asian Americans and NH/PIs. Research centers have the infrastructure and capacity to design and conduct studies as well as involve communities and train the next generation of researchers. For example, the National Research Center on Asian American Mental Health was first established in 1988 at the University of California, Los Angeles (UCLA) and then moved to the University of California, Davis (UCD). This center has designed and implemented research that has proven essential to identifying the mental health needs of Asian American communities, specifically Chinese Americans, as well as developing ways to measure mental health challenges among Asian Americans and training scholars to address Asian American mental health. Similarly, since 2003, the NYU Center for the Study of Asian American Health (CSAAH) at NYU Grossman School of Medicine has provided funding and research to seed the foundation for ongoing work among Asian American communities. Future investment in establishing and developing additional centers focused on the needs of Asian Americans and NH/PIs is critical to building sustainable community partnerships, spurring minority health and health disparities research, providing alliances for new research and establishing the infrastructure for training junior researchers.

CONCLUSION

The future of Asian American and NH/PI health research, especially in understanding the nuances of the various subpopulations, the differences, and commonalities within and between the populations, depends on how well we can inform and help the next generation of researchers to conduct multidisciplinary research studies. Toward this end, we must commit ourselves to promoting the development of large, multisite etiology studies that examine the influence of various social determinants of health; establishing research centers focused on addressing the health and training needs of diverse Asian American and NH/PI communities while simultaneously building alliances with other racial/ethnic communities; and developing and implementing multisite, multilevel, and multifactorial interventions. This three-pronged approach will ensure our holistic commitment to health equity.

APPENDIX

CASE STUDIES

CASE

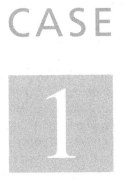

REACH FAR: CULTURALLY ADAPTED, EVIDENCE-BASED HYPERTENSION CONTROL PROGRAMS AMONG ASIAN AMERICANS IN NEW YORK AND NEW JERSEY

DEBORAH K. MIN

Hypertension affects nearly half of adults in the United States and is a major risk factor for cardiovascular disease, the leading cause of death among American adults (Virani et al., 2021). Despite elevated hypertension risk among Asian Americans, there are limited evidence-based programs and policies to improve hypertension control in this disparity population. To address this gap, the NYU Center for the Study of Asian American Health (CSAAH) at NYU Grossman School of Medicine implemented the Racial and Ethnic Approaches to Community Health for Asian Americans (REACH FAR) project. REACH FAR adapted proven evidence-based strategies (EBSs) in hypertension control to better respond to the needs of linguistically and culturally diverse Asian American communities in New York and New Jersey. This case study presents key aspects of the program's design, process evaluation, and achievements, with a view toward providing a model for researchers seeking to tailor programming to better address the needs of diverse immigrant and underserved communities nationwide.

Applied Population Health Approaches for Asian American Communities, First Edition. Edited by Simona C. Kwon, Chau Trinh-Shevrin, Nadia S. Islam, and Stella S. Yi.
© 2023 John Wiley & Sons, Inc. Published 2023 by John Wiley & Sons, Inc.
Companion Website: www.wiley.com/go/kwon/asianamerican

PROGRAM DESIGN

REACH FAR was implemented during 2014–2017 in Asian Indian, Bangladeshi, Filipino, and Korean neighborhoods across the NYC metropolitan area, stretching into New Jersey. To design REACH FAR, CSAAH spearheaded a multisector coalition that included the NYC Department of Health and Mental Hygiene (Health Department) and four community-based organizations (CBOs). The coalition's work was guided by two key objectives: (1) improve healthy eating options for Asian Americans through a nutrition strategy; and (2) increase access to hypertension prevention and control programs for Asian Americans through a clinical-community linkage strategy. REACH FAR employed a community-based participatory research (CBPR) approach to adapt and implement proven EBSs to contribute to both of the program's strategies. As described in greater detail in Chapter 8, CBPR is a methodology through which researchers engage with populations of interest and partner with community stakeholders to help them articulate their own priorities and design research to address community needs (Israel et al., 1998). Coalition partners worked collaboratively to identify and further engage 12 faith-based organizations (FBOs) (including Christian churches, Sikh gurdwaras, and Islamic mosques), 8 restaurants, and 6 ethnic grocery stores in health promotion and disease prevention strategies.

At the outset of the program, REACH FAR staff provided implementation sites with technical assistance, training, and resources. At FBOs, both of the REACH FAR program strategies were implemented. First, when serving communal meals to congregants, FBOs adhered to policies set by the New York City Food Standards (https://www1.nyc.gov/site/doh/health/health-topics/healthy-workplaces.page) to improve the availability of healthy food options. Second, FBOs offered a clinical-community linkage component, represented by Keep on Track (KOT), a blood pressure monitoring program developed by the Health Department (Kwon et al., 2017). At restaurants and grocery stores, sites implemented policies adapted from the Health Department's Shop Healthy program (https://www1.nyc.gov/site/doh/health/neighborhood-health/shop-health.page) and menu labeling initiatives, both of which aimed to support REACH FAR's first strategy of improving access to healthy eating options. Of the total 26 sites that initially agreed to participate in REACH FAR, 20 sites completed the 24-month program. A detailed summary of REACH FAR program components by strategy and implementation site is presented in Table A1.1.

CULTURAL ADAPTATIONS OF EBSs

Cultural adaptation is defined as "the systematic modification of an evidence-based [program] to consider language, culture, and context in such a way that is compatible with the [community's] cultural patterns, meanings and values" and is becoming more and more important as the U.S. population becomes increasingly diverse (Bernal et al., 1995). Guided by the Ecological Validity Model (EVM), which specifies eight domains for cultural adaptation (language, persons, metaphors, content, concepts, goals, methods, and context), REACH FAR adapted EBSs for hypertension control (Kwon et al., 2017). These adaptations are presented in Table A1.2. To support the adaptation process, a CBPR approach was paired with social marketing techniques in order to increase acceptability of new ideas. Social marketing applies principles from the commercial sector to influence audiences to engage in beneficial behavioral change for health promotion (Harris et al., 2012; Kotler & Zaltman, 1971; Nelson et al., 2008).

PROCESS EVALUATION

While program evaluations typically assess the impact of culturally adapted health education and behavior modification programs on health outcomes, research regarding the implementation process is limited, particularly with respect to programs focused on Asian American communities (Ferdinand et al., 2012; Gore et al., 2020; Leyva et al., 2017; Mensah et al., 2018; Nierkens et al., 2013). Knowledge about program acceptability is needed to inform both the dissemination of culturally adapted hypertension control EBSs as well as future research and program design (Mueller et al., 2015). To address this gap, we focused uniquely on the 20 implementation sites that successfully completed the program, aiming to identify site characteristics and other factors that might facilitate success in integrating health education and behavior modification programming within culturally and linguistically distinct communities. Applying the Consolidated Framework for Implementation Research

TABLE A1.1 REACH FAR Program Components

Program components	Intervention options for implementing sites
Nutrition strategies and Keep on Track blood pressure monitoring program	
FBOs 12 sites enrolled; 11 sites completed the program.	- Adopt at least one nutrition policy change out of six related to food and beverages served at on-site communal meals. For example, offer choices of fruit, leafy green salad or fresh vegetable, whole grain options, low-fat milk or yogurt, and low-sodium dressings and condiments. Make water available at no charge during meals. - Hold monthly hypertension screenings so participants can have their blood pressure checked and recorded by a program volunteer, receive one-on-one health counseling, and receive culturally tailored and translated program handouts to improve healthy behavior. Program volunteers to advise participants to take their blood pressure medication as directed by their health provider.
Strategies adapted from NYC's Shop Healthy program and menu labeling initiative	
Restaurants 6 sites enrolled; 3 sites completed the program.	- Implement at least one of six strategies related to menu labeling and options, such as highlighting healthy menu choices, expanding healthier menu options, offering lower pricing or discounts for healthier options, decreasing access to high-sodium products, and decreasing portion sizes.
Grocery stores 8 sites enrolled; 6 sites completed the program.	- Implement at least one of four strategies to increase sales of healthier foods through price incentives, product placement, product promotion and advertising, and greater product choices.
Total participating sites = 26 Of the 26 initially enrolled sites, 20 completed the full program (24 months).	

Source: Gore (2020) / with permission of Oxford University Press.

(CFIR) – a framework discussed in detail in Chapter 5 – CSAAH conducted semi-structured interviews with 15 implementation site leaders from among the 20 sites that completed the program. We focused on understanding the perceptions of site leaders and champions about adopting, adapting, and sustaining the program at the inner (organization) and outer (community or health care) settings to inform future translation and sustainability (Gore et al., 2020). Findings showed that REACH FAR resonated with sites in which:

1. Leaders perceived that unhealthy dietary habits and lifestyles were prevalent in their communities (intervention characteristics);

2. Historically, sites had engaged in health programs as a public service mission (inner setting) and leaders identified with this mission (individuals' characteristics);

3. Site leaders strived to adapt programs to respond to community preferences (outer setting) without compromising core objectives (inner setting); and

4. Leaders noted that that program sustainability could be impeded by staff and volunteer turnover (inner setting) but enhanced by reinforcing programs through community networks (outer setting).

TABLE A1.2   **Cultural Adaptations Using the Ecological Validity Model for REACH FAR Strategies**

Culturally-sensitive domain	Key adaptations	Examples from strategy 1 (nutrition/food access)	Examples from strategy 2 (KOT program)
Language	All program materials were translated to four languages.	For all communities, translation of nutrition posters.	Translation of blood pressure "tracking" card.
Persons	Community and FBO leaders were engaged for program and policy implementation.	Among Korean churches, kitchen staff delivered nutrition education.	For all communities, volunteer trainers were members of FBOs.
Metaphors	Asian- and, where relevant, Asian ethnic subgroup-specific idioms and colloquial phrases were incorporated into materials and training.	For all communities, outreach materials addressed Asian condiments and spice mixes as a key source of dietary sodium.	For all communities, the metaphor of "Blood Pressure Control—It's in Your Court," which community partners expressed would not resonate with Asian individuals, was removed.
Content	Cultural values framed goals and activities (e.g., the importance of traditional and cultural foods and dishes was explicitly acknowledged).	For all communities, outreach materials highlighting the importance of consuming fresh produce were adapted to include images of traditional Asian fruits and vegetables common across subgroups (e.g., bitter melon, guava, cabbage, starfruit).	Training materials and health education materials were adapted to include images of Asian men and women, in both traditional and mainstream dress.
Concepts	The goal of maintaining one's individual health for the health of the family, to promote family harmony, and to support collectivism was integrated.	Among the Sikh community, incorporated the concept of *seva* (service) in promotion of healthy foods to serve during *langar* (shared communal meals) in *gurdwaras* (places of worship).	For all communities, training materials incorporated counseling for participants that emphasized engaging in health promotion activities with family and social networks.
Goals	Program goals were bolstered with messaging and framing around collectivism and group harmony.	For the Filipino community, health education materials incorporated Bible scripture and utilized Bible study guide templates to discuss healthy eating.	Similarly, Bible scripture and study guide templates were applied to promotion of blood pressure monitoring.

Methods	Program activities or procedures were adapted. Given strong leadership and respect for faith leaders, incorporated guidelines and protocols to enhance faith leadership engagement in the program.	To reach South Asian Muslims, nutrition policies in mosques were implemented to align with the month of Ramadan, when FBOs provide daily *iftar* (breakfast) at sundown to celebrate the breaking of fast by incorporating healthy food options during the meal. In Korean and Filipino churches and Sikh gurdwaras, changes were introduced at weekly meal services and adapted if meals were prepared on-site or donated by congregants.	For all communities, FBO leaders were encouraged to enroll in the KOT study and to incorporate project information through FBO-wide announcements.
Context	Contextual issues were incorporated into program and policy procedures.	For all communities, healthy traditional foods or traditional foods with heart-healthy modifications were promoted.	For all communities, FBO congregants were linked to health providers that accepted a variety of insurance types and offered low-cost, sliding fee scales.

Source: Adapted from Kwon (2017).

The findings suggested that to facilitate implementation of culturally adapted health behavior programs through community sites, interventions should reinforce organizational commitments and social ties of the sites.

CONCLUSION

REACH FAR presented a unique opportunity for a multisector coalition to confront hypertension disparities in the Asian Indian, Bangladeshi, Filipino, and Korean communities in New York and New Jersey. Since the completion of the program in 2017, information and programming developed as part of REACH FAR has been translated to new settings in the NYC metropolitan region. For example, researchers worked to integrate program components into NYU Langone's Community Service Plan (CSP), which is a coordinated effort implemented by NYU Langone's Department of Population Health through the Family Health Centers at NYU Langone – primary care centers located throughout the NYC metropolitan area. As part of this effort, REACH FAR's nutrition strategy was translated for implementation in additional mosques throughout the city. When the novel coronavirus (COVID-19) pandemic impacted health programming, volunteers working in these mosques further adapted the REACH FAR strategic approach and used their training to pivot their roles and activities to address food security in their communities.

EBSs to improve policy, systems, and environmental outcomes are critical tools for mitigating health disparities. REACH FAR demonstrated that community settings – including FBOs, restaurants, and ethnic grocery stores – can be leveraged successfully to implement culturally adapted EBSs to reach underserved Asian American immigrant communities. REACH FAR adds to the knowledge base of ways that health researchers and clinicians may build bridges between the health system and diverse racial and ethnic communities with unique linguistic and cultural attributes. Toward that end, our development process can be used to guide cultural adaptations of EBSs for other immigrant and underserved communities.

REFERENCES

Bernal, G., Bonilla, J., & Bellido, C. (1995). Ecological validity and cultural sensitivity for outcome research: issues for the cultural adaptation and development of psychosocial treatments with Hispanics. *Journal of Abnormal Child Psychology* 23(1): 67–82. https://doi.org/10.1007/BF01447045

Ferdinand, K. C., Patterson, K. P., Taylor, C., Fergus, I. V., Nasser, S. A., & Ferdinand, D. P. (2012). Community-based approaches to prevention and management of hypertension and cardiovascular disease. *Journal of Clinical Hypertension* (Greenwich, Conn.) 14(5): 336–343. https://doi.org/10.1111/j.1751-7176.2012.00622.x

Gore, R., Patel, S., Choy, C., Taher, M., Garcia-Dia, M. J., Singh, H., Kim, S., Mohaimin, S., Dhar, R., Naeem, A., Kwon, S. C., & Islam, N. (2020). Influence of organizational and social contexts on the implementation of culturally adapted hypertension control programs in Asian American-serving grocery stores, restaurants, and faith-based community sites: a qualitative study. *Translational Behavioral Medicine* 10(6): 1525–1537. https://doi.org/10.1093/tbm/ibz106

Harris, J. R., Cheadle, A., Hannon, P. A., Forehand, M., Lichiello, P., Mahoney, E., Snyder, S., & Yarrow, J. (2012). A framework for disseminating evidence-based health promotion practices. *Preventing Chronic Disease* 9: E22.

Israel, B. A., Schulz, A. J., Parker, E. A., & Becker, A. B. (1998). Review of community-based research: assessing partnership approaches to improve public health. *Annual Review of Public Health* 19: 173–202. https://doi.org/10.1146/annurev.publhealth.19.1.173

Kotler, P., & Zaltman, G. (1971). Social marketing: an approach to planned social change. *Journal of Marketing* 35(3): 3–12.

Kwon, S. C., Patel, S., Choy, C., Zanowiak, J., Rideout, C., Yi, S., Wyatt, L., Taher, M. D., Garcia-Dia, M. J., Kim, S. S., Denholm, T. K., Kavathe, R., & Islam, N. S. (2017). Implementing health promotion activities using community-engaged approaches in Asian American faith-based organizations in New York City and New Jersey. *Translational Behavioral Medicine* 7(3): 444–466. https://doi.org/10.1007/s13142-017-0506-0.

Leyva, B., Allen, J. D., Ospino, H., Tom, L. S., Negrón, R., Buesa, R., & Torres, M. I. (2017). Enhancing capacity among faith-based organizations to implement evidence-based cancer control programs: a community-engaged approach. *Translational Behavioral Medicine* 7(3): 517–528. https://doi.org/10.1007/s13142-017-0513-1.

Mensah, G. A., Cooper, R. S., Siega-Riz, A. M., Cooper, L. A., Smith, J. D., Brown, C. H., . . . Pérez-Stable, E. J. (2018). Reducing Cardiovascular Disparities Through Community-Engaged Implementation Research: A National Heart, Lung, and Blood Institute Workshop Report. *Circulation Research* 122(2): 213–230. https://doi.org/10.1161/CIRCRESAHA.117.312243

Mueller, M., Purnell, T. S., Mensah, G. A., & Cooper, L. A. (2015). Reducing racial and ethnic disparities in hypertension prevention and control: what will it take to translate research into practice and policy? *American Journal of Hypertension* 28(6): 699–716. https://doi.org/10.1093/ajh/hpu233

Nelson, D. E., Gallogly, M., Pederson, L. L., Barry, M., McGoldrick, D., & Maibach, E. W. (2008). Use of consumer survey data to target cessation messages to smokers through mass media. *American Journal of Public Health* 98(3): 536–542. https://doi.org/10.2105/AJPH.2006.090340

Nierkens, V., Hartman, M. A., Nicolaou, M., Vissenberg, C., Beune, E. J., Hosper, K., van Valkengoed, I. G., & Stronks, K. (2013). Effectiveness of cultural adaptations of interventions aimed at smoking cessation, diet, and/or physical activity in ethnic minorities. a systematic review. *PloS One* 8(10): e73373. https://doi.org/10.1371/journal.pone.0073373.

Virani, S. S., Alonso, A., Aparicio, H. J., Benjamin, E. J., Bittencourt, M. S., Callaway, C. W., . . . American Heart Association Council on Epidemiology and Prevention Statistics Committee and Stroke Statistics Subcommittee (2021). Heart Disease and Stroke Statistics–2021 Update: A Report From the American Heart Association. *Circulation* 143(8): e254–e743. https://doi.org/10.1161/CIR.0000000000000950.

CASE

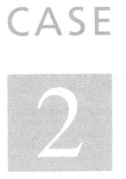

AN INTEGRATIVE DATA APPROACH TO STUDY LUNG CANCER AMONG AA AND NH/PI FEMALES

SCARLETT LIN GOMEZ, IONA CHENG, MINDY C. DeROUEN

Asian American (AA) and Native Hawaiian and Pacific Islander (NH/PI) females who have never smoked experience a disproportionately high burden of lung cancer. While an estimated 15% of all female lung cancer cases in the United States occur among never-smokers, previous reports based on select case series have suggested that up to 70% of lung cancer cases among AA and NH/PI females occur among never-smokers (Gomez et al., 2011). Yet examining lung cancer among AA and NH/PI never-smoking females has been hindered by a lack of population-level incidence data stratified by sex, race and ethnicity, and smoking status. Developing a single database documenting lung cancer incidence rates by smoking status that is sufficiently large to allow for detailed analyses of AA and NH/PI ethnic groups is central to understanding and reducing the lung cancer burden among AA and NH/PI females. In addition, while there are putative risk factors for lung cancer among those who have never smoked (i.e., passive smoking, air pollution, radon, family history of lung cancer, and cooking oil fumes), the degree to which these and other suspected lung cancer risk factors contribute to lung cancer among AA and NH/PI females who have never smoked remains largely unknown (Sisti and Boffetta, 2012; Subramanian and Govindan, 2007; Sun et al., 2007). Much of our knowledge to date on Asian American females is based on studies conducted in Asia, limiting our understanding of risk factors in the development of this disease in the United States.

Integrative data analysis, which involves combining data to enrich the number of observations and/or number of explanatory variables, takes advantage of existing resources (i.e., observational health care data initially collected for non-research purposes) and may be used to examine rare diseases among small populations. Applying this methodology, we assembled a large-scale, multilevel electronic health record (EHR)-based cohort with the purpose of facilitating research on the etiology of lung cancer among AA and NH/PI ethnic groups (Figure A.1.1). The cohort includes female and male individuals of any race or ethnicity and is designed

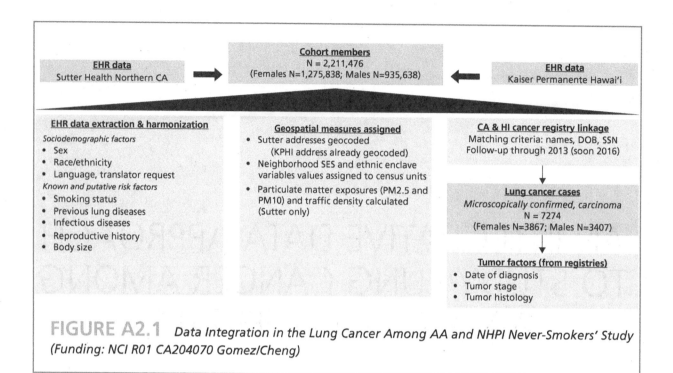

FIGURE A2.1 *Data Integration in the Lung Cancer Among AA and NHPI Never-Smokers' Study (Funding: NCI R01 CA204070 Gomez/Cheng)*

specifically to quantify the burden and risk of lung cancer by smoking status and sex among single and multiracial AA and NH/PI ethnic groups. The cohort dataset contains EHR data from two large health care systems linked to their respective statewide cancer registries and geospatial data. The health care systems—Sutter Health (in northern California) and Kaiser Permanente Hawai'i—were selected because of their robust AA and NH/PI patient populations and the high quality of their EHR datasets.

Sutter Health is a not-for-profit multispecialty health care delivery system, with five medical foundations, 150 ambulatory medical clinics, and more than 4 million patients and 10 million outpatient visits per year. Serving 23 northern California counties, Sutter patients make up 36% of the catchment area population (Palaniappan et al., 2009). Kaiser Permanente Hawai'i is a not-for-profit, integrated health care delivery system with over 245,000 members, one 285-bed acute care inpatient facility, 20 outpatient clinics on the islands of Oahu, Maui, and Hawai'i, and numerous independent primary care providers on Kauai, Lanai, and Molokai. In both health care systems, patients may self-report multiple race and ethnicity categories. For this study, we prioritized small AA and NH/PI populations and distinguished between single and multiple races. All Sutter Health cohort members were linked to the California Cancer Registry, and Kaiser Permanente Hawai'i cohort members were linked to the Hawai'i Tumor Registry to identify incident lung cancers occurring during the follow-up period (from cohort entry through December 31, 2013). In addition to EHR and cancer registry data, patients' addresses at or close to cohort entry were geocoded to facilitate linkage to contextual-level factors, including air pollution and neighborhood social environment measures. Compared to census and cancer registry data for the catchment area, our cohort and diagnosed cases overrepresent AA and NH/PIs, females, and younger individuals and underrepresents White and Hispanic groups.

The full pooled cohort comprised 2,211,476 individuals (1,275,838 females and 935,638 males, including 49,983 NHs, 31,506 PIs, and 352,076 Asian Americans, representing 2.26%, 1.42%, and 15.92% of the overall cohort, respectively). The pooled cohort included 7,274 incident lung cancer diagnoses (3,867 females and 3,407 males) occurring in the follow-up period (2000–2013). There were 1,228 lung cancers diagnosed among AA and NH/PIs, including 328 NHs, 81 PIs, and 819 Asian Americans. There were 889,870 female who never smoked (69.7% of females in the cohort). Among AA and NH/PIs, 198,208 females (79.3%) never smoked. Across all racial and ethnic groups, Asian Indian American females had the highest proportion of those who never smoked (94.7%) and NH females the lowest proportion (54.8%). Among lung cancer cases among females, prevalence of never-smoking ranged from a low of 11.2% among females with non-Asian

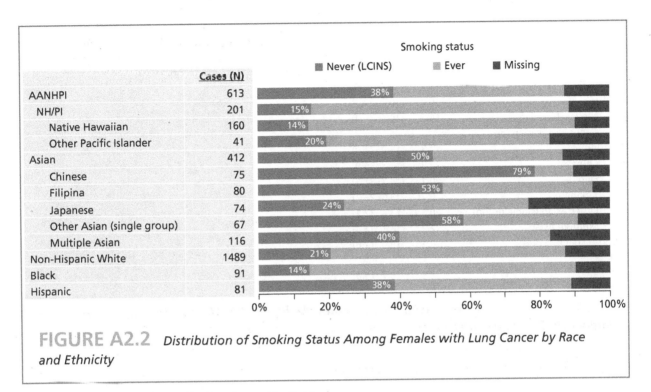

FIGURE A2.2 *Distribution of Smoking Status Among Females with Lung Cancer by Race and Ethnicity*

Notes: AANHPI = Asian American, Native Hawaiian, and Pacific Islander

American or NH/PI multiple races/ethnicities and 15.4% among NHs to a high of 85.7% among Asian Indian and 78.7% among Chinese American females (Figure A1.2).

Age-adjusted incidence rates (AAIR) represent the number of cases per 100,000 population at risk. We calculated AAIR by dividing the number of lung cancer cases by the corresponding person-years of follow-up in our cohort in 15-year age groups, standardizing these age-specific incidence rates to the U.S. 2000 population, summing over the age groups, and multiplying by 100,000 (Figure A1.3). Ninety-five percent confidence intervals were calculated using the Fay and Feuer method (Fay and Feuer, 1997), with the modification by Tiwari et al. for the upper confidence level (Tiwari et al., 2006). The age-adjusted lung cancer incidence rate among never-smoking AA and NH/PIs as an aggregate group was 17.1 per 100,000 (95% CI: 14.9, 19.4). However, incidence rates of lung cancer among those who never smoked varied widely among AA and NH/PIs groups, ranging from 6.4 (95% CI: 3.6, 10.0) among Japanese American females to 22.8 (95% CI: 17.3, 29.1) among Chinese American females. Incidence of lung cancer among female NH/PIs who never smoked was 15.2 (95% CI: 10.2, 21.2).

The assembly of an EHR-based cohort enriched for AA and NH/PI populations coupled with small-area geospatial data linked to high-quality cancer registry data provided a unique and valuable opportunity to address unanswered questions about the burden of lung cancer among AA and NH/PI never-smoking females. Yet researchers conducting future studies should be aware of the challenges of implementing this approach. As the protection of human subjects and data privacy are paramount concerns for study subjects, health care organizations, and research institutions, adequate time must be allocated to address data use permissions for each participating party such that a shared research and public health goal may be achieved. The use of EHR data for research purposes, such as defining race and ethnicity and smoking status, requires careful evaluation and logic checks of structured data, while the pooling of EHR data across different health care systems requires in-depth data harmonization. Local expertise and knowledge of the complexities and nuances of the health care system is critical to meaningful dataset development and use. The follow-up of an EHR cohort requires clear definition of timelines and data collection points and understanding of the tracking of health care encounters within the system. Finally, linking EHR data to secondary data sources requires robust methods such as the careful selection of address information (linkage of geospatial data) and stringent criteria in probabilistic matching (linkage to cancer registry data).

	AAIR	95% CI	Age-adjusted incidence rate (per 100,000)
AANHPI	17.1	(14.9, 19.9)	
NH/PI	15.2	(10.2, 22.5)	
Native Hawaiian	16.7	(10.5, 26.4)	
Other Pacific Islander	~		
Asian	17.5	(15.0, 21.0)	
Chinese	22.8	(17.3, 35.9)	
Filipina	20.1	(14.1, 31.5)	
Japanese	6.4	(3.6, 28.7)	
Other Asian (single group)	20.3	(13.4, 32.1)	
Multiple Asian	22.2	(16.1, 32.4)	
Non-Hispanic White	10.1	(9.0, 11.6)	
Black	~		
Hispanic	8.5	(5.7, 13.0)	

FIGURE A2.3 *Age-Adjusted Incidence Rates (AAIR) per 100,000 and 95% Confidence Intervals (CI) of Lung Cancer Among Females Who Have Never Smoked*

Notes: AANHPI = Asian American, Native Hawaiian, and Pacific Islander

REFERENCES

Fay, M. P., & Feuer, E. J. (1997). Confidence intervals for directly standardized rates: a method based on the gamma distribution. *Statistics in Medicine, 16*(7), 791–801. https://doi.org/10.1002/(sici)1097-0258(19970415)16:7<791::aid-sim500>3.0.co;2-#

Gomez, S. L., Chang, E. T., Shema, S. J., Fish, K., Sison, J. D., Reynolds, P., Clément-Duchêne, C., Wrensch, M. R., Wiencke, J. L., & Wakelee, H. A. (2011). Survival following non-small cell lung cancer among Asian/Pacific Islander, Latina, and Non-Hispanic white women who have never smoked. *Cancer Epidemiology, Biomarkers & Prevention*: a publication of the American Association for Cancer Research, cosponsored by the American Society of Preventive Oncology, *20*(3), 545–554. https://doi.org/10.1158/1055-9965.EPI-10-0965

Palaniappan, L. P., Wong, E. C., Shin, J. J., Moreno, M. R., & Otero-Sabogal, R. (2009). Collecting patient race/ethnicity and primary language data in ambulatory care settings: a case study in methodology. *Health Services Research, 44*(5 Pt 1), 1750–1761. https://doi.org/10.1111/j.1475-6773.2009.00992.x

Sisti, J., & Boffetta, P. (2012). What proportion of lung cancer in never-smokers can be attributed to known risk factors? *International Journal of Cancer, 131*(2), 265–275. https://doi.org/10.1002/ijc.27477

Subramanian, J., & Govindan, R. (2007). Lung cancer in never smokers: a review. *Journal of Clinical Oncology*: official journal of the American Society of Clinical Oncology, *25*(5), 561–570. https://doi.org/10.1200/JCO.2006.06.8015

Sun, S., Schiller, J. H., & Gazdar, A. F. (2007). Lung cancer in never smokers—a different disease. Nature reviews. *Cancer, 7*(10), 778–790. https://doi.org/10.1038/nrc2190

Tiwari, R. C., Clegg, L. X., & Zou, Z. (2006). Efficient interval estimation for age-adjusted cancer rates. *Statistical Methods in Medical Research, 15*(6), 547–569. https://doi.org/10.1177/0962280206070621

CASE

USING DATA TO DEFINE AND EXPLORE HEALTH STATUS IN ASIAN AMERICAN ETHNIC ENCLAVES IN NEW YORK CITY

SUNGWOO LIM, LIZA KING

This case study describes our work to develop a robust definition of Asian enclaves in New York City (NYC) and investigate associations between living in an Asian enclave and chronic disease outcomes among Asian American adults (Lim et al., 2017). An ethnic enclave is a geographical area where a particular ethnic group is spatially clustered and socially and economically distinct from the majority group. Living in an ethnic enclave has been hypothesized to protect immigrants from potential health hazards because individuals residing among their own ethnic community benefit from having family ties in the neighborhood, sharing a familiar culture, and potentially finding work through those connections (Logan et al., 2002). Ethnic enclaves may also provide easy access to groceries and restaurants, allowing residents to retain traditional diets, and offer familiar social and physical environments to residents, providing fertile grounds for the development of community-oriented businesses, community organizations, and civic institutions (Zhou and Lin, 2005; Zhou and Cho, 2010). Living in ethnic enclaves may also allow residents to access services and resources (e.g., legal assistance, health care providers, retailers) within their own community, thereby avoiding discrimination and its associated stressors that they may encounter in broader American society (Zhou and Lin, 2005) (Shell et al., 2013).

However, research examining associations between enclave residence and health status among Asian Americans remains limited, and results are difficult to interpret. In some studies, both smoking and dietary behaviors among enclave residents reflected rates in the countries of origin (Li et al., 2013; Yi et al., 2014). For example, smoking rates among Asian men living in Sunset Park, Brooklyn, were twice as high as rates among Asian men in NYC overall (Li et al., 2013). These studies suggest that health behaviors are indeed impacted by

Applied Population Health Approaches for Asian American Communities, First Edition. Edited by Simona C. Kwon, Chau Trinh-Shevrin, Nadia S. Islam, and Stella S. Yi.
© 2023 John Wiley & Sons, Inc. Published 2023 by John Wiley & Sons, Inc.
Companion Website: www.wiley.com/go/kwon/asianamerican

enclave residence. In line with this hypothesis, a California-based study found an association between living in an ethnic enclave and limited health care access among Asian Americans (Chang and Chan, 2015). However, several studies conducted in NYC found no associations between enclave residence and health status. For instance, Janevic et al. (2014) found no evidence for a protective effect of enclave residence on prevalence of gestational diabetes among Asian Americans in NYC, while Osypuk et al. (2009) found no evidence for a supportive effect of enclave residence on consumption of fruits and vegetables among recent Chinese immigrants.

This mixed evidence may be due to methodological challenges. A key example is confounding, which makes it difficult to identify true neighborhood-level impacts from the effect of individual behaviors on health outcomes. Another important limitation is the inconsistent definition of the parameters constituting an ethnic enclave. Notably, there is a lack of standard cut-points for defining residential segregation for Asian Americans, even though cut-points have been established for use in studying residential segregation for Black and Latino communities (Glaeser and Vigdor, 2001). The diversity of Asian Americans presents a further and unique challenge to defining enclaves. Even if residential segregation for Asian Americans could be studied in aggregate, most datasets do not disaggregate information by ethnic subgroup.

To address these methodological challenges in our work in NYC, we used propensity score matching to control for observed differences between enclave residents and nonresidents and investigated associations between ethnic enclave residence and self-reported health outcomes. To define an Asian American enclave, we used U.S. 2010 Census tract-level race/ethnicity data to calculate dissimilarity and isolation indices, using the majority non-Hispanic White (White) population as our comparison group.

The dissimilarity index measures the proportion of Asian Americans in a particular area that would need to move out of that area in order to achieve an even distribution of White and Asian American populations (Massey and Denton, 1988). For example, if an area were scored with a dissimilarity index of 0.75, 75% of Asian Americans living in that area would need to move to other areas of NYC to balance the proportions of the two racial/ethnic groups (Asian American and White) in the city overall.

The isolation index measures the degree of interaction between Asian American residents in a particular area as compared with interactions between Asian American and White residents in that area (Glaeser and Vigdor, 2001; Massey and Denton, 1988). For example, if the isolation index were 0.60, we would interpret that estimate as indicating that the proportion of Asian American residents in that area exceeds that of Asian Americans in NYC overall by 60% on average, and Asian American residents are more likely to interact with each other. Both indices, ranging from 0 to 1, were calculated across all census tracts and had a positive correlation (correlation coefficient = 0.27, p-value = 0.04).

Census tract level indices were then summed to community district levels, and enclaves were identified at that level. In NYC, there are 59 NYC community districts, which are local jurisdictions represented by community boards (the most local level of city government) and recognized by local residents as distinct neighborhoods. Because there is no established cut-point for Asian American versus White spatial segregation, we graphically examined how NYC community districts were located in terms of the two indices calculated. We then defined community districts where both indices were much higher than others as an Asian American enclave. To capture concentration of ethnic groups in each census tract—another dimension of segregation—and to validate our selection of census tracts as potential enclaves, we used American Community Survey (ACS) data to calculate the percent of Asian American residents, percent of residents speaking Asian languages at home, and percent of residents speaking English less than "very well" in NYC census tracts.

After identifying all neighborhoods that met these criteria and designating them as Asian enclaves, we proceeded to examine health outcomes for clusters of residents in those neighborhoods. In NYC, the primary data source for health outcomes is the Community Health Survey (CHS), a random-digit dial annual telephone survey of 9,000 noninstitutionalized NYC adults. From 2009 to 2012, the NYC CHS sampled approximately 36,000 NYC adults, of which 2,863 reported their race as Asian American. Because CHS data only collected ZIP codes to identify neighborhood of residence, we mapped ZIP code tabulation areas to community districts. Health outcomes included self-reported status of current smoking, hypertension, diabetes, and general health (excellent/very good/good vs. fair/poor). To describe underlying characteristics that might confound associations between enclave residence and health outcomes, we included information about demographics, health care access, and some health behaviors, such as physical activity in the past 30 days.

Descriptive statistics were calculated to describe demographic and health care access characteristics for ethnic enclave residents and nonresidents. We then calculated the likelihood of living in an ethnic enclave (propensity scores) using logistic regression with ethnic enclave residence (dependent variable) and demographic and health care access variables (independent variables). Following DuGoff and colleagues' approach (2014), we also included the survey weight as a predictor of the propensity score model to strengthen external validity (Dugoff et al., 2014). We created six strata based on propensity scores; subsequently, ethnic enclave residents and nonresidents who shared similar propensity scores were matched within the same stratum. Using propensity score-matched data, we then estimated the association between ethnic enclave residence and health outcomes via log-linear Poisson regression models.

Five NYC community districts across three of the city's five boroughs were identified as Asian American enclaves: Chinatown, in Manhattan; Fresh Meadows, Flushing and Elmhurst, in Queens; and Sunset Park, in Brooklyn. All five neighborhoods had high scores of both the dissimilarity and isolation indices (>0.35) and were clustered from other neighborhoods. Of these neighborhoods, a majority of the residents in three of these neighborhoods were Asian American, and more than half of the Asian American residents in each neighborhood spoke an Asian language and reported limited English proficiency. Unfortunately, despite growing evidence for the importance of disaggregated data to describe health among Asian Americans, we were not able to disaggregate Asian American enclaves by Asian American ethnic group (Islam et al., 2010; Osypuk et al., 2009; Yi et al., 2014).

Nearly one-third (31%) of Asian American adults in NYC lived in one of these five ethnic enclaves. Asian Americans living in an ethnic enclave were more likely to be of low socioeconomic status ($p < 0.01$) and less likely to have health insurance ($p = 0.03$) as compared with those not living in an enclave. Ethnic enclave residents were also more likely to speak foreign languages at home and receive flu vaccinations in the past 12 months, whereas there was no significant difference between the two groups in employment, nativity, years of living in the United States, body mass index (BMI), or physical activity. Total servings of fruit/vegetables on average were slightly higher among ethnic enclave residents versus nonresidents (2.8 vs. 2.6, $p = 0.04$).

Residents of Asian American enclaves had significantly lower crude prevalence of excellent/very good/good general health status as compared with nonresidents (65% vs. 73%, $p < 0.01$), but there was no difference in prevalence of current smoking, diabetes, or hypertension. Stratified by sex, men living in an Asian American ethnic enclave were more likely to smoke than nonresidents (25% vs. 14%, $p = 0.03$). For women, crude prevalence of positive perception of general health status was lower among enclave residents relative to nonresidents (63% vs. 73%, $p < 0.01$).

After controlling for individual-level characteristics, enclave residents were more likely to report positive perception of general health status compared with non-enclave residents (PR = 1.06), at borderline significance (95% CI = 0.98, 1.15). Adjusted prevalence estimates of current smoking, hypertension, and diabetes were not associated with living in an ethnic enclave. In stratified analyses, ethnic enclave residence was associated with current smoking for men (PR = 1.42), at borderline significance (95% CI = 0.98, 2.05). All the other chronic health outcomes investigated in this analysis were not associated with enclave residence after adjusting for confounders.

In sum, our findings do not support the hypothesis that ethnic enclave residence impacts chronic disease outcomes among Asian Americans in NYC. However, this case study details a novel analytic approach to identifying Asian American ethnic enclaves by employing spatial measures of dissimilarity, isolation, and concentration in combination with sociodemographic characteristics and individual-level health behaviors. By using the NYC CHS dataset to investigate underlying characteristics associated with ethnic enclave residence among Asian American adults, we were able to control for potential individual-level confounders that could impact associations between ethnic enclave residence and health outcomes.

One key limitation of this study is that we were not able to examine data by Asian ethnic group. It is possible that smaller Asian American populations may experience an effect of ethnic enclave residence that we were unable to detect due to aggregation of larger Asian American groups with those smaller, and potentially more isolated, populations. However, our work represents a step forward in adapting new methodologies to identify health disparities among Asian Americans and other racial/ethnic minority groups.

REFERENCES

Chang, E., & Chan, K. S. (2015). Variations in Asian Americans: How Neighborhood Concordance Is Associated With Health Care Access and Utilization. *American Journal of Public Health, 105*(1), 66–68. https://doi.org/10.2105/AJPH.2014.302275

Dugoff, E. H., Schuler, M., & Stuart, E. A. (2014). Generalizing observational study results: applying propensity score methods to complex surveys. *Health Services Research, 49*(1), 284–303. https://doi.org/10.1111/1475-6773.12090

Glaeser E. L., & Vigdor, J. L. (2001). Racial Segregation in the 2000 Census: Promising News. The Brookings Institution Survey Series. Center on Urban and Metropolitan Policy. Available at http://www.brookings.edu/es/urban/census/glaeser.pdf.

Islam, N. S., Khan, S., Kwon, S., Jang, D., Ro, M., & Trinh-Shevrin, C. (2010). Methodological issues in the collection, analysis, and reporting of granular data in Asian American populations: historical challenges and potential solutions. *Journal of Health Care for the Poor and Underserved, 21*(4), 1354–1381. https://doi.org/10.1353/hpu.2010.0939

Janevic, T., Borrell, L. N., Savitz, D. A., Echeverria, S. E., & Rundle, A. (2014). Ethnic enclaves and gestational diabetes among immigrant women in New York City. *Social Science & Medicine, 120,* 180–189. https://doi.org/10.1016/j.socscimed.2014.09.026

Li, S., Kwon, S. C., Weerasinghe, I., Rey, M. J., & Trinh-Shevrin, C. (2013). Smoking among Asian Americans: acculturation and gender in the context of tobacco control policies in New York City. *Health Promotion Practice, 14*(5 Suppl), 18S–28S. https://doi.org/10.1177/1524839913485757

Lim, S., Yi, S. S., Lundy De La Cruz, N., & Trinh-Shevrin, C. (2017). Defining ethnic enclave and its associations with self-reported health outcomes among Asian American adults in New York City. *Journal of Immigrant and Minority Health, 19*(1), 138–146. https://doi.org/10.1007/s10903-015-0334-6

Logan, J. R., Zhang, W., & Alba, R. D. (2002). Immigrant enclaves and ethnic communities in New York and Los Angeles. *American Sociological Review, 67,* 299–322.

Massey, D.S., & Denton, N. A. (1988). The dimensions of residential segregation. *Social Forces, 67*(2), 281–315.

Osypuk, T. L., Diez Roux, A. V., Hadley, C., & Kandula, N. R. (2009). Are immigrant enclaves healthy places to live? The multi-ethnic study of atherosclerosis. *Social Science & Medicine, 69*(1), 110–120. https://doi.org/10.1016/j.socscimed.2009.04.010

Shell, A. M., Peek, M. K., & Eschbach, K. (2013). Neighborhood Hispanic composition and depressive symptoms among Mexican-descent residents of Texas City, Texas. *Social science & medicine, 99,* 56–63. https://doi.org/10.1016/j.socscimed.2013.10.006

Yi, S. S., Ruff, R. R., Jung, M., & Waddell, E. N. (2014). Racial/ethnic residential segregation, neighborhood poverty and urinary biomarkers of diet in New York City adults. *Social Science & Medicine, 122,* 122–129. https://doi.org/10.1016/j.socscimed.2014.10.030

Zhou M, & Lin M. (2005). Community transformation and the formation of ethnic capital: immigrant Chinese communities in the United States. *Journal of Chinese Overseas, 1*(2), 260–284.

Zhou M, & Cho M. (2010). Noneconomic effects of ethnic entrepreneurship: a focused look at the Chinese and Korean enclave economies in Los Angeles. *Thunderbird International Business Review, 52*(2), 83–96.

CASE

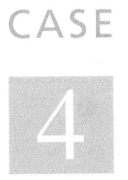

THE DREAM INITIATIVE: AN ITERATIVE APPROACH TO ADDRESSING SOUTH ASIAN HEALTH NEEDS IN NEW YORK CITY

SADIA MOHAIMIN, JENNIFER ZANOWIAK, SHAHMIR H. ALI, SHINU MAMMEN, MD TAHER, GULNAHAR ALAM, MD JALAL UDDIN, SIDRA ZAFAR, SABIHA SULTANA, NADIA S. ISLAM

DREAM OVERVIEW

The Diabetes Research, Education, and Action for Minorities (DREAM) Initiative is a diabetes prevention and management intervention for South Asian patients in New York City (NYC) primary care practices. Launched in 2018 across a network of 18 practices and delivered by seven community health workers (CHWs), this project represents the evolution of a decade of community-engaged research led by the Center for the Study of Asian American Health (CSAAH) at NYU Grossman School of Medicine to meet the disproportionate noncommunicable disease burden faced by South Asians (Islam et al., 2018; Lim, Wyatt, Chauhan, et al., 2019; Lim, Wyatt, Mammen, et al., 2019; Lopez et al., 2017). This case study highlights specific considerations for developing, implementing, evaluating, and scaling up CHW-led interventions for South Asian populations.

A key feature of the DREAM Initiative is its iterative incorporation of lessons learned and best practices of past CHW-led interventions implemented by members and collaborators of the DREAM research team. This process began with the design and implementation of the DREAM Project, a diabetes management program designed specifically for the NYC Bangladeshi American community. First implemented in 2008, the DREAM Project was a six-month CHW-led group-based educational intervention that included one-on-one visits and regular follow-up appointments implemented across clinical and community settings (Islam et al., 2018).

Applied Population Health Approaches for Asian American Communities, First Edition. Edited by Simona C. Kwon, Chau Trinh-Shevrin, Nadia S. Islam, and Stella S. Yi.
© 2023 John Wiley & Sons, Inc. Published 2023 by John Wiley & Sons, Inc.
Companion Website: www.wiley.com/go/kwon/asianamerican

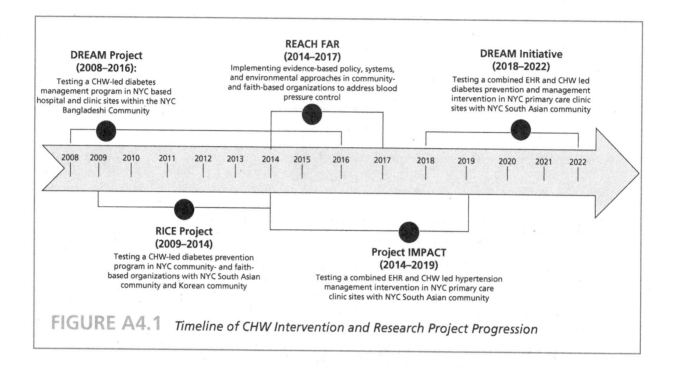

FIGURE A4.1 *Timeline of CHW Intervention and Research Project Progression*

Incorporating findings and lessons learned from the DREAM Project, the research team built successive initiatives for different South Asian communities in NYC that focused on diabetes-related health concerns within those populations (Figure A3.1).

- The DREAM Project (2008) and RICE Project (2009) served as foundational studies for engaging the community in research, with an emphasis on understanding community needs, assets, and priorities, and building trusted, strong partnerships with community institutions, including faith-based and community organizations.

- REACH FAR (2014) leveraged these partnerships to foster community capacity-building for hypertension prevention and management through community-level training and policy-based changes within pharmacies, groceries, restaurants, and faith-based organizations. Additionally, REACH FAR addressed an existing gap in access to culturally tailored, in-language health education resources and partnered with the local health department to develop hypertension materials for diverse Asian American communities, including South Asians.

- Project IMPACT (2014) improved clinical-community linkages through provider- and practice-level trainings, incorporation of culturally and linguistically appropriate health materials within electronic health records (EHRs), and integration of CHWs within the primary care team.

The DREAM Initiative represents a culmination of these projects and serves as a sustainable model of chronic disease prevention through large-scale partnerships and community integration.

Methodology

The design of the DREAM Initiative, which uses a staggered, two-arm randomized controlled trial (RCT) design with a waitlist-controlled group (Lim, Wyatt, Mammen, et al., 2019), was informed largely by lessons learned from smaller community interventions. The DREAM Project, implemented in 2008, served as a principal source of information. Rooted in principles of community-based participatory research (CBPR), the DREAM Project was developed from formative research conducted in collaboration with community organizations that included focus groups and health needs assessments – a process that identified the need for a culturally and linguistically appropriate program for diabetes control and management. To ensure continuous feedback about community members' health and well-being needs, the project was led by a coalition of 15 partners that included community-based organizations (mainly grassroots social services and community advocacy organizations), community leaders, academic researchers, primary care providers, and health educators dedicated to addressing growing health disparities experiences by the NYC Bangladeshi American community (Islam et al., 2012). It was this coalition that expressed concerns about the ethics of employing a traditional RCT study design, given that this configuration would require recruitment of a control group that would not receive the educational intervention. Because the intervention had been shown to have clear benefits for participants and pose no discernable risks to their health or well-being, stakeholders cautioned that withholding the intervention from control group participants could be deemed unethical. As a result, the coalition adopted a study design in which randomization occurred only after the first educational session was delivered to the entire sample. Following that session, one group of participants immediately received the remaining intervention components (i.e., the intervention group) while the other group received the intervention components six months after intervention group (i.e., the waitlist-controlled group). This design ensured all participants would have access to study resources (Islam et al., 2014).

Additional considerations for the study design were informed by lessons learned through Project IMPACT (2014), a clinical-community linkage initiative that combined interventions utilizing health information technology (i.e., EHR-based interventions) and CHW coaching to improve hypertension control among South Asian patients in 15 NYC primary care practices (Lopez et al., 2017). Project IMPACT used a stepped-wedge quasi-experimental design to ensure that all eligible patients with uncontrolled hypertension received the complete intervention while, simultaneously, researchers were able to assess the effectiveness and feasibility of individual intervention components. In the first phase, researchers implemented and evaluated physician-led EHR-based interventions in the participating practices; in the next phase, CHWs identified eligible patients with uncontrolled hypertension via participating practices' EHR systems and then led the coaching and education sessions with enrolled patients. All participants received the first education session, after which they were randomized to receive the coaching and education sessions at different timepoints. To allow for comparison of outcomes among randomized groups, blood pressure measures were collected by the CHWs at baseline, 6 months, and 12 months and via the EHR. Throughout this process, best practices emerged regarding EHR-based recruitment and data collection, integration of CHW-led components within clinic workflows, and effective provider-CHW communication strategies. These best practices informed protocol development for the DREAM Initiative.

As the project was scaled up, specific challenges related to participant recruitment and data collection that resulted in undue CHW caseload burden in both the DREAM and IMPACT projects were addressed by DREAM Initiative researchers. First, eligible participants identified via the practice EHR were randomized to treatment and control groups, and CHWs were only provided with lists of eligible treatment group participants for recruitment. This procedure reduced the number of patients that CHWs were required to contact. Utilizing an innovative "matching" technique, control group participants identified via EHR and never contacted by the CHW were matched on demographic and clinical characteristics to ensure comparability across treatment and control groups and reduce bias. Second, CHW-administered surveys were eliminated for the control group. Instead, researchers collected control group data through the EHR. Additionally, the midpoint (3-month) time point was eliminated to reduce the data collection burden. Finally, researchers delayed the waitlist-control summary intervention session until after all intervention participants received the full intervention. This change reduced the CHWs' workload by introducing a phased implementation, allowing CHWs to focus their efforts on intervention clients before attending to the control group.

Theory and Components

The overarching DREAM Initiative integrated the Chronic Care Model (CCM) to guide implementation and will employ the RE-AIM (Reach, Efficacy/Effectiveness, Adoption, Implementation, Maintenance) framework for evaluation (Glasgow, Vogt, & Boles, 1999; Hung et al., 2007). The CCM is comprised of six components: health system/organizational support, clinical information systems, delivery system design, decision support, self-management support, and community support. Four of these components were integrated into the study design. Decision support and clinical information systems were incorporated by integrating clinical decision support tools into the EHR (e.g., provider alerts for South Asian adult patients with body mass index (BMI) > 23, establishment of registries for patients meeting criteria for pre-diabetes). The patient self-management component was included through the delivery of culturally and linguistically adapted health coaching to participants via one-on-one meetings (e.g., home visits) to foster trust-building and focus on individual needs. Finally, to

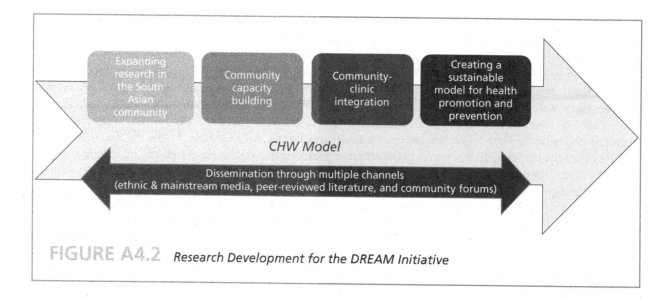

FIGURE A4.2   *Research Development for the DREAM Initiative*

formalize community linkages to clinical systems as part of the delivery system design component, the DREAM Initiative partnered with Healthify, an electronic social service referral network, to enhance direct referrals to culturally sensitive social services (Healthify). Healthify enables CHWs to track the status of a referral service from start to finish, ensuring that CHWs know when a referral to a social service provider has been delivered. The DREAM Initiative research team played a critical role in making recommendations to Healthify for the inclusion of South Asian-serving organizations within the network. Indeed, while the CHW model remained a constant in the DREAM initiative, this model was integrated with lessons learned through past interventions, insights gained from a CBPR-based development strategy, theory-driven implementation and evaluation considerations, and partnering with local service networks (Figure A3.2).

While not yet implemented, RE-AIM will be used to evaluate strengths and weaknesses of the DREAM Initiative's health promotion strategies. Specifically, RE-AIM will be used to assess the effectiveness of in-person and telephone counseling sessions and group education classes.

Stakeholders and Partners

Expanding on the successful engagement of partners involved in the DREAM Project, RICE Project, and REACH FAR coalitions, the DREAM Initiative convened a community advisory board (CAB) consisting of South Asian community-based organizations. CAB members meet quarterly to review health education materials and advise the research team on the cultural appropriateness of patient engagement strategies. For example, CAB members have requested that health promotion and education materials include imagery depicting diverse South Asian communities (e.g., inclusion of a man wearing a *pagri* to represent a Sikh family) and suggestions of how community members may make healthy food choices within South Asian restaurants, such as selecting grilled vegetable or chicken options or forgoing whole milk *lassi* drinks. CAB organizations also provide spaces for health promotion activities, including health education workshops, exercise workshops, and cooking demonstrations, and assist the research team with translations. DREAM Initiative stakeholders play a pivotal role in research dissemination by actively engaging and disseminating project information to local South Asian media outlets, community members, and organizational clientele. Finally, CAB member organizations serve as important referral sites for CHWs linking patients to social services.

More broadly, the original DREAM Project coalition and its ongoing partnerships with community-based organizations, faith-based organizations, primary care clinics, hospitals, and ethnic media outlets have helped to promote the project on an ongoing basis and created greater awareness of the pervasive issue of diabetes within the South Asian community. Formative survey data from the DREAM Project highlighted the importance of in-language health information sources for the Bangladeshi community – specifically, Bengali language newspapers – which motivated the research team to establish partnerships with ethnic print media, such as *Bangla Patrika* and *Thikana* (Islam et al., 2016).

These findings from the early days of the DREAM Project informed broader media efforts with various in-language resources to reach additional communities throughout the DREAM Initiative. For example, researchers worked with TV84, a nonprofit Punjabi-language television channel, to support health-related reporting and health-promoting messaging. Stakeholders also noted the importance of building and maintaining community trust and connections throughout the study period. In line with stakeholder recommendations, the research team sought buy-in from institutions to support CHWs by recruiting respected physicians who could serve as "champions" (i.e., liaisons between CHWs and the community) for the project. Cultural competency among health care providers was increased by educating health care teams on customs and practices found across diverse South Asian groups. One component of this effort was developing and disseminating educational materials for a clinical audience that described the needs of diverse NYC South Asian populations. For example, researchers shared data drawn from a sample of South Asian taxi drivers showing that they are at higher risk of elevated cholesterol, overweight/obesity, and a sedentary lifestyle. In parallel, connections between the research team and the community were strengthened through engagement in strategy sessions with the CAB to identify channels for enhancing community pride, such as hosting community events to celebrate "graduation" from the DREAM Initiative, incorporating traditional songs and poems in DREAM-related activities and materials, inviting community leaders and elected officials to affiliated events, and sharing project-related success stories and photos in ethnic media outlets.

Principles

Aligning with the key considerations for developing interventions in Asian American communities identified in Chapter 5, a number of South Asian cultural and social dynamics were addressed by the DREAM Initiative research team to enhance the intervention's success. These dynamics included family, gender, community, religion, holidays, language, immigration, and geography. Researchers also took into account the need to apply a framework of intersectionality and an awareness of the impact of the model minority stereotype on the lived experiences of South Asians. Table A3.1 presents examples of how these factors were addressed within the intervention model and CHW descriptions of their work within each dynamic.

TABLE A4.1 **Cultural Dynamic Components within the DREAM Initiative**

Cultural dynamic	Incorporation within the DREAM intervention	Supporting statements by CHWs
Family	– Enlisting family member buy-in in participant enrollment, as family members are key decision makers – Using home visits as an opportunity to build rapport with family members and support for the participant throughout the intervention (e.g., heart-healthy meals, physical activity) – Encouraging family members to join intervention sessions, including children – Assisting a participant's family members with social service needs, medications, etc.	*"We have to make sure we have the trust of the entire family."* *"The home visit is the key to connecting with the participant."* *"I always invite them to bring their husband, wife, or kids [to a health education class or session]. Sometimes what happens is that when the wife comes to a session, the husband doesn't know and doesn't value that class. But when both people come, they realize this is important for their family members."*

(Continued)

TABLE A4.1 (Continued)

Cultural dynamic	Incorporation within the DREAM intervention	Supporting statements by CHWs
Gender	– Creating women- and men-only sessions – Engaging participants' spouses to join as a "couple" – Pairing male CHWs with a female lay health worker to assist with exercise demonstrations for female participants – Addressing traditional South Asian gender norms/bias using positive affirmations – Building self-efficacy among women participants (e.g., teaching them how to travel to appointments alone)	*"Lots of women participants don't want to do the session with men. I have to consider and think about their comfort zone."* *"When I call a man, I look for a woman, too [to connect to]. I try to ask a woman or someone else to join." (female CHW)* *"Rather than saying 'you always make women cook' [to men], I encourage them to cook and give the example of male chefs at five-star hotels [restaurants]. . .I tell them, 'If they can do it, you can do it too.'"*
Community	– Understanding cultural nuances within subgroups or communities (e.g., alcohol acceptance, dietary practices, religious norms, etc.) – Accommodating the logistical needs associated with scheduling sessions with low-income workers and members of traditional communities (e.g., coordinating with nightshift workers or homemakers who structure days around their children's school schedules, conducting one-on-one visits in community spaces, providing travel incentives to reduce financial barriers to participation)	*"In one community, if I ask about drinking [alcohol], they don't hesitate to answer. But when you ask a similar question in another community, the women will look at you like 'Are you seriously asking me this?' So, I say, 'I am sorry, it is part of a series of questions I have to ask.' So you have to know differences between communities."* *"When working with a community of taxi drivers, you have to be very flexible. They work 60–70 hours a week. So, I have to keep my schedule open seven days for them."* *"When I invite family to a session, I always give them a MetroCard [provided by our program too]. If a family member can bring the participant to the center, then they feel okay that they don't have to spend a dollar."*
Religion	– Considering different religious practices within a group setting – Being cognizant of religious restrictions (e.g., proscriptions against certain types of meats or other foods) – Giving examples related to religion during one-on-one interactions – Scheduling intervention sessions around daily prayer times or holidays – Drawing from religious principles when teaching stress-reduction methods (e.g., mindfulness meditation) – Including culturally appropriate images with an emphasis on modesty	*[CHW speaking about classes with a mixed religious group] "I start off my class by saying, 'Hello, Assalamwalaikum and Namaskar."* *[CHW speaking about classes with a mixed religious group] "I never mention 'beef.' I always keep it general and say 'red meat.'"* *"I give religious examples. I say, just like you pay attention to Baghban, God, or Allah when praying, you should pay attention similarly when you exercise."*

Holidays	– Understanding religious holidays and implications for study participation and health behaviors (e.g., scheduling considerations, helping participants to prepare for fasting, or other changes to eating routines) – Working with leadership at community mosques to offer healthier foods during religious holidays – Providing health education materials on healthy eating/fasting during religious holidays (e.g., Ramadan)	*"If they are going to a festival or celebrating, I tell them they should choose healthy food, rather than the usual rich food."* *"We stop our sessions [during religious/cultural holidays] because we have to consider that it is enjoyment time for them. . .they are busy shopping, organizing food, and attending prayers."*
Language	– Ensuring translations are appropriate, easy to understand, and convey the original meaning of the English words or message – Assigning CHWs to patients based on shared culture so that linguistic and cultural nuances are accommodated (e.g., being aware of the various dialects of a single South Asian language) – Providing education materials in English so that English-speaking children and family members may help parents understand and because participants may not read in their native language	*"Language along with cultural knowledge is very important. If you speak Punjabi fluently, you might not be able to deliver the message in the same way from someone who understands the cultural background and sensitivities of the culture. . .if a participant mentions chutney and you don't know what that is, then it is hard to suggest better culturally appropriate foods."* *"Sometimes we can't use them [translated materials] and need to switch gears. Some participants don't read [due to their education level]. That is when we work with them individually to find someone to help them at home [with our culturally adapted material]. Sometimes it's their children, grandchildren, spouse, or even the neighbor. . .if I teach the family, they don't need me every time"* *"With men, they will say yes to tobacco use if we just ask about paan. But for women, we have to ask about paan and follow up and ask about jorda [tobacco substance similar to tobacco] to start the conversation."*
Immigration	– Understanding immigration-related fears and ensuring a safe space within the program – Providing immigration assistance to participants or family members when requested (e.g., referrals to legal or social services)	*"From the beginning, I explain that this is a confidential group – you don't have to talk about immigration status at all here."* *"I have to make sure they are not distressed from these issues...I often do one-on-one counseling with them, I refer them to a lawyer to help with immigration needs."*

(Continued)

TABLE A4.1 **(Continued)**

Cultural dynamic	Incorporation within the DREAM intervention	Supporting statements by CHWs
Geography	– Mapping of geographical location and resources in the area that impact health (e.g., parks/walking paths, healthy food options, pharmacies, faith-based organizations, community centers) – Engaging community resources and institutions for project collaboration (e.g., making referrals)	*"Learning about the neighborhood your participant is in is important. I need to know where the Gurdwara is, where the pharmacies are. . ."*
Intersectionality	– Finding unique ways, through one-on-one meetings and individualized support, to engage members who have intersecting identities (e.g., strategizing ways to privately connect with a participant from a low-income family who shares a mobile phone with family members, older immigrants need technical assistance from children/grandchildren)	*[CHW speaking of a husband and wife that had language barriers and lower education levels that affected health care access] "For the man, it was easy for him to go to the doctor [alone] whenever he need[ed to do so]. For the wife, it was difficult [to go alone] because she's a woman and needs to be home to cook [due to cultural/societal expectations]. . .The husband's mindset was, 'I am the man, I am the one that decides if my wife goes to treatment or not' and the wife just focuses on what husband says. It was not only because of language issues, not only because of women [gender] issues, it is all together. . .[To help the woman], my first step was to build trust by speaking to them together [during one-on-ones], and later shifted to only the wife and helped her [become self-sufficient]."*
Model Minority	– Identifying community priorities, collecting disaggregated data, and raising awareness of disease disparities within specific Asian American groups	*"It helped when we did a community needs assessment and saw the issue of diabetes. Then the community felt like this was an issue. Otherwise, we are always grouped with everyone else and it is hard to tell."*

The DREAM Initiative is currently in its final wave of implementation and data collection, which is set to conclude in 2022. Due to the novel coronavirus (COVID-19) pandemic, the DREAM Initiative adapted its intervention in March 2020 to a remote model, utilizing tailored strategies developed by research team members working in collaboration with CHWs to address the needs of individuals facing digital barriers. A program evaluation conducted in August 2020, found that the transition to an online curriculum resulted in high levels of fidelity, retention, and patient satisfaction. Additionally, the DREAM Initiative has expanded beyond NYC with the launch of DREAM Atlanta, a replication of the DREAM Initiative being implemented in Atlanta, Georgia. The DREAM Atlanta team receives training and technical assistance from the DREAM Initiative research team to replicate the NYC-based study in Atlanta's South Asian community, addressing hypertension and diabetes management among individuals with both conditions.

REFERENCES

Glasgow, R. E., Vogt, T. M., & Boles, S. M. (1999). Evaluating the public health impact of health promotion interventions: the RE-AIM framework. *Am J Public Health, 89*(9), 1322–1327. doi:10.2105/ajph.89.9.1322

Healthify. https://www.healthify.us/

Hung, D. Y., Rundall, T. G., Tallia, A. F., Cohen, D. J., Halpin, H. A., & Crabtree, B. F. (2007). Rethinking prevention in primary care: applying the chronic care model to address health risk behaviors. *Milbank Q, 85*(1), 69–91. doi:10.1111/j.1468-0009.2007.00477.x

Islam, N., Riley, L., Wyatt, L., Tandon, S. D., Tanner, M., Mukherji-Ratnam, R., . . . Trinh-Shevrin, C. (2014). Protocol for the DREAM Project (Diabetes Research, Education, and Action for Minorities): a randomized trial of a community health worker intervention to improve diabetic management and control among Bangladeshi adults in NYC. *BMC Public Health, 14*, 177. doi:10.1186/1471-2458-14-177

Islam, N. S., Patel, S., Wyatt, L. C., Sim, S.-C., Mukherjee-Ratnam, R., Chun, K., . . . Kwon, S. C. (2016). Sources of health information among select Asian American immigrant groups in New York City. *Health Communication, 31*(2), 207–216. doi:10.1080/10410236.2014.944332

Islam, N. S., Tandon, D., Mukherji, R., Tanner, M., Ghosh, K., Alam, G., . . . Trinh-Shevrin, C. (2012). Understanding barriers to and facilitators of diabetes control and prevention in the New York City Bangladeshi community: a mixed-methods approach. *Am J Public Health, 102*(3), 486–490. doi:10.2105/ajph.2011.300381

Islam, N. S., Wyatt, L. C., Taher, M. D., Riley, L., Tandon, S. D., Tanner, M., . . . Trinh-Shevrin, C. (2018). A culturally tailored community health worker intervention leads to improvement in patient-centered outcomes for immigrant patients with type 2 diabetes. *Clinical Diabetes, 36*(2), 100–111. doi:10.2337/cd17-0068

Lim, S., Wyatt, L. C., Chauhan, H., Zanowiak, J. M., Kavathe, R., Singh, H., . . . Islam, N. S. (2019a). A culturally adapted diabetes prevention intervention in the New York City Sikh Asian Indian community leads to improvements in health behaviors and outcomes. *Health Behavior Research, 2*(1), 4. doi:10.4148/2572-1836.1027

Lim, S., Wyatt, L. C., Mammen, S., Zanowiak, J. M., Mohaimin, S., Goldfeld, K. S., . . . Islam, N. S. (2019b). The DREAM Initiative: study protocol for a randomized controlled trial testing an integrated electronic health record and community health worker intervention to promote weight loss among South Asian patients at risk for diabetes. *Trials, 20*(1), 635. doi:10.1186/s13063-019-3711-y

Lopez, P. M., Zanowiak, J., Goldfeld, K., Wyka, K., Masoud, A., Beane, S., . . . Islam, N. (2017). Protocol for project IMPACT (improving millions hearts for provider and community transformation): a quasi-experimental evaluation of an integrated electronic health record and community health worker intervention study to improve hypertension management among South Asian patients. *BMC Health Serv Res, 17*(1), 810. doi:10.1186/s12913-017-2767-1

CASE

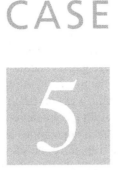

ALZHEIMER'S DISEASE/ ALZHEIMER'S DISEASE-RELATED DEMENTIAS

JENNIFER A. WONG

The current healthy aging research literature is constrained by a paucity of published work related to Alzheimer's disease and Alzheimer's disease and its related dementias (AD/ADRD) that is specifically focused on Asian American and Native Hawaiian and Pacific Islander (NH/PI) populations (Đoàn et al., 2019; Shah & Kandula 2020; Wong et al., 2019). Relatedly, AD/ADRD disparities in Asian Americans and NH/PIs in the United States are magnified by a dearth of clinical-community resources supporting culturally competent and timely AD/ADRD diagnosis and services.

In 2018, the NYU Center for the Study of Asian American Health (CSAAH) at NYU Grossman School of Medicine established a Healthy Aging Research Track to address critical research and knowledge gaps in health interventions that aim to support the prevention, early identification, and treatment of AD/ADRD among Asian American and NH/PI populations. To initiate our work, CSAAH conducted a series of mixed-methods research activities to inform and develop the Healthy Aging Research Track's research agenda, including engagement of our extensive base of national and local community partners to gain a deeper understanding about AD/ADRD in this diverse and growing population. Engaging with Asian American and NH/PI community leaders is critical to prioritizing a strategic, relationship-focused, community-engaged research agenda to understand, address, and reduce AD/ADRD disparities among Asian American and NH/PI communities. Findings from this preliminary work helped to establish a baseline understanding of Asian American and NH/PI communities' familiarity with and needs related to AD/ADRD to better guide CSAAH's community partnership work and research initiatives to comprehensively support AD/ADRD prevention, early identification, and treatment in Asian Americans and NH/PIs.

Applied Population Health Approaches for Asian American Communities, First Edition. Edited by Simona C. Kwon, Chau Trinh-Shevrin, Nadia S. Islam, and Stella S. Yi.
© 2023 John Wiley & Sons, Inc. Published 2023 by John Wiley & Sons, Inc.
Companion Website: www.wiley.com/go/kwon/asianamerican

SCOPING REVIEW

CSAAH conducted an environmental scan and scoping review of peer-reviewed, interdisciplinary published literature on AD/ADRD in Asian Americans and NH/PIs (Lim et al., 2020; Lim et al., 2019). Scoping review findings identified significant research and knowledge gaps related to AD/ADRD symptoms and risk factors, as well as misconceptions about AD/ADRD as part of the natural aging process. Studies show elevated levels of stigma around the topic of Alzheimer's disease, dementia, and related issues, with nuances related to how stigma manifests within the family, among caregivers, or within the greater community.

Very few studies include NH/PI or South Asian populations and very few studies present disaggregated data by Asian American or NH/PI ethnic group. To better understand these topics in the research literature, key themes from the assessment of the literature were used to develop an interview guide for a series of key informant interviews.

KEY INFORMANT INTERVIEW SERIES

CSAAH conducted a series of key informant interviews ($n = 11$) with Asian American and NH/PI older adult service providers to elucidate population-specific attitudes, existing programs and services, and needs related to AD/ADRD, and to gain consensus on key priority research areas identified in the initial scoping review. Semi-structured, in-depth, one-hour interviews were completed in-person or via phone with 11 Asian American and NH/PI older adult-serving regional community experts from May to August 2019. Research team members structured interview guide questions to identify and assess the following:

1. Community-level barriers and facilitators to understanding and addressing healthy aging and AD/ADRD health and disparities research;

2. Asian American and NH/PI cultural and social considerations (community knowledge, attitudes, and norms) related to the topics of healthy aging and AD/ADRD;

3. Effective strategies or priorities to address and raise awareness of AD/ADRD in these communities;

4. Innovative or emerging social networks or media channels to promote and disseminate AD/ADRD health-related information resources and study results.

Interview participants were identified through recommendations from members of our National Advisory Committee on Research (NAC), a formal advisory body that CSAAH regularly convenes, described in more detail in the next section. NAC representatives were asked to identify two to three local experts embedded in regional communities serving Asian American or NH/PI older adults. Themes from the key informant interviews informed CSAAH's use of a consensus-building activity, a modified Delphi technique, held with CSAAH's NAC as well as our Scientific Committee (SC), a second formal advisory body that is comprised of academic and scientific stakeholders.

MODIFIED DELPHI TECHNIQUE WITH COMMUNITY AND RESEARCH STAKEHOLDERS

CSAAH's NAC is a formal advisory group comprised of community leaders and champions representing 14 community-based organizations, social service, and advocacy agencies, federally qualified health centers, health care professional organizations, and academic representatives with a long history of implementing successful strategies to promote the health of Asian American and NH/PI communities across the United States. CSAAH co-leads the NAC with partners from the Asian & Pacific Islander American Health Forum (APIAHF), the oldest and largest health advocacy organization working with Asian American and NH/PI communities across the United States. The NAC informs CSAAH's health disparities research agenda, research training and dissemination activities, and community engagement and capacity-building activities to foster community-initiated research. CSAAH's SC, consisting of six academic and professional stakeholders, provides scientific feedback on health disparities research and research initiatives for greater sustainability. CSAAH and APIAHF convene the NAC and SC jointly, three times a year virtually or in-person, as a collaborative advisory partnership to inform our center's community engagement and dissemination work to advance Asian American and NH/PI community research capacity and health equity.

CSAAH selected the Delphi method as a community-based participatory research and consensus-building approach for use with our NAC and SC members to triangulate research priorities for our Healthy Aging health disparities research agenda with interview and scoping review findings. The Delphi technique is a validated, systematic method useful for generating consensus with experts on a particular research question (de Villiers et al., 2005). Participants, or experts, contribute to a series of intensive questionnaires and structured feedback sessions over several rounds; input is "pooled" to generate reliable, group-derived decisions or agreed-upon consensus positions (Benson et al., 2020; Coleman et al., 2013; Hasson et al., 2000; Rideout et al., 2013).

CSAAH has successfully applied this consensus and appraisal method and found it to be effective for exploring priorities for public health across diverse health topic areas and in gaining group agreement with communities and multisector stakeholders, including with our NAC (Grieb et al., 2017; Kwon et al., 2017; Rideout et al., 2013). An iterative Delphi approach streamlines the rich feedback-gathering process and inspires cross-pollination of ideas from NAC members' professional and personal knowledge of regional community priorities and needs, resource strengths, and preferred channels for communication across distinct Asian American and NH/PI subgroup populations. Furthermore, this approach helps participant members come to agreement through in-person, robust discussions that foster sharing of ideas and facilitate the emergence of meaningful solutions for community-facing research training products and healthy information-sharing tools.

CSAAH led the NAC and SC in a two-round Delphi approach to prioritize CSAAH's healthy aging research initiatives and inform Asian American and NH/PI community engagement approach planning. Two rounds were sufficient to gain alignment with this representative collective of community leaders and stakeholders in determining top priority research areas. The focus of the consensus-building activity was to clarify NAC- and SC-prioritized recommendations for:

- Research topics for CSAAH's Healthy Aging research agenda as related to AD/ADRD, and

- Technical assistance and training activities and key communication methods or strategies for CSAAH to develop to support community partners' AD/ADRD research and programming

NAC and SC members were invited to respond to and rate priorities in an anonymous online survey distributed via email in Phase One of the Delphi. A four-question survey asked participants to prioritize three out of seven research focus areas derived from key informant interview themes. Three additional open-ended survey questions measured participants' familiarity with existing Asian American and NH/PI community-focused resources and programs aimed at supporting healthy aging and ADRD, training or tool needs to build community AD/ADRD support capacity, and effective community dissemination channels or strategies to support AD/ADRD health-information sharing in Asian American and NH/PI communities. The web-based survey was open for a four-week period, with several reminder emails sent to encourage participant feedback.

NAC and SC members were informed that survey feedback would be presented at an in-person meeting within two weeks after survey close; prior to that meeting, a trained study team member reviewed and prepared survey results to allow for a well-structured, focused group discussion. The Phase Two discussion portion of the Delphi technique was included as a key agenda item during a regularly scheduled group meeting with NAC and SC members. During the discussion, participants were presented with the prioritized seven research focus areas and the additional survey question inputs and then asked to clarify or adjust their rankings after reviewing the group results. CSAAH and APIAHF staff collaboratively guided the discussion to hone in on NAC- and SC-prioritized research topic recommendations for CSAAH's research agenda on healthy aging related to AD/ADRD, generate recommendations, and drive group agreement on top-priority research topic areas and health education trainings for development that would support community organizations' work and research capacity as related to AD/ADRD. NAC and SC members narrowed the priority research focus areas to three key topics, presented in Table A5.1.

In general, the qualitative data from the NAC and SC member group discussion validated survey findings and added nuance to the interview themes. Findings supported the need for basic AD/ADRD health information tailored to the needs of Asian American and NH/PI communities, such as culturally adapted trainings for caregivers on how to speak to older adult family members about aging (including AD/ADRD). NAC and SC input

TABLE A5.1   Priority Research Areas Defined by NAC and SC through Modified Delphi Approach

Research topic area prioritized by NAC & SC	Specific recommendations for future research and health education derived from the Delphi approach
Value of social support and social networks	**Leverage community assets and existing strengths related to social support and social networks.** NAC and SC members placed critical importance on strengthening and utilizing social supports and networks within Asian American and NH/PI communities. Social networks are important not only for the individual (patient with AD/ADRD) but also for caregivers, family members, and the greater community. The NAC spoke of the value in sharing AD/ADRD stories to address cultural stigma about the topic and to derive strategies to support aging individuals within local or ethnic/cultural communities.
Engagement with the health care system	**Integrate strategies for direct clinical–community linkages and better engagement with the health care system.** NAC and SC stressed the need for training, culturally congruent and in-language information for audiences with low English proficiency, low literacy, or low health literacy, and guidance on how to find, utilize, and engage with services within the U.S. health care system.
Need for AD/ADRD education	**Develop culturally and linguistically relevant education and information about AD/ADRD to raise individual- and community-level awareness.** There is a general lack of knowledge and awareness about AD/ADRD across communities and ethnic groups. There are also few in-language, culturally adapted resources detailing healthy aging for these populations. NAC and SC members agreed that education about AD/ADRD as a health topic as well as AD/ADRD prevention, resources, care strategies, and social support options are needed.

identified tools for external researchers to develop or offer as resources and research support to community organizational partners. For example, members suggested ways of developing training for staff and providers in community-based organizations and federally qualified health centers to help them address end-of-life care in ways that were supportive and relevant both to their organizational missions as well as to the culture and needs of community members and patients. NAC and SC input from the Delphi approach underscored important contextual factors specific to community organizations serving Asian Americans and NH/PIs, including the need for tailored, culturally appropriate information-sharing approaches to allow staff to engage effectively in conversations with diverse, under-resourced community audiences with low English proficiency about healthy aging and AD/ADRD. Members recommended that the trainings focus information toward both direct-service staff as well as higher-level personnel and that in-person, short-duration programs would be the most effective and accessible to NAC and SC member organizational staff.

Findings also highlighted the need for future research and health education efforts focused on raising Asian American and NH/PI individual- and community-level awareness about AD/ADRD and leveraging existing community assets to integrate effective engagement strategies to access AD/ADRD services within the health care system. Community partner engagement in developing CSAAH's Healthy Aging research agenda provided much-needed complexity to describing community preferences and values in the types of AD/ADRD health information needed and confirmed preferred communication channels to best deliver that information to Asian American and NH/PI communities of focus to support their needs.

REFERENCES

Benson, H., Lucas, C., & Williams, K. A. (2020). Establishing consensus for general practice pharmacist education: A Delphi study. *Currents in Pharmacy Teaching and Learning, 12*(1), 8–13. https://doi.org/10.1016/j.cptl.2019.10.010

Coleman, C. A., Hudson, S., & Maine, L. L. (2013). Health literacy practices and educational competencies for health professionals: A consensus study. *Journal of Health Communication, 18*(sup1), 82–102. https://doi.org/10.1080/10810730.2013.829538

de Villiers, M. R., de Villiers, P. J. T., & Kent, A. P. (2005). The Delphi technique in health sciences education research. *Medical Teacher, 27*(7), 639–643. https://doi.org/10.1080/13611260500069947

Đoàn, L. N., Takata, Y., Sakuma, K.-L. K., & Irvin, V. L. (2019). Trends in clinical research including Asian American, Native Hawaiian, and Pacific Islander participants funded by the us national institutes of health, 1992 to 2018. *JAMA Network Open, 2*(7), e197432. https://doi.org/10.1001/jamanetworkopen.2019.7432

Grieb, S. D., Pichon, L., Kwon, S., Yeary, K. K., & Tandon, D. (2017). After 10 years: A vision forward for progress in community health partnerships. *Progress in Community Health Partnerships: Research, Education, and Action, 11*(1), 13–22. https://doi.org/10.1353/cpr.2017.0002

Kwon, S. C., Tandon, S. D., Islam, N., Riley, L., & Trinh-Shevrin, C. (2018). Applying a community-based participatory research framework to patient and family engagement in the development of patient-centered outcomes research and practice. *Translational Behavioral Medicine, 8*(5), 683–691. https://doi.org/10.1093/tbm/ibx026

Lim, S., Mohaimin, S., Min, D., Roberts, T., Sohn, Y.-J., Wong, J., Sivanesathurai, R., Kwon, S. C., & Trinh-Shevrin, C. (2020). Alzheimer's disease and its related dementias among Asian Americans, Native Hawaiians, and Pacific Islanders: A scoping review. *Journal of Alzheimer's Disease, 77*(2), 523–537. https://doi.org/10.3233/JAD-200509

Lim, S., Roberts, T., Wong, J., Mohaimin, S., Sohn, Y.-J., Sivanesathurai, R., Kwon, S. C., & Trinh-Shevrin, C. (2019). Systematic review and gap analysis on Alzheimer's disease in Asian Americans, Native Hawaiians, and Pacific Islanders. *Innovation in Aging, 3*(Supplement_1), S117–S117. https://doi.org/10.1093/geroni/igz038.431

Rideout, C., Gil, R., Browne, R., Calhoon, C., Rey, M., Gourevitch, M., & Trinh-Shevrin, C. (2013). Using the Delphi and snow card techniques to build consensus among diverse community and academic stakeholders. *Progress in Community Health Partnerships: Research, Education, and Action, 7*(3), 331–339. https://doi.org/10.1353/cpr.2013.0033

Shah, N. S., & Kandula, N. R. (2020). Addressing Asian American misrepresentation and underrepresentation in research. *Ethnicity & Disease, 30*(3), 513–516. https://doi.org/10.18865/ed.30.3.513

Wong, R., Amano, T., Lin, S.-Y., Zhou, Y., & Morrow-Howell, N. (2019). Strategies for the recruitment and retention of racial/ethnic minorities in Alzheimer disease and dementia clinical research. *Current Alzheimer Research, 16*(5), 458–471. https://doi.org/10.2174/1567205016666190321161901

CASE

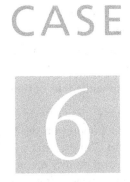

MANHATTAN DETENTION CENTER

YI-LING TAN

Rikers Island is home to New York City (NYC)'s largest correctional institution. It has a reputation for abuse and neglect of inmates, of whom the majority (85%) are pretrial defendants. In 2017, Mayor Bill de Blasio announced an $8 billion plan to close the Rikers Island jail complex and build four smaller new facilities in Manhattan, Brooklyn, Queens, and the Bronx. A federal building at 80 Centre Street on the periphery of Chinatown was selected to be the proposed site of the new 40-story "borough-based jail" in Manhattan and city environmental impact reviews were conducted for that site. Due to mounting resident protests over the scale of the project and the lack of transparency and community consultation, the site of the proposed jail was hurriedly changed to the current Manhattan Detention Center at 125 White Street in Chinatown without conducting a new environmental impact review or further community engagement. In the new city plans, the Manhattan Detention Center, which consist of two towers, would be demolished to build a larger, 29-story high-rise jail facility.

Community stakeholders immediately expressed multiple concerns about the new site of the proposed jail in Chinatown. They were particularly concerned about the impact of the years-long urban construction process on the health of vulnerable, low-income older adults with limited English proficiency living at the Chung Pak complex, which shares a wall with the current Manhattan Detention Center. Based on its prior history of collaborative work in Chinatown, the NYU Center for the Study of Asian American Health (CSAAH) at NYU Grossman School of Medicine was approached as an academic partner by a coalition of neighborhood activists and advocacy groups (i.e., Neighbors United Below Canal Street, the Chinatown Core Block Association, Abacus Federal Savings Bank, and Hamilton-Madison House) to understand the impact of long-term construction on the health of older adults and to identify evidence-informed mitigation strategies to protect vulnerable older residents in Chinatown.

Over nine months in 2019, CSAAH staff responded to the coalition's concerns through a community-engaged process consisting of the following:

- A high-level scoping review of the environmental and psychosocial health impact of long-term construction and evidence-based mitigation strategies;

Applied Population Health Approaches for Asian American Communities, First Edition. Edited by Simona C. Kwon, Chau Trinh-Shevrin, Nadia S. Islam, and Stella S. Yi.
Companion Website: www.wiley.com/go/kwon/asianamerican

- Key informant interviews of academic experts on priority topic areas such as geriatric health, mental health, environmental medicine, and urban planning;

- In-person meeting of community stakeholders and content experts to prioritize evidence-informed and culturally relevant mitigation strategies; and

- A report summarizing the results and recommendations of the scoping review, key informant interviews, and the meeting.

The report on the impact of long-term construction on the health of older adults in Chinatown was condensed into a one-page summary, translated into Chinese, and widely disseminated to policymakers, city planning officials, community-based organizations, community members, and the media (Tan et al., 2019). CSAAH staff participated in public information and community visioning sessions about the proposed jail. Additionally, CSAAH staff submitted testimonies as part of the environmental and land use review of the jails and advised city planning officials to take into account the health of the older adults living at Chung Pak (Sanders, 2019).

The report was submitted as part of an evidence package in a lawsuit brought against the city by a coalition partner, Neighbors United Below Canal Street. The Manhattan Supreme Court ruled in favor of the community coalition bringing the lawsuit and cited the report as a key factor in its decision to bar construction from moving forward until new reviews and approvals were completed. Additionally, the judge agreed with the coalition that the health of older adults in the community was not adequately taken into consideration during the city's environmental and land use review process (Chinatown mega-jail plan blocked by community lawsuit, 2020).

CSAAH continues to respond to community concerns around the Manhattan Detention Center even after the 2019 meeting and the favorable ruling in the lawsuit. Part of the recommended mitigation strategies discussed during the meeting involved the independent monitoring of noise pollution and air quality. Through a new initiative, Sound Health of UnderServed NeighborHoods (SHUSH), researchers at CSAAH and the NYU Center for Urban Science and Progress (CUSP) installed three noise sensors on the rooftop of Chung Pak in order to collect baseline ambient noise levels prior to the start of construction at the Manhattan Detention Center. The objective of the collaboration was to provide an independent source of noise data for community stakeholders, citizen scientists, and policymakers to support advocacy and civic engagement efforts. SHUSH researchers monitor the data from the noise sensors and translate them into simple charts and plain language for ease of community dissemination. The data were shared with community groups and policymakers during a community noise forum; more of the noise data are publicly available on the SHUSH website (www.soundsofchinatown.com).

CSAAH is currently exploring new forms of community engagement and collaboration around the Manhattan Detention Center. Multiple researchers are evaluating the impact of long-term construction on Chinatown's food ecology, food industry employment, and impact on food and vegetable consumption among Chinatown residents through agent-based modeling (Kim, 2020). CSAAH is also working with community members to identify new and ongoing concerns around the Manhattan Detention Center.

The city continues to appeal the decision and move ahead with construction through other mechanisms.

REFERENCES

Chinatown mega-jail plan blocked by community lawsuit. (2020, September 28, 2020). *The Village Sun*. Retrieved from https://thevillagesun.com/chinatown-mega-jail-plan-blocked-by-community-lawsuit

Kim, M. (2020, November 20, 2020). *Asian American Businesses Face Distinct Challenges Amid Coronavirus Pandemic*. Retrieved from https://www.kqed.org/forum/2010101880896/asian-american-business-face-distinct-challenges-amid-coronavirus-pandemic

Sanders, A. (2019, August 23, 2019). Concerns raised over health of seniors near proposed Manhattan jail. *New York Daily News*. Retrieved from https://www.nydailynews.com/news/politics/ny-health-concerns-seniors-manhattan-jail-proposal-20190823-ferd7fcw5vg2pcog75giwqugx4-story.html

Tan, Y.-L., Wong, J., Pan, J., & Kwon, S. (2019). *The Long-Term Impact of Construction on the Health of Older Adults in New York City's Chinatown*. (2019). New York: NYU Center for the Study of Asian American Health. Retrieved from https://constructionandolderadults.wordpress.com/report/

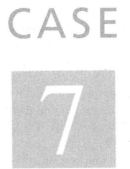

CASE

FORGING PARTNERSHIPS

LAN N. ĐOÀN, STELLA S. YI, JENNIFER A. WONG, MATTHEW K. CHIN, SIMONA C. KWON

Establishing Asian American, Native Hawaiian, and Pacific Islander Community Partnerships for Rapid Response to COVID-19: the Forging Partnerships Project

The novel coronavirus (COVID-19) pandemic has ravaged racialized populations, highlighting the vulnerabilities of groups that are disproportionately burdened with chronic conditions because of structural inequities, including limited health care access, greater occupational exposure to COVID-19 infection, racism and discrimination, and low socioeconomic status (Flagg et al., 2020; Rubin-Miller et al., 2020; Sze et al., 2020). The Forging Partnerships project, funded by the national Centers for Disease Control and Prevention (CDC) Office of Minority Health (OMH), is focused on addressing these inequities among Asian Americans and Native Hawaiians and Pacific Islanders (NH/PIs). This case study describes the CDC's rationale for convening this collaborative, describes the project's goals and activities, and describes the NYU Center for the Study of Asian American Health (CSAAH) at NYU Grossman School of Medicine's role as an academic research partner within the coalition of community project partners.

More than 24 months into the pandemic, Asian American and NH/PI communities have been largely excluded from the national dialogue and research literature detailing the impact of COVID-19 on communities of color. COVID-19 related disparities experienced by these communities have been pieced together through social media, news media (Ramachandran, 2020), blog posts (Chang et al., 2020; Chin et al., 2021; Yan et al., 2020), and pre-print sites (i.e., where complete but not yet peer-reviewed manuscripts are posted for distribution to the broader health sciences field) (Marcello et al., 2020; Quach et al., 2020). For example, NBC Asian America was able to report on the disproportionate COVID-19 mortality among Chinese adults and high COVID-19 test positivity among South Asians in New York City (NYC) based on a pre-print (Marcello et al., 2020; Ramachandran, 2020). Furthermore, the pandemic has brought to the forefront ongoing challenges for mitigating negative COVID-19-related health outcomes for Asian Americans and NH/PIs, including: extension of the model minority stereotype on health, poor quality of available racial/ethnic data, limited collection and reporting of disaggregated racial/ethnic data, difficulties related to pivoting to conduct community-based participatory research virtually, and insufficient resources to support and fairly compensate community partners for their expertise and time (Yi et al., 2021).

Applied Population Health Approaches for Asian American Communities, First Edition. Edited by Simona C. Kwon, Chau Trinh-Shevrin, Nadia S. Islam, and Stella S. Yi.
© 2023 John Wiley & Sons, Inc. Published 2023 by John Wiley & Sons, Inc.
Companion Website: www.wiley.com/go/kwon/asianamerican

The overarching goal of Forging Partnerships is to establish a collaborative network of partner organizations to enhance the CDC's ability to identify and respond to the needs of Asian American and NH/PI communities that have emerged or worsened as a result of COVID-19. More specifically, the partnering organizations are charged with developing culturally and linguistically appropriate, community-facing COVID-19 education materials based on the CDC's COVID-19 resources and recommendations. The project was developed in response to calls for coordinated public health crisis response for COVID-19 preparedness and response activities as well as in order to enhance the public health infrastructure to rapidly respond to public health emergencies. CSAAH is one of 17 partnering organizations leading this initiative. CSAAH's role in this project is to identify and harness available disaggregated data on COVID-19 infection, hospitalization, and mortality for focused prevention efforts and health equity assessments; conduct rapid assessments of the impact of COVID-19 on individuals and families, addressing jobs and income, what individuals need the most help with during the pandemic, and health behaviors related to COVID-19, including testing, likelihood of opting to receive the COVID-19 vaccine, and access to care; collaborate with partner organizations to disseminate project materials; and pilot and assess lessons learned to mitigate the impact of COVID-19 in high-risk Asian American and NH/PI populations.

Asian Americans are plagued by the model minority stereotype and, consequently, are not seen as a community of color that experiences health disparities (Yi, 2020) – observations that are illustrated by the exclusion of Asian Americans from clinical research studies (Borno et al., 2020), allocation of funding (Đoàn et al., 2019), policy recommendations (National Academies of Sciences, Engineering, and Medicine, 2020a), and outreach and engagement efforts for vulnerable populations (NIH, 2020). The inconsistency in measurement and lack of standardization around racial/ethnic data collected and reported at the national, regional, and local levels have hampered an accurate depiction of high- and at-risk Asian American and NH/PI groups. The Forging Partnerships project has underscored the need to amplify Asian American and NH/PI COVID-19-related disparities into national discourse, particularly during a global pandemic. Intentional and strategic collaborations, as well as quick dissemination of information and alerts to a broad array of stakeholders, including news media, scientists, policymakers, and community stakeholders, is central to leading and supporting public health emergency preparedness and response.

The Forging Partnerships initiative is led by the Asian & Pacific Islander American Health Forum (APIAHF), the oldest and largest national health advocacy organization focused on informing policy, mobilizing communities, and strengthening programs and organizations to improve the health of Asian Americans and NH/PIs, in collaboration with organizations in sectors including public health, social services, civic engagement, and primary care: CSAAH, Association of Asian Pacific Community Health Organizations (AAPCHO), Asian Pacific Islander American Public Affairs (APAPA), Buddhist Tzu Chi Medical Foundation, Coalition for Asian American Children and Families (CACF), National Asian Pacific American Bar Association (NAPABA), National Council of Asian Pacific Americans (NCAPA), NICOS Chinese Health Coalition, Pacific Islander Community Association of Washington (PICA-WA), Pacific Islander Center of Primary Care Excellence (PI-CoPCE), Pacific Islander Health Partnership (PIHP)/ Southern California Pacific Islander COVID-19 Response Team (SoCal PICRT), Papa Ola Lōkahi, Philippine Nurses Association of America Foundation (PNAAF), Progressive Vietnamese American Organization (PIVOT), Southeast Asia Resource Action Center (SEARAC), and Vietnamese American Roundtable (VAR). These partnering organizations are responsible for coordinating and implementing a community-tailored COVID-19 health education and infection risk prevention campaign. At the time of writing, approximately 350 organizations and 65 individuals have been engaged in this process to establish new and strengthen ongoing partnerships with local Asian Americans and NH/PI-serving organizations. Lead organization members of this partnership serve as both access and dissemination points for collaboratively developed, CDC-informed educational materials related to COVID-19 contact tracing, testing, access to testing and care, and vaccination. Key priority subpopulations of this project include individuals residing in multigenerational homes, essential and frontline health workers, and individuals with prediabetes and diabetes.

Trust is assessed and discussed regularly among participating partner organizations to ensure the effective and multidirectional exchange of ideas among this group of stakeholders. This collaborative energy also ensures that the group is able to hold each organization accountable to ensure the project's principles and values remain community-centered throughout the project period. For instance, transparency of the project process and production of deliverables was evaluated on an ongoing basis to ensure that Asian American and NH/PI communities were included in the decision-making process and to build trust and strengthen partnerships. The Forging

Partnerships project has resulted in the transcreation of COVID-19 related educational campaigns and strategies (e.g., videos, pamphlets) for Asian American and NH/PI communities in more than 15 languages and reflect shared, community-centered solutions (https://www.aa-nhpihealthresponse.org).

Forging Partnerships project partners contribute to strengthening collaboration and completing project deliverables, as well as to coordinating efforts to bring attention to Asian American and NH/PI health disparities exacerbated by the COVID-19 pandemic. The project partners also worked to inform federal COVID-19 related planning and priority setting to include Asian American and NH/PI communities. For instance, when the National Academies of Sciences, Engineering, and Medicine (NASEM) released the "Discussion Draft of the Preliminary Framework for Equitable Allocation of COVID-19 Vaccine" (Draft Framework), on September 1, 2020, for public comment for four days, the Forging Partnerships network was able to put together response statements rapidly with strong support from Asian American- and NH/PI-serving organizations. The Discussion Draft was a set of recommendations on the development and deployment of the COVID-19 vaccine distribution system in the United States, in which COVID-19-related disparities were identified among all racial/ethnic minority populations except for Asian American and NH/PI communities (National Academies of Sciences, Engineering, and Medicine, 2020b). APIAHF and CSAAH, along with nine national Asian American and NH/PI health response partners (including community partners from the Forging Partnerships project); the National Pacific Islander Covid-19 Response Team (NPICRT); and the Filipinx/a/o Covid-19 Resource and Response team submitted response statements advocating for the federal government to explicitly address the documented disparities in the overall Asian American and NH/PI population as well in specific subgroups, like Filipino health workers.

The collective effort in submitting response statements successfully resulted in the inclusion of NH/PI populations in the final recommendations for the equitable allocation of the COVID-19 vaccine (National Academies of Sciences, Engineering, and Medicine, 2020a). Asian American and NH/PI organizations, including those involved in the Forging Partnership initiative, mobilized a coordinated submission of statements through existing communication networks, underscoring the value and strength of trust across the partners as well as the impact of collective, strategic advocacy. This network has continued submitting statements throughout the pandemic in response to the federal COVID-19 response. Examples include a letter to the members of the COVID-19 Advisory Board for the Biden-Harris Transition, led by the Filipinx/a/o Covid-19 Resource and Response team, and a letter to policymakers to ensure the equitable distribution of COVID-19 vaccines to Asian American and NH/PI communities, led by the National Council of Asian Pacific Islander Physicians (NCAPIP).

CSAAH has a unique role within the coalition of Forging Partnerships partners. As the only National Institutes of Health (NIH) National Institute on Minority Health and Health Disparities (NIMHD)-funded Specialized Center of Excellence focused on Asian American health disparities research and evaluation, CSAAH's strength lies in our familiarity with community-engaged, community-led research data resources, tools, and evaluation analyses, to support the COVID-19 data needs of the Forging Partnerships project. Thus, CSAAH provides foundational research expertise for project partners as the academic research partner. In this role, CSAAH faces the challenge of maintaining a delicate balance in several regards, including harmonizing the need to pursue a research agenda with ensuring true community benefit; acknowledging and addressing power and ethical dynamics around ownership, sharing, and reporting of data; and recognizing and resolving tensions and community mistrust of academia, federal agencies, and those outside of the community. One of CSAAH's priorities is to utilize qualitative and quantitative data and to leverage fellow partners' extensive networks, partnerships, and capacity for outreach to identify Asian American and NH/PI populations at high risk for COVID-19-related morbidity and mortality. This work aims to improve the availability and completeness of disaggregated data for specific Asian American and NH/PI populations. As part of the Forging Partnerships project, CSAAH worked with partner organizations to identify existing and planned data collection efforts related to COVID-19 among Asian American and NH/PI populations nationwide:

- Eleven primary data collection efforts related to COVID-19, including national and regional surveys (Figure A7.1);

- Two national and three regional datasets available for secondary data analyses within which high-risk Asian American and NH/PI subgroups may be identified;

- Twelve other primary data collection efforts that are not intended specifically for COVID-19 assessment but contain COVID-19-related questions that may prove useful to researchers.

Survey	Partnering Organization	Population and Sample Size	Geography and Start Date
CSAAH-led			
DREAM (Diabetes Research, Action, and Education for Minorities) Project		Indian, Bangladeshi, Indo-Caribbean, Nepali, Pakistani 530 adults age 18+ years	NYC, NY. May 2020
Older Adult Community Health Resources and Needs Assessment (CHRNA)		Arab, Asian Indian, Bangladeshi, Chinese, Korean, Mexican, Russian 1,750 adults age 50+ years	NYC, NY. February 2022
North-South Survey/ NIH Community Engagement Alliance (CEAL) Common Survey 2	Icahn School of Medicine at Mt Sinai; Institute for Family Health	Asian, Arab, foreign-born 1,050 adults age 18+ years	U.S. (Northeast, South, Midwest). December 2021
National Rapid Needs Assessment	Asian Pacific Islander American Public Affairs (APAPA), Buddhist Tzu Chi Medical Foundation, Coalition for Asian American Children and Families (CACF), National Asian Pacific American Bar Association (NAPABA), NICOS Chinese Health Coalition, Pacific Islander Community Association of Washington (PICA-WA), Philippine Nurses Association of America Foundation (PNAAF), Pacific Islander Health Partnership (PIHP), Papa Ola Lōkahi, Asian & Pacific Islander American Health Forum (APIAHF)	Arab, Chinese, Filipino, Japanese, Korean, Marshallese, Micronesian, Native Hawaiian, Nepali, Samoan, South Asian, Tongan, Vietnamese 1,000 adults age 18+ years	U.S. January 2022
Community-led, CSAAH advising			
Regional CHRNAs	Asian Pacific Community in Action (APCA); Center for Pan Asian Community Services (CPACS); National Tongan American Society (NTAS)	Chinese, Filipino, Hawaiian, Korean, Marshallese, Micronesian, Taiwanese, Tongan, Samoan, Vietnamese 1,110 adults age 18–75 years	Phoenix, AZ; Atlanta, GA; Salt Lake City, UT. April 2021
NYC COVID-19 CHRNA	CACF; Chinese-American Planning Council (CPC)	Arab, Burmese, Cambodian, Chinese, Filipino, Japanese, Korean, Lao, Latinx, South Asian, Vietnamese 1,355 adults age 18+ years	NYC, NY. May 2021

Survey	Partnering Organization	Population and Sample Size	Geography and Start Date
SEARAC Rapid Needs Assessment	Southeast Asia Resource Action Center (SEARAC)	Cambodian, Hmong, Lao, Vietnamese, NH/PI, Southeast Asian 250 adults age 18+ years	U.S. February 2022
CSAAH-partnered			
AA & NH/PI COVID-19 Needs Assessment	DePaul University; Pacific Islander Center of Primary Care Excellence (PI-CoPCE); Asian American Psychological Association	CHamoru, Chinese, Fijian, Filipino, Korean, Marshallese, Native Hawaiian, Samoan, South Asian, Vietnamese 5,000 adults age 18+ years	U.S. January 2021
Eastern Virginia CHRNA	Eastern Virginia Medical School	Chinese, Filipino 800 adults age 18+ years	Eastern VA. February 2022
Health and Life Study of Koreans	University of Michigan	Korean 600 adults age 18+ years	U.S. February 2022
Existing data – aggregate data will be provided			
Speak UP on COVID-19	Mount Sinai	American Indian/Alaskan Native, Black, Chinese, Filipino, Korean, Japanese, Latinx, NH/PI, South Asian, white 10,000 adults age 18+ years	NYC, NY. April 2020

FIGURE A7.1 *Forging Partnerships Primary Data Collection Efforts*

Relatedly, CSAAH also became involved in national conversations with the Asian American & NH/PI COVID-19 Policy & Research Team, a group formed in May 2020, in response to the COVID-19 pandemic. This group is comprised of high-profile researchers and highly leveraged policy professionals from throughout the nation who meet regularly to discuss databases and other sources of information to monitor the COVID-19 experience in Asian American and NH/PI communities. Multiple layers of community-engaged research projects and partnership continue to shape and strengthen CSAAH individual- and coalition-level contributions to addressing COVID-19 in underserved populations.

CSAAH has leveraged our partnerships to coordinate primary data collection efforts in order to harmonize COVID-19-related measures and demographic questions across tools (Figure A7.1) to better capture the COVID-19 experience in Asian American and NH/PI populations nationally. The urgency of the toll of COVID-19 on Asian American and NH/PI communities has required flexibility and thoughtful coordination with other research and community efforts to avoid overburdening Asian American and NH/PI communities that have experienced multiple losses and grief throughout the pandemic.

For example, CSAAH engaged community members and community-based organizations in many conversations throughout the survey development process to gain consensus on relevant measures and to vet the final surveys. Survey development relied on the review and assessment of existing instruments both nationally (e.g., the PhenX Toolkit, a collection of quantitative and qualitative measures for **Phen**otypes and e**X**posures; the U.S.

Census Bureau Household Pulse survey) (U.S. Census Bureau, 2021) and locally (e.g., the Mount Sinai Speak UP on COVID-19 survey in NYC) to maximally integrate survey measures across datasets in future work. Harmonized data will generate a sample size of about 15,000 Asian American and NH/PI individuals, addressing approximately 30 questions across 11 survey domains.

Survey measures included in the final survey instrument were vetted by community partners to ensure that community perspectives were embedded into the survey tool and to enhance survey design and acceptability in the target population. Specifically, engaging community members in tool development increases the likelihood of participants from target communities completing the full survey questionnaire and engaging in the survey process. This unprecedented national coordination across these different groups allows for methodological and cost efficiencies, such as sharing linguistic translations, design of new surveys focused on Asian American and NH/PI populations not being reached by other efforts, and importantly, conscious efforts to not overwhelm the Asian American and NH/PI community with multiple surveys.

Findings from the Forging Partnership project have been shared directly with the CDC contacts to inform the national COVID-19 response and are informing the development, adaptation, and dissemination of culturally appropriate strategies to reduce COVID-19 morbidity and mortality disparities in Asian American and NH/PI subgroups and regional communities. This approach of leveraging existing and new data collection efforts, guided and informed by community partners who have "boots on the ground" and direct interactions with Asian American and NH/PI communities, may serve as a guide for improving collection of disaggregated racial/ethnic data and centering data collection, reporting, and dissemination efforts on health equity and community needs.

REFERENCES

Borno, H. T., Zhang, S., & Gomez, S. (2020). COVID-19 disparities: An urgent call for race reporting and representation in clinical research. *Contemporary Clinical Trials Communications, 19*. https://doi.org/10.1016/j.conctc.2020.100630

Chang, R. C., Penaia, C., & Thomas, K. (2020, August 27). *Count Native Hawaiian and Pacific Islanders in COVID-19 Data—It's an OMB Mandate*. Health Affairs Blog. https://doi.org/10.1377/hblog20200825.671245

Chin, M., Đoàn, L. N., Chong, S. K., Wong, J. A., Kwon, S. C., & Yi, S. S., (2021, May 24). Asian American Subgroups And The COVID-19 Experience: What We Know And Still Don't Know. *Health Affairs Blog*. https://www.healthaffairs.org/do/10.1377/hblog20210519.651079/full/

Đoàn, L. N., Takata, Y., Sakuma, K.-L. K., & Irvin, V. L. (2019). Trends in clinical research including Asian American, Native Hawaiian, and Pacific Islander Participants funded by the US National Institutes of Health, 1992 to 2018. *JAMA Network Open, 2*(7), e197432. https://doi.org/10.1001/jamanetworkopen.2019.7432

Flagg, A., Sharma, D., Fenn, L., & Stobbe, M. (2020, August 21). *COVID-19's Toll on People of Color Is Worse Than We Knew*. The Marshall Project. https://www.themarshallproject.org/2020/08/21/covid-19-s-toll-on-people-of-color-is-worse-than-we-knew

Marcello, R. K., Dolle, J., Grami, S., Adule, R., Li, Z., Tatem, K., Anyaogu, C., Ayinla, R., Boma, N., Brady, T., Cosme-Thormann, B. F., Ford, K., Gaither, K., Kanter, M., Kessler, S., Kristal, R. B., Lieber, J. J., Mukherjee, V., Rizzo, V., . . . Team, N. Y. C. H. + H. C.-19 P. H. D. (2020). Characteristics and outcomes of COVID-19 patients in New York City's Public Hospital System. *MedRxiv*, 2020.05.29.20086645. https://doi.org/10.1101/2020.05.29.20086645

National Academies of Sciences, Engineering, and Medicine. (2020a). *Framework for Equitable Allocation of COVID-19 Vaccine*. The National Academies Press. https://doi.org/10.17226/25917

National Academies of Sciences, Engineering, and Medicine. (2020b). *Discussion Draft of the Preliminary Framework for Equitable Allocation of COVID-19 Vaccine*. https://www.nap.edu/resource/25917/25914.pdf

National Institutes of Health (NIH) (2020, September 16). *NIH funds community engagement research efforts in areas hardest hit by COVID-19*. https://www.nih.gov/news-events/news-releases/nih-funds-community-engagement-research-efforts-areas-hardest-hit-covid-19

Quach, T., Đoàn, L. N., Liou, J., & Ponce, N. (2020). Simultaneously blamed and ignored: barriers, behaviors, and impact of COVID-19 on Asian Americans. *JMIR Preprints*. https://doi.org/10.2196/preprints.23976

Ramachandran, V. (2020, December 17). South Asian, Chinese New Yorkers among the hardest hit by Covid, study shows. NBC News. https://www.nbcnews.com/news/asian-america/south-asian-chinese-new-yorkers-among-hardest-hit-covid-study-n1251457

Rubin-Miller, L., Alban, C., Artiga, S., & Sullivan, S. (2020). COVID-19 Racial Disparities in Testing, Infection, Hospitalization, and Death: Analysis of Epic Patient Data, *KFF* [Issue Brief]. https://www.kff.org/report-section/covid-19-racial-disparities-in-testing-infection-hospitalization-and-death-analysis-of-epic-patient-data-issue-brief/

Sze, S., Pan, D., Nevill, C. R., Gray, L. J., Martin, C. A., Nazareth, J., Minhas, J. S., Divall, P., Khunti, K., Abrams, K. R., Nellums, L. B., & Pareek, M. (2020). Ethnicity and clinical outcomes in COVID-19: A systematic review and meta-analysis. *EClinicalMedicine, 29*. https://doi.org/10.1016/j.eclinm.2020.100630

U.S. Census Bureau. (2021). *Household Pulse Survey: Measuring Social and Economic Impacts during the Coronavirus Pandemic*. https://www.census.gov/programs-surveys/household-pulse-survey.html

Yan, B., Ng, F., & Nguyen, T. T. (2020). *High Mortality from COVID-19 among Asian Americans in San Francisco and California* [Research Brief]. UCSF School of Medicine and Asian American Research Center on Health (ARCH). https://asianarch.org/press_releases/Asian%20COVID-19%20Mortality%20Final.pdf

Yi, S. S. (2020). Taking Action to Improve Asian American Health. *American Journal of Public Health, 110*(4), 435–437.

Yi, S. S., Đoàn, L. N., Choi, J. K., Wong, J. A., Russo, R., Chin, M., Islam, N. S., Taher, M. D., Wyatt, L., Chong, S. K., Trinh-Shevrin, C., & Kwon, S. C. (2021). With no data, there's no equity: Addressing the lack of data on COVID-19 for asian american communities. *EClinicalMedicine, 41*. https://doi.org/10.1016/j.eclinm.2021.101165

CASE

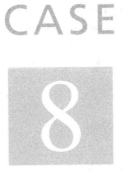

HOPE CLINIC: HOUSTON'S MEDICAL HOME FOR ASIAN AMERICANS

ANDREA CARACOSTIS

Since 2002, the Asian American Health Coalition of the Greater Houston Area (AAHC)'s dba HOPE Clinic (HOPE Clinic) has provided a wide range of health-related services for ethnically diverse, medically underserved residents of Houston, Texas. Prior to establishing HOPE Clinic, AAHC emerged in 1994 as an organization dedicated to improving the health of Houstonians of Asian descent, especially those facing linguistic and cultural barriers. Although HOPE Clinic was established to serve that population, the organization has evolved over time into a place where anyone in need can feel welcome and be assured of receiving quality healthcare services, regardless of their race/ethnicity, culture/beliefs, language, gender, age, ability to pay, or any other factor. HOPE Clinic's mission is *"to improve the health of residents in greater Houston through culturally and linguistically appropriate services."* Even as HOPE Clinic has expanded to serve this increasingly diverse patient population, AAHC has remained a leader in serving the Asian American and Pacific Islander (PI) populations, identifying unmet health care needs, and developing programs, systems and services to address them.

"THE AMERICAN FUTURE IS HERE IN HOUSTON, NOW"

Dr. Stephen L. Klineberg, a longtime professor of sociology at Houston's Rice University, shared this quote with an audience at the Houston Asia Society nearly a decade ago (Asia Society, 2012). Characterizing the rapid demographic transformation of Houston into a multiethnic urban center, Dr. Klineberg emphasized the uniqueness of Houston, which boasts the most evenly distributed ethnic composition of any urban population in the United States, with no majority ethnic group. If any single area of the city provides evidence for Dr. Klineberg's characterization, it is that of southwest Houston, located in Harris County. Within this almost 53-square-mile

Applied Population Health Approaches for Asian American Communities, First Edition. Edited by Simona C. Kwon,
Chau Trinh-Shevrin, Nadia S. Islam, and Stella S. Yi.
© 2023 John Wiley & Sons, Inc. Published 2023 by John Wiley & Sons, Inc.
Companion Website: www.wiley.com/go/kwon/asianamerican

269

TABLE A8.1 **Ethnic Composition of the Population in the HOPE Clinic Service Area as Compared to Local, County, State, and National Populations, 2019**

	White	Black*	Asian American & PI	Hispanic	Other**
United States	60.70%	12.31%	5.62%	18.01%	3.35%
Texas	41.95%	11.78%	4.82%	39.34%	2.11%
Harris County	29.59%	18.57%	6.97%	42.94%	1.93%
Metro Area	36.15%	16.87%	7.71%	37.29%	1.99%
HOPE Clinic Service Area	15.48%	23.35%	13.69%	46.60%	1.64%

*A large percentage of the patients who marked Black are African, not African American.
**Other includes mostly refugees from the Middle East.
Source: 5-year estimates, Table DP05, 2019.

area, over 43% of the residents were born outside of the United States (as compared to 13% nationally, 16.5% statewide, and 25.3% in Harris County as a whole) (Table A8.1). Home to "Asia Town," southwest Houston has street signs in English, Vietnamese, and Chinese. Businesses and residents in the area have ethnic origins in almost every country in Asia, as well as in Africa, the Caribbean, and Latin America.

AAHC: EARLY ACHIEVEMENTS

In June 1994, following a Southeast Asian Health Symposium held in Houston, four Asian American women founded the AAHC to serve as a liaison between Asian American and mainstream communities in Houston, providing the dual purpose of helping residents of Asian descent to navigate the complex maze of processes and procedures inherent in the U.S. healthcare system and helping health care providers navigate complex cultural and linguistic barriers in order to provide more relevant and effective care to Asian American patients. AAHC's work centered on the following goals:

1. Ensure an effective, comprehensive, linguistically and culturally competent system of health services.
2. Provide health promotion, education, and information/referral services.
3. Advocate for Asian American health issues.
4. Foster network-building between Asian Americans and health care providers.
5. Be inclusive of all Asian American ethnic groups.

In its first decade, AAHC accomplished numerous important steps to prioritize and promote Asian American health issues, both within and beyond Houston. Importantly, AAHC served as an integral participant and partner in various health-related assessments of underserved Asian American populations. For example, in 1997, the Opening Doors Project, funded by the Robert Wood Johnson and Henry J. Kaiser Foundations, and sponsored by the Association of Asian Pacific Community Health Organizations (AAPCHO), showed that Houston respondents had very low awareness of basic preventive health practices: 63% of females reported never having had a Pap smear to test for cervical cancer; 14% of Chinese women and 25% of Vietnamese women had never even heard of this test. Additionally, 72% of Vietnamese women and 43% of Chinese women reported never having performed a breast self-exam, and over 70% of women over age 40 had never had a mammogram.

In 2001, AAHC achieved designation as an independent 501(c)(3) nonprofit organization. Shortly thereafter, in 2002, AAHC worked with the Chinese Community Center (CCC) and the Chinese Baptist Church to establish Project HOPE (Helping Other People through Encouragement) as a volunteer health clinic to provide basic primary care services during four hours each month to medically underserved, low-income families and senior citizens, primarily of Asian descent. AAHC provided administrative and fiscal oversight, while the Chinese Community Center (CCC) provided one large room to serve as a clinical site and the Chinese Baptist Church provided volunteer physicians and other health professionals to staff the clinic. Project HOPE was expanded to operate as a community health center focusing on meeting the cultural and linguistic needs of vulnerable, medically underserved, foreign-born, Asian, and refugee populations.

FROM VOLUNTARY NONPROFIT TO FEDERALLY QUALIFIED HEALTH CENTER

AAHC's board made the decision early on that in order to provide long-term health access to their community, they needed to become a Federally Qualified Health Center (FQHC). Thus, they sought expertise to help them achieve that goal, and AAHC's health services expanded exponentially over the next years. Through focused grant writing and fundraising efforts, AAHC successfully garnered funding to expand service hours to eight hours per month and to support a variety of programming to address specific health-related concerns. For example, the AAHC Phoenix Project was launched in 2003 to provide breast cancer education, screening, patient navigation services, diagnostics, and breast cancer treatment for Asian American women in various Asian languages at the HOPE Clinic site.

A major cataclysm impacted HOPE Clinic's growth and sense of urgency when, on August 29, 2005, Hurricane Katrina struck Louisiana and resulted in an influx of more than 50,000 evacuees seeking shelter in Houston. Known for its cultural and linguistic orientation to the Asian population, HOPE Clinic coordinated and ensured the provision of care for over 3,000 Vietnamese evacuees from the neighboring state. As a result, AAHC provided clinical care to more than 8,000 evacuees (9,093 patient encounters) in 2005, a phenomenal feat for such a small organization.

This success led to further responsibilities and expansion. One example of this expansion was the Diabetes Awareness and Education in the Community (DAEC) Project, also known as The Asian American Diabetes Education Project, or DEP – a joint program between the Texas Department of Health (TDH), AAHC, and the Harris County Hospital District. This consortium of partners worked together successfully to demonstrate the urgent need for diabetes education and screening among Houston residents of Vietnamese and Chinese descent. By documenting low levels of diabetes-related awareness in these populations, AAHC and its partners were awarded a TDH/Texas Diabetes Council grant to develop and implement the Asian Diabetes Outreach Program. This initiative provided culturally and linguistically appropriate information and education on diabetes prevention and control to Asian Americans. Based on successful early results, the program was subsequently supported by the National Asian Women's Health Organization (NAWHO).

AAHC also worked with the Department of State Health Services to transform its clinical initiatives into a federally qualified health center (FQHC). In 2007, AAHC expanded its clinical operating hours to 32 hours per week and restructured its board of directors. Importantly, the board recognized the need for a safety net health provider to meet the needs of the entire population in the catchment area of the clinic, beyond people of Asian and PI descent. Accordingly, the board changed the name of the organization from "Asian American Health Coalition of Greater Houston" to "HOPE Clinic."

In line with this shift in mission, HOPE Clinic relocated its services to a 4,000-square-foot facility to accommodate a full-time comprehensive health center. Dr. Andrea Caracostis was hired as CEO and tasked with converting the nonprofit clinic into a fully-fledged FQHC. In December 2008, HOPE Clinic received the designation of FQHC Look-Alike and, in 2012, HOPE Clinic received its first H30 grant from the federal Health Resources and Services Administration (HRSA), as a full FQHC.

MAINTAINING A SPECIAL COMMITMENT TO ASIAN AMERICAN HEALTH

Since receiving its FQHC designation, HOPE Clinic has continually expanded to meet the needs of specific culturally and linguistically underserved, vulnerable populations, including Asians, Hispanics, and refugee/

immigrant populations, while also providing quality care and increasing access for other low-income English-speaking groups. In parallel, HOPE Clinic has maintained its special commitment to identifying and serving the unique needs of Asian American and PI populations. For example, even prior to achieving FQHC designation, in 2008, HOPE Clinic secured a four-year W. K. Kellogg Foundation capacity-building and community outreach grant that allowed the organization to lead a community-wide collaborative aimed at reducing health disparities among Asian Americans and PIs in Houston. The grant provided funding for capacity-building activities to strengthen smaller community-based organizations delivering frontline services and expand advocacy and policy efforts that impact the health of Asian Americans and PIs.

One of the health conditions of concern identified through this process was hepatitis B virus infection rates among people of Asian descent. HOPE Clinic assumed a leadership role and sought assistance from different national organizations and foundations for the creation of the Houston B-Free program. As part of the program, HOPE Clinic created an advisory council to coordinate hepatitis B screening, education and treatment activities, and, ultimately, developed a strategic plan to create the B-Free Houston HBV program, which now manages over 600 active hepatitis B patients. Houston B-Free represented a major step for HOPE Clinic, transforming its work from clinical provision of services and small-scale outreach to a leadership role in driving advocacy, tailored service provision, professional training, and education for Asian American and Pacific Islander populations. HOPE Clinic addressed hepatitis B virus not only from the clinical point of view, but also by taking a holistic approach, advocating for free adult immunizations and new CDC screening guidelines as well as developing a hepatitis B training for primary care providers to facilitate replication of the HOPE Clinic model all around the country.

In 2014, HOPE Clinic opened a second site in West Houston and increased its scope of practice to include labor and delivery services at the local hospital. This important step was taken in response to emerging evidence that Asian American and PI patients struggled to navigate hospital services and receive timely care due to language barriers. Ultimately, this expansion has proven to be a catalyst for growth and has cemented the HOPE Clinic as a medical home for Asian American and PI families. A third clinical site was launched in 2016 to better serve the Vietnamese community, with a full range of health-related services including dental, vision, and mental health services. Currently, this clinic is operating at full capacity.

Most recently, in 2019, HOPE Clinic opened the first community-based graduate medical education program in Houston in Obstetrics, Gynecology, and Family Medicine. With the goal of expanding the pool of health care providers who understand the needs of multi-ethnic, -linguistic, and -cultural communities and who find passion in serving communities of color, HOPE Clinic partnered with Hospital Corporation of America (HCA) to open a first-of-its-kind residency program focusing on Asian American and PI health and underserved communities. HOPE Clinic envisions this program as the seed from which to grow future health care leaders who are sensitive and committed to preserving communities' distinct roots and cultures.

NEXT STEPS

HOPE Clinic's experience is certainly not unique. Nonetheless, HOPE Clinic has been one of the fastest-growing FQHCs in Houston. Its strong grassroots origins were critical in allowing the organization to keep its focus on the Asian American and PI communities while simultaneously expanding to serve the broader populations. Another strength of the model was implementing a strong needs assessment early on, which allowed the organization to establish robust baseline data to inform the development of its business plan. HOPE Clinic focused on high quality of care by hiring excellent providers, while also prioritizing seamless continuity of care. Together, these two aspects helped the clinic attract and retain a diverse payor mix, which contributed to HOPE Clinic's financial success and allowing the organization to attract insured and uninsured patients alike. During the summer of 2021, HOPE Clinic will be breaking ground on a 70,000-square-foot clinic and wellness center. This building will serve as a legacy for future generations as a center that celebrates the diversity of Houston and the contributions of the Asian American and PI communities to our city.

REFERENCE

Asia Society. (2012, April 13). Houston most ethnically diverse city in United States, study finds. https://asiasociety.org/texas/houston-most-ethnically-diverse-city-united-states-study-finds

CASE

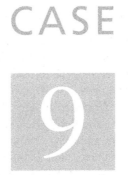

THE CHINATOWN-INTERNATIONAL DISTRICT OF SEATTLE/ KING COUNTY

MARGUERITE J. RO, NADINE L. CHAN

OVERVIEW

Asian Americans and Native Hawaiians/Pacific Islanders (NH/PIs) played a prominent role in the development of Seattle and its surrounding areas in King County, Washington. Asian Americans and NH/PIs helped build the marina docks and railroads that spurred the growth of trade in the Pacific Northwest. From the canneries to the farmlands, Asian Americans and NH/PIs helped build these industries and fought alongside other communities of color to obtain rights, particularly for laborers and immigrants. Today, the approximately 462,000 Asian Americans and NH/PIs (20.5% of King County's total population) who reside in King County continue to build on the rich legacy left by individual and collective contributions of many Asian American and NH/PI community leaders.

Carrying on this strong history of community activism, Asian Americans and NH/PIs have worked collectively, at multiple levels and across sectors, to protect and preserve the Chinatown-International District (CID), the historical and cultural hub for the Asian American and NH/PI community. This work has included assuring the health and well-being of CID residents. Uniquely, the CID has pan-Asian roots stemming from early Japanese, Chinese, and Filipino immigrants who arrived in the late 1800s and early 1900s. After the fall of Saigon in 1975, a wave of Vietnamese and other Southeast Asians arrived to build Seattle's Little Saigon portion of the CID. With the growth of the Asian American and NH/PI population, Asian American and NH/PI leaders and community organizations have continued to play an active role in the region's multilevel, multisector initiatives. Two snapshots of these initiatives are provided below.

Applied Population Health Approaches for Asian American Communities, First Edition. Edited by Simona C. Kwon, Chau Trinh-Shevrin, Nadia S. Islam, and Stella S. Yi.
© 2023 John Wiley & Sons, Inc. Published 2023 by John Wiley & Sons, Inc.
Companion Website: www.wiley.com/go/kwon/asianamerican

BUILD HEALTH CHALLENGE (BUILD)

Funded by a group of regional and national philanthropies, BUILD (www.buildhealthchallenge.org) is a collaborative, cross-sector approach to improve health. BUILD Seattle Chinatown-International District (2016–2017) was a partnership between CID neighborhood partners [InterimCDA (lead), the Seattle Chinatown International District Preservation and Development Authority (SCIDpda), Chinatown International District Business Improvement Area (CIDBIA), International Community Health Services (ICHS) and Yesler Community Collaborative (YCC)], Swedish Health Services, and Public Health–Seattle King County (the local health department). Notably, the CID neighborhood partners represent a range of sectors and include a community development organization, a federally qualified health center, and a community preservation and district authority that have a history of working together to address Asian American and NH/PI community concerns.

Together, the BUILD Seattle CID partners share a vision for a CID that is healthy, safe, and livable for residents, businesses, and community members. A cornerstone of the initiative was the development of the "2020 Healthy Community Plan," which serves as a roadmap for their efforts. Another critical element was gathering data and information that captured the perspectives of CID residents. These efforts – the plan, the data gathering, and the community engagement – built momentum for the initiative that gained the attention of key decision-makers, including the Seattle City Council. Recognizing the public health implications of public safety issues impacting this neighborhood, the Council allocated half a million dollars directly to the neighborhood, demonstrating the Council's commitment to supporting culturally competent public safety practices, improvements in public spaces, and investments in community-gathered data. Over a two-year period, BUILD Seattle CID conducted health promotion and education activities; received funding to address public safety concerns; worked with businesses to address sanitation issues; and strengthened relationships that can serve as the basis for future efforts.

COMMUNITIES OF OPPORTUNITY (COO)

"Multisector partnerships that put racial equity and community leadership at their center can create pathways to healthy communities" (Wysen, 2019). Supported by the Seattle Foundation and King County government, Communities of Opportunity (www.coopartnerships.org) was launched in 2014 to create greater health, social, economic, and racial equity in King County so that all people thrive and prosper, regardless of race or place. COO invests in geographic and cultural communities that have experienced the greatest inequities to develop and implement community-driven solutions in the areas of health, economic opportunity, housing, and community connection. COO community partners are working to create inclusive communities where low-income people and people of color are able to fully participate in and benefit from the transformation of their communities. This vision means changing traditional ways of implementing policies and projects: people and communities most affected by community transformation projects must be engaged in planning and decision-making processes to support their self-determination. To ensure that COO is community-driven, community members make up the majority of COO's Governing Group. This group assures that equity is integrated in the entire COO process, including the selection of investments, governance committee representation, COO staffing, and performance metrics. COO seeks to produce a major impact that cannot be achieved by any one sector alone. Through multisector efforts, COO is explicitly taking advantage of and leveraging areas of intersection (i.e., housing, health, and the economy) for the benefit of all.

Although COO is not an Asian American- or NH/PI-specific initiative, the engagement of Asian American and NH/PI community leaders and community organizations is an important feature of this collective effort to drive larger policy and systems improvements across King County. An example is the work of the Friends of Little Saigon (FLS), a grassroots organization with the mission "to preserve and enhance Little Saigon's cultural, economic, and historic vitality" and is one of the COO partners under COO's Institutional Systems and Policy Change strategy. FLS has been actively addressing the issues of displacement and gentrification in the CID, as well as working to meet the needs of immigrants and refugees. FLS has partnered with many of the CID organizations listed above and is a member of several critical taskforces (e.g., City of Seattle's Equitable Development Initiative Advisory Committee, City of Seattle's Race and Social Equity Taskforce, the CID Public Safety Taskforce).

As part of COO, FLS has increased the visibility of the issues that Little Saigon is facing and created opportunities for the voices of the Vietnamese immigrant and refugee community to be heard. As a result of the organization's work to develop new partnerships and relationships with real estate developers and city agencies, FLS participated in the development of new historic review guidelines and facilitated the adoption of an executive order to ensure the CID benefited from a Community Preference policy. The policy encourages nonprofit housing developers receiving city money to offer a portion of their affordable units to communities with ties to the neighborhood, particularly those with a high risk of displacement. In other words, the Community Preference policy provides an opportunity for residents in high-displacement neighborhoods, such as the CID, to return and stay in their neighborhood.

In sum, the CID provides an example of a pan-Asian, cross-sectoral effort to benefit individual Asian and NH/PI ethnic groups as well as the Asian American and NH/PI population as a whole. The CID also demonstrates a successful effort through which Asian American and NH/PI community leaders joined with other communities of color to raise issues related to racism, economic injustice, and residential displacement within mainstream political and economic structures.

REFERENCE

Wysen, K. (2019). Listen and be ready to shift: how racial equity and community leadership launched "Communities of Opportunity." *J Public Health Manag Pract., 27*(1): E48–E56.

CASE

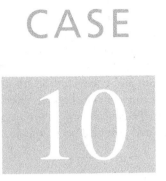

PATH FOR WOMEN: IMPROVING ACCESS TO BREAST AND CERVICAL CANCER SCREENING FOR THAI WOMEN IN LOS ANGELES

MARY ANNE FOO

In 2000, the Orange County Asian and Pacific Islander Community Alliance (OCAPICA) began a 15-year journey to improve breast and cervical cancer screening among Southeast Asian and Pacific Islander (PI) women. Funding was first secured through the California Breast Cancer Research Program, followed by grants from The California Endowment through the CDC Foundation, Susan G. Komen, and the Centers for Disease Control and Prevention. Although the program covered multiple Asian American and Native Hawaiian and Pacific Islander (NH/PI) populations, this case study will highlight the program's model of implementing multi-sector, multi-level approaches to health promotion with the Thai community in Los Angeles, California. Specifically, we will describe how a program with only one staff member vastly increased cancer screening among Thai women, supported health systems to transform to be more accessible, involved the Thai media in health advocacy, and supported small ethnic businesses and spiritual centers to be program champions for breast and cervical cancer.

OCAPICA's Promoting Access to Health (PATH) for Women program was a community-based participatory research program implemented over 15 years with the goal of identifying influences and systemic changes that could improve access to breast and cervical cancer screening for Asian American and NH/PI women. During this time, more than 200,000 community members were educated about breast and cervical health and more than 12,000 women received mammograms and Pap tests. PATH for Women was a collaboration of multiple community-based organizations and universities. The study population was recruited in Southern California, while control groups were recruited in Northern California. From this research, multiple influences were found to improve cancer screening via health promotion efforts with the Thai community.

Applied Population Health Approaches for Asian American Communities, First Edition. Edited by Simona C. Kwon, Chau Trinh-Shevrin, Nadia S. Islam, and Stella S. Yi.
© 2023 John Wiley & Sons, Inc. Published 2023 by John Wiley & Sons, Inc.
Companion Website: www.wiley.com/go/kwon/asianamerican

The PATH for Women program focused on Thai women who were very low income and working in low-wage jobs as garment, massage parlor, nail salon, and restaurant workers. These women had to work all the time in order to earn enough to pay their rent and help support their families. About half of the women were also undocumented. The women had little time, if any, to go to a health care provider, and most did not have a medical home. A Thai Health Navigator was hired for the program and conducted health promotion and education activities, patient navigation services, and training for health care providers about making their facilities and services more accessible. The Thai Health Navigator also started a cancer support group, a pool from which 24–38 cancer survivors became very active as program champions and provided peer support to other Thai women.

PROGRAM DEVELOPMENT

During the planning phase of the program, an extensive 100+ question baseline survey was implemented. Conducted as an interview, the survey was administered to 742 Thai women. Each survey took about two hours to conduct. Notable results included the findings that a majority of women felt that they would only need a mammogram if they felt symptoms (71.3%); breast cancer can be cured by traditional healers (25.5%); that one only needs to have a mammogram when one feels a breast lump (77.8%); and there is little one can do to prevent breast cancer (70.4%) (Dang et al., 2010).

Our research questions focused on the key individual, interpersonal, and community factors needed in a breast and cervical cancer health promotion and patient navigation program; the culturally appropriate and tailored strategies needed to support cancer screenings and navigation through the cancer care continuum; and the specific trainings and capacity building needed to support community health navigators to be successful (Nguyen et al., 2011).

The program utilized the socioecological model (intrapersonal, interpersonal, institutional, community, and public policy factors) and the House model (informational, instrumental, affective, and appraisal support) to inform the need to involve multi-sector and multi-level resources to lead to system and policy change (Nguyen et al., 2011).

Multisector partners and collaborators on the program were built throughout the program. These included the worksites of the Thai women and their supervisors, small business owners, local policy makers (city council, county supervisors, state policymakers, planning commissions, parks and recreation leaders), health care systems and institutions (hospitals, clinics, county health systems, Medicaid managed care systems, social services), health care providers and administrators, public transportation, community partners (housing, legal, social services, mental health), spiritual centers (Thai temples and their leadership), the Thai Consulate General and the Thai Consulate office, and mainstream breast and cervical cancer programs.

Multilevel approaches focused on transformation and a systems approach:

- At the individual level – promoting health and knowledge change with Thai community members (women and their family members);

- At the community level – gaining champions from Thai media, Thai community organizations and leaders, Thai worksites, and small businesses; and

- At the policy systems change level – county and city health and social service system, local hospitals and community clinics in the geographic areas of the Thai community, local policymakers representing Thai Town and the geographic regions of the Thai community.

ACTIVITIES AND ACHIEVEMENTS

Individual awareness change occurred via saturation of the community with health promotion messages and education about breast and cervical cancer in Thai women. Outreach and education occurred on a daily basis with workers at beauty salons, massage parlors, restaurants, and garment factories. As knowledge increased among the Thai women, more women wanted to be screened and get assistance. Our patient navigation program expanded and our program began to provide support to women to make medical appointments, deliver medical interpretation services, provide transportation, provide education, and explain medication and treatment plans to increase adherence, for example. Navigation and support occurred throughout the cancer care continuum, from screening to treatment, recovery, and palliative care.

With a vast increase in the number of Thai women wanting screening, health care institutions took notice. The appointments and front office staff of several of the county clinics and hospitals partnered with our Thai Health Navigator to create special screening days strictly for her Thai patients. A Nurse Practitioner and Breast Surgeon who worked at several hospitals and county locations befriended and partnered with our Thai Health Navigator to educate our cancer survivors. These two health care providers became our program champions and spoke to the health care institutions and systems about our partnership. Several hospitals started to sponsor and support our cancer support groups at their locations, provided community benefit funds for the cancer support group, assigned health care providers to conduct education and answer questions, assigned special days to focus on the Thai patients, and provided bus passes, parking permits, and personnel clearance for our Health Navigator to be able to navigate women to other hospital and clinic resources.

Our program administrators met with the hospital and clinic administrators to discuss how the partnership helped the health care institutions to meet their community benefit requirement, improved their efficacy and patient-provider communication, and supported achievement of screening and treatment goals. Demonstrating mutual benefits secured a longer-term partnership with the health care systems and facilitated additional improvements in access for our Thai community members.

As part of these improvements, all of the hospitals and health care systems worked with the Thai Health Navigator to have their signage and policies translated into Thai. The health care institutions and providers also saw an improvement in patient-provider communication and understanding of cultural issues impacting screening and education; thus, the institutions requested the Thai Health Navigator to join health care providers and interns in their morning rounds. One hospital invited the Health Navigator to be a member of their Tumor Board.

As the health care system became more accessible to the Thai women, the Health Navigator focused on increasing the community members' self-efficacy to navigate the health care systems for themselves. This included teaching the women how to make appointments, how to work with the pharmacists to understand their medication regimens, and how to access public transportation. The county's public transportation system was very helpful and allowed us to take the women on free field trips on the buses to show them the routes, introduce them to the bus drivers, and teach them how to transfer between buses. The county and cities' parks and recreation departments gave us free community space and community policing for safety so the support group could do exercise and walks.

The Thai media, including television and newspaper, and the Thai Consulate General published weekly articles and announcements promoting the program and the cancer support groups. Business owners that learned of the program through these channels offered financial donations and space in which the cancer support groups could meet. Local restaurants sponsored a gathering, fashion show, and celebration of the cancer survivors, which was highlighted in the media. A Thai music video producer saw this story and organized a music benefit for the program featuring Thai musical artists, incorporating the survivors into the program, and producing a video show to honor the survivors and raise additional funds for the program. Health care providers and policymakers joined the gathering, along with 600 community members, to celebrate and promote the program.

Finally, with all the promotion and involvement of others, worksites including owners and supervisors started to hear about the program and requested our Health Navigator and survivors to conduct education for their employees. It was the first time that garment factories, beauty salons, restaurants, and massage parlors gave us access to their employees and granted paid breaks for their workers to listen to our education. Eventually, the employers allowed the women time off to go to appointments for screenings. The specialized screening dates and appointments for Thai women at the local clinics and hospitals allowed community members to get quicker appointments. This pleased the worksites because the employees did not need to take off an entire day from work to attend their screening appointments.

Working with multi-sector and multi-level resources greatly supported our health promotion work in cancer screening, allowing us to develop our program in line with Thai community needs to both increase of cancer prevention and treatment for Thai women as well as effect longer-term system and policy changes. Our program may serve as a model for other ethnic communities seeking to increase culturally and linguistically appropriate delivery of cancer screening and treatment services for their members within mainstream health care institutions.

REFERENCES

Dang, J., Lee, J., & Tran, J. (2010). Knowledge, attitudes, and beliefs regarding breast and cervical cancer screening among Cambodian, Laotian, Thai, and Tongan women. *J Cancer Educ., 25*(4): 595–601. doi:10.1007/s13187-010-0082-1

Nguyen, T.U., Tran, J.H., Kagawa-Singer, M., & Foo, M.A. (2011). A qualitative assessment of community-based breast health navigation services for Southeast Asian women in Southern California: recommendations for developing a navigator training curriculum. *American J Public Health, 101*(1):87–93. doi:10.2105/AJPH.2009.176743

CASE

11

PARTNERING WITH OLDER ADULT REFUGEES FOR BETTER HOME HEALTH CARE DELIVERY

TINA R. SADARANGANI, SARAH M. MINER, LARISSA R. BURKA

PROBLEM STATEMENT

Since 2007, approximately 84,800 Bhutanese refugees have been resettled in the United States (United Nations High Commission on Refugees, 2015). Approximately 6.6% of these refugees are older Bhutanese adults (International Organization of Migration, 2008) and represent a particularly vulnerable group. Compared with other refugee groups, refugees from Bhutan are significantly less likely to be employed, have much lower median household incomes, have significantly lower educational attainment, and have very low English proficiency (Capps and Newland, 2015). Furthermore, middle-aged and older refugees have special vulnerabilities. As compared to younger age groups, these individuals tend to have even lower levels of education, fewer opportunities to develop skills once they arrive in the country of resettlement, and be less likely to seek help (Choi et al., 2015; International Center at Temple University, 2011).

In addition to poverty, low levels of education, and limited English proficiency, older refugees' health is negatively affected by other factors. Older refugees have disproportionately low levels of health literacy, limiting their ability to obtain, process, and understand the basic health information needed to make appropriate decisions around their healthcare needs (Capps and Newland, 2015). Low health literacy, along with low literacy and low English proficiency, limits older Bhutanese refugees' ability to understand medication labels and treatment plans and, consequently, negatively impacts their adherence to provider-directed medication regimens and care plans. Like other refugee groups, Bhutanese older adults also struggle with both mental and physical chronic illnesses. Refugees' experiences fleeing their countries of origin and residing in refugee camps include significant and repeated traumatic events that lead to serious mental health risks (Thapa et al., 2003).

Applied Population Health Approaches for Asian American Communities, First Edition. Edited by Simona C. Kwon, Chau Trinh-Shevrin, Nadia S. Islam, and Stella S. Yi.
© 2023 John Wiley & Sons, Inc. Published 2023 by John Wiley & Sons, Inc.
Companion Website: www.wiley.com/go/kwon/asianamerican

Additionally, the Bhutanese population is impacted disproportionately by anemia and B$_{12}$ deficiency (CDC, 2021). In this case study, we examine how participatory action research (PAR) was used to address these mental and physical health issues and support health management in older Bhutanese refugees, as well as among refugees from other ethnic groups.

INTERVENTION

This PAR collaboration began in 2012 in Rochester, New York, as a joint effort between HCR Home Care, a Rochester-based home health agency with 40 years of experience serving older adults, and Refugees Helping Refugees (RHR), a nonprofit organization providing health and social services to diverse refugee populations in the Rochester region. Rochester is a welcoming hub for newly resettled refugees. Over the last 35 years, nearly 15,000 refugees have been resettled in Rochester (Catholic Family Center, 2021). In addition to the Bhutanese community, Rochester is also home to Cuban, Somali, and other refugee populations.

To better respond to the needs of the older adult refugee community, HCR Home Care established a two-year (2013–2014) community-engaged partnership with RHR. Among the goals of this formal partnership were to facilitate connections with refugee populations, implement strategies for better coordination and delivery of home health care to older adult refugees in the region, and better understand issues and barriers affecting home health care service delivery in refugee communities.

The initiative began with meetings and informal data collection between members of the HCR Home Care health care team, RHR staff members, other local refugee advocacy and resettlement organizations, and health care providers. These meetings resulted in a shared understanding that home health care aligned with many of the health and social needs of older adult refugees. Discussions also revealed barriers to delivering home health care among refugee populations, including refugee families refusing services, not understanding home health services, not trusting home care providers, and refusing to open the door when HCR Home Care providers would attempt to initiate services.

With this shared understanding of potential benefits and barriers, HCR Home Care and RHR agreed to work together to improve access to services for older adult refugees and enhance the service experience for patients as well as home care staff. The organizations set up regular meetings for discussion and information sharing and invited a community health worker (CHW) from the refugee community to participate. Initially, HCR Home Care had one Bhutanese staff member who agreed to fill the CHW role; subsequently, RHR assisted HCR Home Care to recruit and hire additional CHWs from other refugee communities. The CHWs' role was to arrange and participate in visits with the home health care team and refugee patients, provide language assistance and guidance on cultural matters, educate the refugee community about home health care services, and identify and advocate for community members who may benefit from home health care.

ASSESSMENT

To assess the outcomes of the collaboration, HCR Home Care and RHR worked with researchers from a local university to design and conduct a mixed-methods evaluation study. Throughout the research process, members of HCR Home Care and RHR participated at every level. The process began with a chart review to assess the home health outcomes of older adult refugee clients who received services through the partnership (Miner, Liebel, Wilde, Carroll, Zicari, & Chalupa, 2017). Overall, the partnership provided care connections for older adults from Bhutan as well as from Somalia, Burma, Liberia, Vietnam, Cambodia, and Burundi. Using a limited set of measures to assess changes in health outcomes, researchers found that receipt of home health care positively impacted the health of the older adult refugee population. Older adult refugee clients' health status improved as much as – and, in some cases, more than – the health status of other distinct populations served by the agency and were equal to or surpassed state and national averages for home health outcomes. A qualitative research study was also implemented to explore the perceptions of older adults and their caregivers about home health care (Miner, Liebel, Wilde, Carroll, & Omar, 2017). Because of limited linguistic and other resources, the qualitative study was conducted by the Somali CHW exclusively among Somali older adults and caregivers. However, the findings were presented to a focus group of Burmese and Bhutanese older adults.

RESULTS

This intervention generated valuable cultural and clinical insights regarding the older adult Asian refugee population. For HCR Home Care staff, working with RHR facilitated a better understanding of refugee issues. Home care staff were better able to understand the resettlement process for Bhutanese older adult refugees and how this process affected their former and current health needs, their health literacy, and their family relationships and structures. HCR Home Care staff found that families often struggled with the concept of chronic illness and the need for lifelong self-management of chronic conditions among older adults. With Bhutanese families, HCR Home Care staff found that although the son of the older adult client was often chosen as the spokesperson, the daughter-in-law frequently managed the medications and served as principal caregiver for the older adult client. With the assistance of the CHW, staff focused on educating clients and their families about medications, including why they must be taken daily irrespective of symptomology and why medications could not "cure" illnesses like diabetes or hypertension. Mental health issues were prevalent, and trauma-informed care was essential for all family and client interactions, guiding the development of the plan of care, scheduling of home visits, and all aspects of working with families. Working with RHR also helped to facilitate understanding among HCR Home Care staff that Bhutanese families rarely considered the option of placing older adults in institutions for care. Older adults were often perceived as the most important members of the community, and families described both a desire and an expectation to care for them at home. Families also refused home health aide services because they preferred the agency to advocate and facilitate their connection to programs that would pay a family member to care for the older adult in the home. This information facilitated communication and interaction between home care staff and families and resulted in more culturally acceptable and appropriate plans of care for the older adult refugees receiving home health.

KEY TAKEAWAYS

The results of the research, focus group results, and interactions with older adult refugee clients and their families over the course of the two-year project identified a number of key points that were essential to the improved delivery of home health services to older adult refugees. Most importantly, refugee older adults relied on their ethnic community for support and information about available care and services. Using a community engaged approach, the collaboration discovered that the barriers to receiving home care services were often related to a lack of understanding of home health services and that there was a need to better engage community leaders to facilitate trust and information sharing between the home health agency and refugee older adult populations. HCR Home Care staff gained credibility by using community-engaged approaches, collaborating with RHR, and employing a CHW. Critically, the CHW was seen as a trusted and active community member and advocate for older adult refugees. Because of this trust, older adult refugee clients and their families were willing to share information with the CHW that they never would have shared with an unknown health provider or researcher. Conversely, the CHW could interpret and share cultural nuances they detected in the responses of clients and their families to contextualize previous and current health experiences relevant to the success of the home health experience.

The use of PAR in this collaboration was essential to meeting the goals originally established by the partnership. It facilitated trust building by the agency with the older adult refugee community, which, in turn, facilitated the collection of high-quality data in the research process. The information was translated directly into practice at the home care agency and the gathered data informed changes to programming and the delivery of home health services to make them more culturally acceptable and appropriate to the social and health needs of refugee older adults. Ultimately, this not only enhanced the experience of home health for older adult refugees and their caregivers but also improved their health outcomes.

CONCLUSION

Currently, over 12,000 certified home health agencies in the United States care for over 3.4 million patients (MedPAC, 2019). Benefits of home health care include improving and assisting in the understanding and management of illness and disability, improving and/or maintaining functional status, reducing mortality and admission to long term care institutions, and connecting people to community resources (Caffrey, Sengupta, Moss, Harris-Kojetin, & Valverde, 2011; Elkan et al., 2001; Health Quality Ontario, 2013; Liebel, Friedman, Watson, & Powers, 2009; National Association for Home Care and Hospice, 2010; Tappenden, Campbell, Rawdin, Wong, & Kalita, 20122012). To date, nonwhite populations have been understudied in home health care research because their language preference and/or ethnicity has not been tracked in standard home health care data sets. Yet, as the diversity of older Americans increases, the home health care industry must adapt to tailor services to new populations, including Asian Americans. Engaging with individual Asian ethnic communities is essential to ensuring that high-quality, culturally appropriate, in-language home health care services are available and accessible for older adults of diverse Asian backgrounds.

REFERENCES

Caffrey, C., Sengupta, M., Moss, A., Harris-Kojetin, L., & Valverde, R. (2011). Home health care and discharged hospice care patients: United States, 2000 and 2007. *National Health Statistics Reports* (38), 1–27.

Capps, R.A., & Newland, K. (2015). *The Integration Outcomes of US Refugees: Successes and Challenges*, Report for the Migration Policy Institute (MPI). http://www.migrationpolicy.org/research/integration-outcomes-us-refugees-successes-and-challenges

Catholic Family Center. (2021). *Welcoming Refugees & Immigrants*. https://www.cfcrochester.org/our-services/welcoming-refugees-and-immigrants/

Centers for Disease Control. (2021). *Bhutanese Refugee Health Profile*. https://www.cdc.gov/immigrantrefugeehealth/profiles/bhutanese/index.html?CDC_AA_refVal=https%3A%2F%2Fwww.cdc.gov%2Fimmigrantrefugeehealth%2Fprofiles%2Fbhutanese%2Fpriority-health-conditions%2Findex.html#b12

Choi, S., Davis, C., Cummings, S., Van Regenmorter, C., & Barnett, M. (2015). Understanding service needs and service utilization among older Kurdish refugees and immigrants in the USA. *International Social Work, 58*(1), 63–74. https://doi.org/10.1177/0020872812471694

Elkan, R., Kendrick, D., Dewey, M., Hewitt, M., Robinson, J., Blair, M., Williams, D., & Brummell, K. (2001). Effectiveness of home based support for older people: systematic review and meta-analysis. *BMJ (Clinical research ed.), 323*(7315), 719–725.

Gautam, R., Mawn, B. E., & Beehler, S. (2018). Bhutanese older adult refugees recently resettled in the united states: A better life with little sorrows. Journal of Transcultural Nursing, 29(2), 165–171. https://doi.org/10.1177/1043659617696975

Health Quality Ontario. (2013). In-home care for optimizing chronic disease management in the community: an evidence-based analysis. *Ontario health technology assessment series, 13*(5), 1–65.

International Center at Temple University. (2011). 'Needs Assessment of Refugee Communities from Bhutan and Burma', Report for the Southeast Asia Resource Action Center, Philadelphia, PA, May. http://philarefugeehealth.org/wp-content/uploads/2014/03/Final-Report-Needs-Assessment-of-Refugee-Communities-from-Bhutan-and-Burma.pdf

International Organization of Migration. (2008). Cultural profile: The Bhutanese refugees in Nepal. http://www.peianc.com/sitefiles/File/resources/cultural_profiles/Bhutanese-Refugees-in-Nepal.pdf

Liebel, D. V., Friedman, B., Watson, N. M., & Powers, B. A. (2009). Review of nurse home visiting interventions for community-dwelling older persons with existing disability. *Medical care research and review: MCRR, 66*(2), 119–146. doi:10.1177/1077558708328815

MedPAC (2019). Report to the Congress: Medicare Payment Policy. http://www.medpac.gov/docs/default-source/reports/mar19_medpac_ch9_sec.pdf?sfvrsn=0

Miner, S., Liebel, D., Wilde, M.H., Carroll, J., & Omar, S. (2017) "Somali Older Adults' and their Families' Perceptions of Adult Home Health Services". Journal of Immigrant and Minority Health. doi.org/10.1007/s10903-017-0658-5

Miner, S., Liebel, D.V., Wilde, M. H., Carroll, J. K., Zicari, E., & Chalupa, S. (2017). Meeting the needs of older adult refugee populations with home health services. *Journal of Transcultural Nursing, 28*(2), 128–136.

National Association for Home Care and Hospice. (2010). Basic Statistics about Home Care. http://www.nahc.org/assets/1/7/10HC_Stats.pdf

Tappenden, P., Campbell, F., Rawdin, A., Wong, R., & Kalita, N. (2012). The clinical effectiveness and cost-effectiveness of home-based, nurse-led health promotion for older people: a systematic review. *Health Technology Assessment (Winchester, England), 16*(20), 1–72. doi:10.3310/hta16200

Thapa, S.B., van Ommeren, M., Sharma, B., de Jong, J., & Hauff, E. (2003) Psychiatric Disability among Tortured Bhutanese Refugees in Nepal. *American Journal of Psychiatry, 160*: 2032–7.

United Nations High Commission on Refugees. (2015). Resettlement of Bhutanese refugees surpasses 100,000 mark. http://www.unhcr.org.ezproxy.med.nyu.edu/564dded46.html

CASE

12

INDIA HOME

SELVIA SIKDER, SHAARANYA PILLAI

India Home, Inc., is the first professionally staffed, secular community-based organization in the United States solely dedicated to serving South Asian older adults. Founded in 2007 in the New York City (NYC) borough of Queens, the mission of India Home is *to improve the quality of life for vulnerable South Asian seniors who find themselves socially isolated and struggling to access necessary culturally appropriate services*. India Home fulfills its mission by providing a wide range of culturally relevant services to South Asians, including senior center programs, case management, creative aging programs, adult empowerment programs, and advocacy and awareness campaigns. India Home started its programs in 2008, establishing itself in two locations accessible to the South Asian community in the Queens area, reaching 25–50 seniors with its flagship programs. Since then, the organization has established itself in numerous locations throughout Queens, often through partnerships with local community centers and houses of worship. India Home has served over 3,000 South Asian seniors and currently serves an average of more than 500 individual seniors every week. The organization is the largest older adult-serving agency for South Asians in NYC and one of the largest in the United States. Currently, India Home has four senior center locations across Queens, in the neighborhoods of Sunnyside, Kew Gardens, Jamaica, and Jamaica Estates. The organization has served seniors from a diverse range of South Asian cultures, including Bangladeshi, Gujarati, Punjabi, Indo-Caribbean, Tamil, Malayalee, Pakistani, Sindhi, and Sinhala. The members come from many different religious backgrounds as well, including Muslim, Hindu, Christian, Jewish, Jain, and Sikh.

While a key purpose of these centers is to provide culturally tailored services for South Asian older adults, equally important is that the centers create a sense of community and offer a physical location where members may enjoy activities and time with one another, allowing older adults to create social networks and combat the social isolation they are more likely to face as they age. As described in Chapter 11, social support and social

Applied Population Health Approaches for Asian American Communities, First Edition. Edited by Simona C. Kwon, Chau Trinh-Shevrin, Nadia S. Islam, and Stella S. Yi.
Companion Website: www.wiley.com/go/kwon/asianamerican

engagement help to strengthen cognitive function in older age. Senior centers play an important role in increasing social support and engagement for older adults in the general U.S. population but are underused by NYC's South Asian older adults (India Home, 2019). India Home was established to address this service gap by providing in-language, culturally tailored health and social services for this diverse population. Programming has expanded to accommodate the diverse needs and growth of members over time. Examples of India Home's senior center activities include congregate meals, health and wellness programs, community education on legal, financial, and life planning, creative aging, community development programs, and case management. These programs are described below.

Health and Wellness Programs. South Asian immigrants and their unique health needs often are excluded from health discourse in the United States. For example, South Asian immigrants are six times more likely to have diabetes than other seniors, but few primary care providers or centers serving the general population focus resources toward addressing the unique needs of South Asians (Diabetes in South Asians 2019). To address this gap, India Home offers numerous health wellness programs to older adults. One component of this programming is offering health talks in clients' native languages to inform them about opportunities to participate in daily physical activities. These health talks are delivered by professionals (e.g., doctors, registered nurses, certified health educators, nutritionists, community health workers, social workers) who work within the South Asian community and understand the importance of delivering tailored, actionable information to South Asian older adults. Additionally, through peer education sessions led by case workers, clients are able to talk with each other about their experiences and challenges related to specific health conditions, providers, services, and benefits programs (e.g., Medicare, Medicaid). India Home also offers physical activity, yoga, and meditation sessions through which older adults maintain and improve their physical and mental wellness. Also, through a partnership with the NYU Center for the Study of Asian American Health (CSAAH) at NYU Grossman School of Medicine, India Home teaches seniors how to self-monitor blood pressure, diabetes, and other chronic disorders – an important approach for improving and maintaining health and wellness over the long term.

Congregate Meal Program. Every week, India Home provides over 500 nutritious, culturally appropriate hot meals to seniors in group settings. These meals cater to the diverse dietary requirements of this community, including Muslim Halal, Hindu vegetarian, and Jain vegetarian diets. Congregate meals help seniors meet their daily nutritional requirements, which many older adults are unable to maintain in their homes. Through the congregate dining setting, clients also bond and build lasting friendships. Older adults socialize for more than 30 minutes during meals, an interval that has been demonstrated to increase brain activity and decrease the chances of developing brain and cognitive disorders, including Alzheimer's disease and other forms of dementia (Fowler, 2020). Additionally, research has shown that participating in congregate meals reduces the likelihood of hospital admissions for older adults (ACL Staff, 2019).

Case Management Program. India Home's case managers help financially and medically vulnerable older adults access vital services such as benefits and entitlements, food and housing support, immigration services, and health care. Case managers facilitate activities such as health insurance enrollment, cash benefits and entitlement checks, and completion of housing, citizenship, and green card applications, as well as health care visits, medication management, and accessing respite or home care services. A key aspect of the program is providing in-language services for diverse South Asian linguistic groups. Case managers offer translation/interpreter services and provide translated materials to older adults to enhance their understanding of available programs and services, as well as health-related information. Case managers also help clients learn about and access resources provided by other community-based organizations, as well as various agencies in the city, state, and federal level. Not only are older adults empowered with greater awareness and knowledge, but they also learn when and how they may access these resources in times of need.

Creative Aging Program. Through arts and creativity, India Home engages older adults to stay active and healthy. Clients get involved in art classes in which they engage with painting, sketching, and traditional art forms from their cultures. With the cooking and crafts programs, seniors learn and share sustainable, culturally relevant culinary skills, bolster their creativity, and improve their cognitive and motor function. By singing and dancing in culturally relevant mediums, older adults feel a sense of home while also keeping their minds active, helping them to reduce the likelihood of being impacted by dementia and other brain-related disorders.

Adult Empowerment. All seniors served by India Home are immigrants who speak a variety of different languages. Clients who have recently immigrated and have limited English proficiency face difficulties navigating federal and local government systems and accessing public resources due to language barriers. To address this challenge, India Home provides English as a Second Language (ESL)/English to Speakers of Other Languages (ESOL) classes, which help clients to expand their horizons. India Home also helps address low digital literacy in this population by offering technology classes, in which older adults develop basic skills needed for computer and internet use.

Advocacy and Research. Building on India Home's direct services, staff also engage in advocacy and awareness campaigns. These campaigns include providing testimony at city hall and with elected officials, engaging in partnerships with museums, and developing articles for publication in newspapers and online focusing on senior empowerment. Through these campaigns, the voices of underrepresented South Asian and Indo-Caribbean older adults are amplified on issues that directly impact their lives, elevating the needs of this population within the policy landscape so that actionable steps may be identified to address those needs. Recognizing the importance of research to support advocacy, India Home conducted a mixed-methods study in 2017 assessing the needs of South Asian older adults in NYC. Recruitment efforts intentionally excluded India Home members to avoid bias in the study sample. This study included the largest sample ($n = 681$) surveyed to date among this specific group of older adults and employed a questionnaire and focus groups to collect both quantitative and qualitative data. Results highlighted the heterogeneity of the South Asian population and the need for services addressing housing insecurity, low English proficiency, mental health stigma, and gender inequity.

COVID-19 and Beyond. Globally, NYC was the hardest-hit metropolitan area by the novel coronavirus (COVID-19) pandemic, and Queens was one of NYC's hardest-hit boroughs (Honan, 2019). With India Home's older adults already being a vulnerable population in terms of their age, being people of color, and almost all of them residing in Queens, this pandemic had devastating effects on India Home's clients. The organization took a holistic approach to addressing the crisis, quickly implementing a number of programs in response to COVID-19. Examples include delivering culturally appropriate meals and groceries to low-income seniors in their homes three times a week, offering online senior center activities (e.g., educational and nutrition talks; yoga, meditation, and exercise sessions; ESL, technology, citizenship & art classes; group counseling and socialization hours; telephone reassurance check-ins, and remote case management). To ensure older adults' access to virtual programs, India Home provided individualized training to its clients over the phone and through printed materials in-language on how to participate in the online programs. India Home will continue to offer these online resources to encourage connectivity and engagement among its member population.

India Home's holistic approach to addressing the multitude of needs in this population has proven successful, as illustrated by the increased utilization of India Home's services over time. These data contrast with estimates of ongoing underutilization of conventional senior center programs by the South Asian older adult population in NYC and attest to the importance of culturally competent services in serving aging Asian populations.

REFERENCES

ACL Staff, Grove, C., & Moens, R. (2019, March 15). At Senior Centers, Meals Become Gateways to Activities, Services and Connections. Retrieved from https://acl.gov/news-and-events/acl-blog/more-just-meal

Diabetes in South Asians. (2019, January 15). Retrieved from https://www.diabetes.co.uk/south-asian

Fowler, R. (n.d.). Congregate Meals at Senior Centers. Retrieved from http://www.seniorcenterdirectory.com/senior-center-articles/congregate-meals.htm

Honan, K. (2020, April 1). The New York neighborhoods with the most coronavirus cases. *Wall Street Journal.* https://www.wsj.com/articles/the-new-york-neighborhoods-with-the-most-coronavirus-cases-11585781164

India Home (2019). South Asian Seniors in New York City: Needs Assessment. New York, NY https://indiahome.org/wp-content/uploads/2020/10/India-Home-Needs-Assessment-final.pdf

CASE

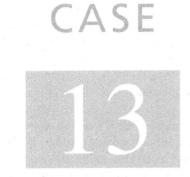

ASIAN IMMIGRANT WOMEN ENGAGING IN SEX WORK IN MASSAGE PARLORS

JOHN J. CHIN, LOIS M. TAKAHASHI

Between October 2014 and July 2016, researchers from Hunter College and University of Southern California interviewed 116 Chinese and Korean women who reported that they at least once in the past had provided sexual services in a massage parlor (MP) setting in New York City or Los Angeles County. Participants constituted a convenience sample recruited through ads in ethnic newspapers, online ads, direct recruitment at MPs, referrals from social service providers, and recruitment at courthouses. Because our study focused specifically on Chinese and Korean MP workers, our sample did not include substantial representation of women who participated in other sectors of the sex industry, such as street-based solicitation, escort businesses, or sex businesses based in private homes. It is also important to note that our sample comprised women who were willing to be interviewed; therefore, the voices of women who may be working in more oppressive or controlled situations may be under-represented.

STIGMA AND SOCIAL ISOLATION

Our findings suggested that the most important problems facing most of these women were the lack of alternative employment and negative experiences with clients and, more often, with the police. Many of the women in our study were undocumented immigrants with very limited English proficiency. Their other choices for earning a living were confined to nail salons, where they would earn low wages and be exposed to toxic chemicals, or restaurants, which offered similarly low wages and demanded back-breaking work.

Applied Population Health Approaches for Asian American Communities, First Edition. Edited by Simona C. Kwon, Chau Trinh-Shevrin, Nadia S. Islam, and Stella S. Yi.

Many of the women were doubly vulnerable because they were both undocumented immigrants and engaging in illegal activities. Especially in the current hostile climate toward immigrants, the women were reluctant to turn to the police for help if they were robbed (a prevalent risk in this cash-based industry) or assaulted, fearing they might themselves be arrested or deported if they drew attention to themselves. In this fraught context, the women were especially in need of support from their co-ethnic communities. However, we found that the women participating in our study were extremely isolated from their communities because of the stigma and shame associated with their work.

Concerns about stigma and shame weighed heavily on the women, affecting their self-esteem and mental health and exacerbating the stress of their difficult work situations. When they discussed stigma and shame, the women tended to focus on their own families and co-ethnic communities, fearing that their families and communities would learn of their profession. Only 8% of the study participants said they had told a family member that their work involves providing sexual services. In general, participants were reluctant to reveal any connection to MP work because community members associated MPs in general with sexual services.

One participant pointed out that churches serving the ethnic community can be particularly stigmatizing because of their tightly knit networks that allow gossip to spread easily. On the other hand, several participants said that churches were among the few organizations from which they sought help to deal with life challenges, such as taking English language classes, suggesting that churches could play an important supportive role for these women. However, the kind of help that MP workers received did not require disclosure of their work, and many feared that disclosing their employment could result in stigmatization and compromise the quality of support that they receive at churches or other religious institutions.

STIGMA, MISINFORMATION, AND HIV RISK

HIV stigma was seen by some MP workers as exacerbating the stigma associated with MP work. Because one of the main modes of transmission of HIV is through sexual activity, sexual activity may, in turn, be associated with HIV. Thus, the women feared being stigmatized by their association with illicit MP work and, therefore, with HIV. The stigma has practical consequences for them since having HIV or being perceived as having HIV would affect their ability to engage in MP work. One illicit MP worker said, "I am afraid of HIV because I want to continue to stay in this field."

HIV stigma and fear of HIV may be a barrier to learning about HIV, which would help the women protect themselves. Some of the study participants said that they had little knowledge about HIV and other sexually transmitted infections, which was reflected in misconceptions or confusion they had about HIV prevention and treatment:

> I don't know any medication. . . .can prevent HIV after dangerous sex. . . .I don't know how much the medical expense in China and United States cost and don't know whether it is free or not. I don't know where I can get free HIV medication and don't know what specialty I need to consult if [I have] HIV.

One way that stigma and fear create barriers is by making it more difficult to discuss HIV and sexually transmitted infections, even within the MP setting. One woman had symptoms of a sexually transmitted infection but did not take any action and was confused about what her symptoms meant. She also noted a general reluctance among her coworkers and the management to discuss such issues:

> Sometimes my genital area was itchy and with yellow and white discharge. Sometimes I had burning sensation when I urinate. . . . I believe HIV and STD can have no symptom but I don't know how long and why they have no symptom. Between coworkers and boss, we will not talk about their own sexual service and sickness.

Without access to accurate health and disease prevention information, study participants used strategies of varying effectiveness to minimize the health risks of their work. Many study participants said they tried to avoid clients who had visible signs of skin trouble. One participant said that she "would refuse to provide service if I saw customers had rash on their genital area." Another participant said that "one time a customer wanted the light dimmed. And then when he disrobed, I saw that he had some lesions or rashes on his skin. I was concerned about getting a disease so [I] refused to continue with services."

Although observable skin conditions could, in some cases, be genuine indicators of a transmittable disease, many women relied on purely impressionistic and subjective indicators. For these women, conscious or unconscious bias dictated the development of a false hierarchy of safer and riskier male clients based on race, odor, and body appearance. For example, one study participant said that she "will refuse to serve customers who *seem* dirty or *look like* have skin diseases or STIs."

Making decisions about which customers to accept based on subjective impressions could potentially elevate risk when positive impressions led to greater willingness to engage in riskier practices. One woman said that "if she felt that the customers look clean and tidy, she is willing not to put on condom and follow what the customers want." One study participant said that "she prefers a nice, tall, handsome white man;" another said that she "only provides sexual services to white men who look attractive." Another participant made distinctions based on socioeconomic class, saying that she "preferred well-educated clients, such as doctors or lawyers."

On the other hand, a number of study participants were familiar with condoms and said that they were able to insist that customers use them. For example, one participant said, "I told a customer who did not want to use condom that he had to wear a condom because I don't want to take a risk of STD or any other disease." Another participant said that she "kicked out customers when they refused [to use a] condom. They are not going to take responsibility for my risk of getting AIDS or any sexual diseases."

Many study participants lacked adequate access to health care, often because of their undocumented immigration status. As summarized by one woman, "I saw a doctor but never have had a regular medical checkup in the United States because I am undocumented." Stigma and its associated social isolation may exacerbate the lack of access to health information and health care experienced by these women, leading to increased prevalence of sexually transmitted infections and low rates of health care utilization. Among the study participants, 7% reported having ever had some type of hepatitis infection; 7% reported having had at least one sexually transmitted infection; 43% had not been tested for HIV; an additional 3% did not know if they had been tested; and 36% had not had a gynecological exam in the last year.

For Asian immigrant sex workers, one approach to reducing stigma and social isolation may be to reframe their experiences and challenges as a labor rights issue and as an aspect of the larger immigrant story of survival, explained by many of the same dynamics that shape other immigrant experiences, rather than a puzzling or embarrassing anomaly. Many of the women used their MP earnings to support their children and families, both in the United States and in their home countries, and yet many of these women did not feel free to talk about their work with friends and family because of stigma. This situation commonly led to feelings of isolation and sadness. The women's vulnerability as workers was exacerbated because they did not receive the same types of social and community support as other types of workers. It is hard to imagine a situation where workers in illicit MPs would be fully embraced by their ethnic communities, but a broader recognition and understanding of illicit MP work within ethnic communities, coupled with labor protections from government, may reduce levels of social isolation and labor exploitation considerably.

INDEX

Please note that page references to Figures will be followed by the letter 'f', to Tables by the letter 't'